Substance Use Disorders, Part II

Editors

RAY CHIH-JUI HSIAO
PAULA D. RIGGS

CHILD AND ADOLESCENT PSYCHIATRIC CLINICS OF NORTH AMERICA

www.childpsych.theclinics.com

Consulting Editor
HARSH K. TRIVEDI

October 2016 • Volume 25 • Number 4

ELSEVIER

1600 John F. Kennedy Boulevard • Suite 1800 • Philadelphia, Pennsylvania, 19103-2899

http://www.theclinics.com

CHILD AND ADOLESCENT PSYCHIATRIC CLINICS OF NORTH AMERICA Volume 25, Number 4
October 2016 ISSN 1056–4993, ISBN-13: 978-0-323-46302-7

Editor: Lauren Boyle
Developmental Editor: Kristen Helm

Child and Adolescent Psychiatric Clinics of North America (ISSN 1056-4993) is published quarterly by Elsevier Inc., 360 Park Avenue South, New York, NY 10010-1710. Months of issue are January, April, July, and October. Business and Editorial Offices: 1600 John F. Kennedy Boulevard, Suite 1800, Philadelphia, PA 19103-2899. Periodicals postage paid at New York, NY and additional mailing offices. Subscription prices are $310.00 per year (US individuals), $544.00 per year (US institutions), $100.00 per year (US students), $360.00 per year (Canadian individuals), $662.00 per year (Canadian institutions), $200.00 per year (Canadian students), $430.00 per year (international individuals), $662.00 per year (international institutions), and $200.00 per year (international students). International air speed delivery is included in all *Clinics* subscription prices. All prices are subject to change without notice. **POSTMASTER:** Send address changes to *Child and Adolescent Psychiatric Clinics of North America*, Elsevier Health Sciences Division, Subscription Customer Service, 3251 Riverport Lane, Maryland Heights, MO 63043. **Customer Service: 1-800-654-2452 (U.S. and Canada); 314-447-8871 (outside U.S. and Canada). Fax:** 314-447-8029. **E-mail:** JournalsCustomer Service-usa@elsevier.com **(for print support) or** journalsonlinesupport-usa@elsevier.com **(for online support).**

Reprints. For copies of 100 or more of articles in this publication, please contact the Commercial Reprints Department, Elsevier Inc., 360 Park Avenue South, New York, New York 10010-1710 Tel.: 212-633-3874; Fax: 212-633-3820, E-mail: reprints@elsevier.com.

Child and Adolescent Psychiatric Clinics of North America is covered in *MEDLINE/PubMed (Index Medicus), ISI, SSCI, Research Alert, Social Search, Current Contents,* and *EMBASE/Excerpta Medica.*

Contributors

CONSULTING EDITOR

HARSH K. TRIVEDI, MD, MBA
President and Chief Executive Officer, Sheppard Pratt Health System; Clinical Professor and Vice Chair of Psychiatry, University of Maryland School of Medicine, Baltimore, Maryland

CONSULTING EDITOR EMERITUS

ANDRÉS MARTIN, MD, MPH

FOUNDING CONSULTING EDITOR

MELVIN LEWIS, MBBS, FRCPSYCH, DCH

EDITORS

RAY CHIH-JUI HSIAO, MD
Associate Professor, Department of Psychiatry and Behavioral Sciences, University of Washington School of Medicine; Co-Director, Adolescent Substance Abuse Program, Seattle Children's Hospital, Seattle, Washington

PAULA D. RIGGS, MD
Professor and Director, Division of Substance Dependence, Department of Psychiatry, University of Colorado School of Medicine, Aurora, Colorado

AUTHORS

AUSTEN R. ANDERSON, BS
Doctoral Student, Department of Public Health Sciences, Miller School of Medicine, University of Miami, Miami, Florida

REBECCA P. BARCLAY, MD
PAL Consultant, Child Psychiatry, Seattle Children's Hospital, Seattle, Washington

MARGARET M. BENNINGFIELD, MD, MSCI
Assistant Professor, Department of Psychiatry and Behavioral Sciences; Medical Director, School Based Mental Health Services, Vanderbilt University Medical Center, Nashville, Tennessee

JACOB T. BORODOVSKY, BA
PhD Student, Health Policy and Clinical Practice, Center for Technology and Behavioral Health, Dartmouth College, Lebanon, New Hampshire

JOSHUA BORUS, MD, MPH
Division of Adolescent/Young Adult Medicine, Boston Children's Hospital, Harvard Medical School, Boston, Massachusetts

ALAN J. BUDNEY, PhD
Professor, Department of Psychiatry, Geisel School of Medicine at Dartmouth, Lebanon, New Hampshire

SHEILA E. CROWELL, PhD
Department of Psychology, University of Utah, Salt Lake City, Utah

MARK D. GODLEY, PhD
Senior Research Scientist, Chestnut Health Systems, Normal, Illinois

CHRISTOPHER J. HAMMOND, MD
Assistant Professor of Child Psychiatry, Behavioral Pharmacology Research Unit, Department of Psychiatry and Behavioral Sciences, Johns Hopkins University School of Medicine, Baltimore, Maryland

ROBERT J. HILT, MD
Associate Professor of Psychiatry, University of Washington, Seattle Children's Hospital, Seattle, Washington

VIVIANA E. HORIGIAN, MD
Associate Professor, Department of Public Health Sciences, Miller School of Medicine, University of Miami, Miami, Florida

RAY CHIH-JUI HSIAO, MD
Associate Professor, Department of Psychiatry and Behavioral Sciences, University of Washington School of Medicine; Co-Director, Adolescent Substance Abuse Program, Seattle Children's Hospital, Seattle, Washington

YIFRAH KAMINER, MD, MBA
Professor of Psychiatry and Pediatrics, Alcohol Research Center, University of Connecticut School of Medicine, Farmington, Connecticut

ERIN A. KAUFMAN, MS
Department of Psychology, University of Utah, Salt Lake City, Utah

AMY HUGHES LANSING, PhD
Postdoctoral Fellow, Department of Psychiatry, Geisel School of Medicine at Dartmouth, Lebanon, New Hampshire

SHARON LEVY, MD
Adolescent Substance Abuse Program, Division of Developmental Medicine, Boston Children's Hospital, Harvard Medical School, Boston, Massachusetts

LISA A. MARSCH, PhD
Professor of Psychiatry, Center for Technology and Behavioral Health, Dartmouth College, Lebanon, New Hampshire

IMAN PARHAMI, MD, MPH
Division of Child and Adolescent Psychiatry, Department of Psychiatry and Behavioral Sciences, Johns Hopkins University School of Medicine, Johns Hopkins Children's Center, Baltimore, Maryland

LORA L. PASSETTI, MS
Research Projects Manager, Chestnut Health Systems, Normal, Illinois

PAULA D. RIGGS, MD
Professor and Director, Division of Substance Dependence, Department of Psychiatry, University of Colorado School of Medicine, Aurora, Colorado

ZACHARY D. ROBINSON, MD
Fellow, Child and Adolescent Psychiatry; Fellow, Children's Hospital Colorado, University of Colorado Hospital, University of Colorado School of Medicine, Aurora, Colorado

ERIN SCHOENFELDER, PhD
Assistant Professor, Department of Psychiatry and Behavioral Sciences, University of Washington School of Medicine, Seattle, Washington

SHANNON SIMMONS, MD, MPH
Acting Assistant Professor, Department of Psychiatry and Behavioral Sciences, University of Washington, Seattle Children's Hospital, Seattle, Washington

CHLOE R. SKIDMORE, MS
Department of Psychology, University of Utah, Salt Lake City, Utah

CATHERINE STANGER, PhD
Associate Professor, Department of Psychiatry, Geisel School of Medicine at Dartmouth, Lebanon, New Hampshire

LIZA SUÁREZ, PhD
Department of Psychiatry, Institute for Juvenile Research, University of Illinois at Chicago, Chicago, Illinois

JOSÉ SZAPOCZNIK, PhD
Professor, Department of Public Health Sciences, Miller School of Medicine, University of Miami, Miami, Florida

SARAH S. WU, PhD
Department of Psychiatry and Behavioral Medicine, Seattle Children's Hospital, Seattle, Washington

Contents

Screening, Brief Intervention, and Referral to Treatment is a quick, effective technique with which to manage substance use in adolescents and young adults. Use of a validated measure for detecting substance use and abuse is significantly more effective than unvalidated tools or provider intuition. There are a variety of validated tools available to use in the adolescent/young adult population, and there are opportunities to increase the efficiency and scalability of screening by using computerized questionnaires. This area continues to evolve rapidly.

Adolescent substance use is a major risk factor for negative outcomes, including substance dependence later in life, criminal behavior, school problems, mental health disorders, injury, and death. This article provides a user-friendly, clinically focused, and pragmatic review of current and evidence-based family treatments, including multisystemic therapy, multidimensional family therapy, functional family therapy, brief strategic family therapy, ecologically based family therapy, family behavior therapy, culturally informed flexible family treatment for adolescents, and strengths-oriented family therapy. Outcomes, treatment parameters, adolescent characteristics, and implementation factors are reviewed.

Although cognitive behavioral therapy (CBT) is widely recognized as the preferred treatment of psychiatric disorders, less is known about the application of CBT to substance use disorders, particularly in adolescence. This article discusses how CBT conceptualizes substance use and how it is implemented as a treatment of adolescent substance abuse. The article draws on several manuals for CBT that implement it as a standalone treatment or in combination with motivational enhancement therapies. Also reviewed are several studies that examined the efficacy of CBT. Finally, the implications are discussed. Numerous starting resources are provided to help a clinician implement CBT.

Multiple interventions for treating adolescents with substance use disorders have demonstrated efficacy, but a majority of teens do not show an enduring positive response to these treatments. Contingency management (CM)-based strategies provide a promising alternative, and clinical research focused on the development and testing of innovative CM models continues to grow. This article provides an updated review on the progress made in this area. It is important to continue to search for more effective models, focus on post-treatment maintenance (reduce relapse), and strive for high levels of integrity and fidelity during dissemination efforts to optimize outcomes.

Providing school-based mental health treatment offers an opportunity to reach a greater number of affected youth by providing services in the setting where youth spend the majority of their time. In some contexts, even a single session of assessment has been linked with significant decreases in substance use; however, more robust treatments are likely needed to sustain these decreases over time. Empirically based individual and group treatments designed for delivery in clinic settings can readily be adapted for implementation in school settings. School-based delivery of substance use services offers an important opportunity to bridge a significant gap in services.

Adolescents who enter treatment for substance use often do not complete the program and do not connect with continuing care services. Most return to some level of substance use. Our review found 10 outcome studies of continuing care treatment. More assertive approaches can increase continuing care initiation rates and rapid initiation of continuing care makes a difference in reducing substance use. Continuing care is appropriate for those who complete treatment and for those who do not. Adaptive treatment designs hold promise for establishing decision rules as to which adolescents need low-intensity continuing care services and which need more intensive care.

Adolescent substance use disorders (SUDs) are a significant public health issue due to the associated morbidity, mortality, and societal cost. While effective for some adolescents, psychosocial interventions generally produce small-to-moderate reductions in substance use. Most youth relapse within 12 months of treatment. One approach to improve outcomes is through adjunctive pharmacotherapy. Medication assisted treatments have been shown to improve adult SUD treatment outcomes, and preliminary studies in adolescents suggest that combining medication with psychosocial interventions may also enhance SUD outcomes for youth. This article presents a comprehensive review and grading of the evidence from studies conducted in adolescents with SUDs.

Research shows that the majority of adolescents with substance use disorders also have other cooccurring psychiatric disorders, which has been associated with poorer treatment outcomes. Despite considerable consensus that treatment of cooccurring disorders should be integrated or concurrent, most such youth do not receive it. In addition to systemic and economic barriers, few studies have been conducted that inform evidence-based integrated treatment approaches. This article provides a review of current research from which empirically derived principles of integrated treatment can originate and which have informed the development of at least one evidence-based model of integrated mental health and substance treatment.

There is a strong, bidirectional link between substance abuse and traumatic experiences. Teens with cooccurring substance use disorders (SUDs) and posttraumatic stress disorder (PTSD) have significant functional and psychosocial impairment. Common neurobiological foundations point to the reinforcing cycle of trauma symptoms, substance withdrawal, and substance use. Treatment of teens with these issues should include a systemic and integrated approach to both the SUD and the PTSD.

Emerging adulthood has heightened risk for substance use. College students experience unique challenges, making them prone to use of alcohol, marijuana, and nonmedical use of prescription drugs. This article reviews rates of college students' substance use, risk factors, and populations at elevated risk. Consequences include legal, academic, and mental health problems; engagement in other risky behaviors; increased rates of injury; and death. Researchers, clinicians, and university administrators must identify those at greatest risk and provide prevention and intervention programs. Despite broad evidence supporting such programs, many students fail to access appropriate treatment. Future research should elucidate treatment barriers.

Preventing or mitigating substance use among youth generally involves 3 different intervention frameworks: universal prevention, selective prevention, and treatment. Each of these levels of intervention poses unique therapeutic and implementation challenges. Technology-based interventions provide solutions to many of these problems by delivering evidence-based interventions in a consistent and cost-effective manner. This article summarizes the current state of the science of technology-based interventions for preventing substance use initiation and mitigating substance use and associated consequences among youth.

Integrated care is a way to improve the prevention, identification, and treatment of mental health difficulties, including substance abuse, in pediatric care. The pediatrician's access, expertise in typical development, focus on prevention, and alignment with patients and families can allow successful screening, early intervention, and referral to treatment. Successful integrated substance abuse care for youth is challenged by current reimbursement systems, information exchange, and provider role adjustment issues, but these are being addressed as comfort with this care form and resources to support its development grow.

CHILD AND ADOLESCENT PSYCHIATRIC CLINICS

AACAP Members: Please go to www.jaacap.org for information on access to the Child and Adolescent Psychiatric Clinics. *Resident* Members of AACAP: Special access information is available at www.childpsych.theclinics.com.

THE CLINICS ARE AVAILABLE ONLINE!
Access your subscription at:
www.theclinics.com

CHILD AND ADOLESCENT PSYCHIATRIC CLINICS

FORTHCOMING ISSUES

January 2017
Health Information Technology for Child and Adolescent Psychiatry
Barry Sarvet and John Torous, Editors

April 2017
Care of Transitional Age Youth
Adele Martel and Catherine Fuller, Editors

July 2017
Early Childhood Mental Health: Empirical Assessment and Intervention—Age 0-6
Mini Tandon, Editor

RECENT ISSUES

July 2016
Substance Use Disorders, Part 1
Ray Chih-Jui Hsiao and Leslie Renee Walker, Editors

April 2016
Prevention of Mental Health Disorders: Principles and Implementation
Aradhana Bela Sood and Jim Hudziak, Editors

January 2016
Adjudicated Youth
Louis Kraus, Editor

AACAP Members: Please go to www.jaacap.org for information on access to the Child and Adolescent Psychiatry Clinics. Resident Members of AACAP: Special access information is available at www.childpsych.theclinics.com.

Erratum

In the July 2016 issue of *Child and Adolescent Psychiatric Clinics of North America* (Volume 25, Issue 3), in the article "Opioid Use Disorders," an error was made regarding an author's name and degree. Gabriela Barnett, MS is incorrectly listed as Gabrielle Barnett, MA.

Child Adolesc Psychiatric Clin N Am 25 (2016) xiii
http://dx.doi.org/10.1016/j.chc.2016.07.001
1056-4993/16/© 2016 Elsevier Inc. All rights reserved.

childpsych.theclinics.com

Erratum

In the July 2016 issue of *Child and Adolescent Psychiatric Clinics of North America* (Volume 25, Issue 3), in the article, "Opioid Use Disorder," an error was made regarding an author's name and degree. Gabriela Herrell, MS is incorrectly listed as Gabriela Herrell, MA.

Child Adolesc Psychiatric Clin N Am 25 (2016) xiii
http://dx.doi.org/10.1016/j.chc.2016.09.001
1056-4993/16/$ – see front matter © 2016 Elsevier Inc. All rights reserved.
childpsych.theclinics.com

Preface

The Changing Landscape of Adolescent Substance Treatment

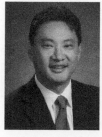 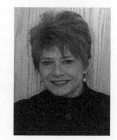

Ray Chih-Jui Hsiao, MD   Paula D. Riggs, MD
Editors

The editors wish to thank the authors who contributed to this issue on the treatment of adolescents with substance use disorders. Taken together, these current research review articles document significant progress in developing more effective treatment for such youth. It is also clear that there is much room for improvement and more work to be done in the context of the changing landscape of national health care reform. The Mental Health and Addiction Parity Act (2008) and the Affordable Care Act (2010) have initiated a cascade of transformational changes that have paved the way for the integration of mental health and addiction treatment into the mainstream medical health care system in the United States in ways that will shape future research and clinical practice.

Integrating addiction treatment into medical settings is appropriate, given that ample research has established the neurobiological basis of addiction and its similarity to other chronic medical conditions such as diabetes and cardiovascular disease. As such, it is important to dispel the residual notion that individuals suffering from addiction must "hit rock bottom" before they are willing to enter treatment. This notion has contributed to the development of interventions and a treatment system that predominantly serve only those at the most severe end of the spectrum.

Progress toward greater integration of addiction treatment in medical settings will help overcome existing barriers to substance treatment referral and improve access to care. Addiction medicine and addiction psychiatry will increasingly be recognized as medical subspecialties, and the treatment and clinical management of patients with addiction will gradually shift toward a chronic disease management model. Increasing public awareness of the medical basis of addiction will help reduce the stigma associated with addiction. This transformation will require the field to develop (a) more effective screening, prevention and earlier interventions for at-risk

Child Adolesc Psychiatric Clin N Am 25 (2016) xv–xvi
http://dx.doi.org/10.1016/j.chc.2016.07.002
1056-4993/16/© 2016 Published by Elsevier Inc.

youth; (b) earlier detection and treatment for youth who have started using/abusing substances to prevent progression to more serious chronic addiction in adulthood; (c) effective interventions for the growing number of patients with medical illnesses complicated by substance use disorders or harmful levels of alcohol, drug, or prescription medication abuse; (d) cost-effective treatment interventions that can be feasibly implemented and sustained in nontraditional practice settings such as schools and primary care medical settings; and (e) more effective and efficient ways to train clinicians and expand the clinical workforce.

Ray Chih-Jui Hsiao, MD
Department of Psychiatry
and Behavioral Sciences
University of Washington School of Medicine
Adolescent Substance Abuse Program
Seattle Children's Hospital
M/S OA.5.154
PO Box 5371
Seattle, WA 98145-5005, USA

Paula D. Riggs, MD
Division of Substance Dependence
Department of Psychiatry
University of Colorado School of Medicine
Mail Stop F478
12469 East 17th Place, Building 400
Aurora, CO 80045, USA

E-mail addresses:
rhsiao@uw.edu (R.C.-J. Hsiao)
paula.riggs@ucdenver.edu (P.D. Riggs)

Screening, Brief Intervention, and Referral to Treatment

Joshua Borus, MD, MPH[a],*, Iman Parhami, MD, MPH[b],
Sharon Levy, MD[c]

KEYWORDS

- Screening, Brief Intervention, and Referral to Treatment • Substance use
- Adolescents • Screening • Alcohol • Substance abuse • Motivational interviewing

KEY POINTS

- Screening, Brief Intervention, and Referral to Treatment is a quick, effective technique with which to manage substance use in adolescents and young adults.
- Use of a validated measure for detecting substance use and abuse is significantly more effective than unvalidated tools or provider intuition. There are a variety of validated tools available to use in the adolescent/young adult population.
- There are opportunities to increase the efficiency and scalability of screening by using computerized questionnaires. This area continues to evolve rapidly.

INTRODUCTION

Substance use is a major driver of morbidity and mortality in adolescents and young adults and a cause of numerous public health problems including elements of mortality (eg, unintentional injury, suicide, motor vehicle accidents) and morbidity (eg, sexual transmitted infections, involvement in violence as either perpetrator or victim,

Dr I. Parhami's preparation of this article was supported in part by the National Institute on Drug Abuse and American Academy of Child and Adolescent Psychiatry Resident Training Research Award in Substance Abuse and Addiction. Dr S. Levy's preparation of this article was supported in part by the Substance Abuse and Mental Health Services Administration (TI025389), NIAAA (AA021913), and the Conrad N Hilton Foundation (20140273).
The authors have no financial relationships to disclose.
[a] Division of Adolescent/Young Adult Medicine, Boston Children's Hospital, Harvard Medical School, 300 Longwood Avenue, Boston, MA 02115, USA; [b] Division of Child and Adolescent Psychiatry, Department of Psychiatry and Behavioral Sciences, Johns Hopkins School of Medicine, Johns Hopkins Children's Center, 733 N Broadway, Baltimore, MD 21205, USA; [c] Adolescent Substance Abuse Program, Division of Developmental Medicine, Boston Children's Hospital, Harvard Medical School, 25 Shattuck Street, Boston, MA 02115, USA
* Corresponding author.
E-mail address: Joshua.borus@childrens.harvard.edu

unprotected intercourse leading to teen pregnancy) for this population. Age of onset of both alcohol and marijuana use is inversely associated with risk of substance use disorder (SUD) development.[1,2] Marijuana use during adolescence has increased in recent years and is associated with an increased risk of mental illness, cognitive decline, and increased risk of opioid addiction.[3–6]

Substance use is most commonly initiated during adolescence. According to a nationally representative survey, 4,336,000 adolescents (or 17.4% of persons age 12–17 in the United States) are estimated to have used illicit drugs including marijuana, cocaine, heroin, hallucinogens, and inhalants or misused prescription medications (ie, medications that were not prescribed to them, or at a higher dose or different route than was prescribed) in 2014.[7] Specifically, 292,000 adolescents smoke cigarettes daily; 257,000 adolescents drink alcohol heavily (drinking 5 or more drinks on the same occasion in the past month); and 1,251,000 (or 5% of all adolescents) meet diagnostic criteria for a substance use related disorder for any illicit drug or alcohol. Substance use may be the most important modifiable health risk behavior of adolescence; consequently, substance use should be identified and addressed.

Both the American Psychiatric Association and the American Academy of Child and Adolescent Psychiatry recommend inquiring about substance use during initial psychiatric evaluations.[8,9] Specifically, the American Academy of Child and Adolescent Psychiatry practice parameter encourages brief interventions or referrals for more intensive services for substance use when warranted, in addition to treatment for the co-occurring psychopathology.[9] Given these recommendations and the availability of effective, brief SUD interventions in pediatric mental health settings, it is compelling for mental health and primary care clinicians to screen and provide brief treatments for SUD.[10–14]

There is a movement to screen and provide brief interventions for adolescent substance use. In 2003, the Substance Abuse and Mental Health Services Administration (SAMHSA) launched an initiative to increase rates of identifying and addressing substance use in routine medical care for both adults and children and developed a framework called Screening, Brief Intervention, Referral to Treatment (SBIRT).[15] In accordance with the broad goal of expanding the medical home to incorporate mental and behavioral health treatment as set forth by the Affordable Care Act, several professional organizations and government agencies recommend incorporating SBIRT into routine health care for adolescents.[15–20] This movement presents both an opportunity and a challenge, as clinicians feel squeezed for time because they are encouraged to cover more material and document more thoroughly at each clinical encounter, a trend seen throughout medicine. For example, a review of American Academy of Pediatrics (AAP) guidelines in 2006 identified 162 recommended verbal health directives for children and families throughout childhood routine health visits.[21] Similarly, family practice doctors estimated they would need to spend 7.4 hours per working day on preventive advice if they were to follow all of their professional recommendations.[22] In this landscape, SBIRT must be quick, inexpensive, and easy to implement.

In 2012, the United States Preventative Services Task Force released guidelines recommending SBIRT to address tobacco and alcohol use as part of routine health care of adults. The United States Preventative Services Task Force has determined that there are insufficient data to support a similar recommendation for the adolescent population, suggesting the need for more research to determine how to best address substance use with adolescents.[23,24] Nonetheless, based on promising data and the low cost and low risk of SBIRT, the AAP released a policy statement in 2011 recommending universal SBIRT for tobacco, alcohol, and other substance use be incorporated into routine health care for adolescents and has produced a clinical report with guidance on SBIRT practice.[17] An updated policy statement from the AAP on SBIRT is currently in press and expected to be published in June 2016.[25]

SCREENING, BRIEF INTERVENTION, REFERRAL TO TREATMENT IN CHILD AND ADOLESCENT PSYCHIATRY

Although SBIRT research has primarily centered on emergency department and primary care settings, addressing substance use in the mental health treatment settings is equally pressing given the frequency of co-occurring SUDs in youth with mental health problems.[26,27] For instance, approximately one-third of adolescents who use illicit drugs in a year and one-quarter of adolescents that meet diagnostic criteria for SUD also meet criteria for major depressive episode in the same year.[28] These findings corroborate those of previous studies that found youth with mental illnesses as varied as ADHD, bipolar disorder, and anxiety disorders to have significantly higher rates of comorbid SUD.[10,29–33] Results from a recent epidemiologic study that surveyed more than 10,000 adolescents found that any prior mental disorder significantly increased the risk of transition from nonuse to first use and from use to problematic use of either alcohol or illicit drugs.[34]

Adolescents with co-occurring disorders may present at a variety of mental health treatment settings.[35–38] Among more than 9000 pediatric psychiatric inpatient admissions, one study found that a quarter were for SUDs.[35] Another SAMHSA report indicated that 43% of adolescents receiving mental health services meet diagnostic criteria for a SUD.[38] Adolescents with co-occurring SUD are more likely to exhibit severe symptoms (multiple psychosocial and family issues, low engagement in treatment, poor retention in treatment, and poor outcomes) and are more likely to meet criteria for SUD in adulthood.[39–41] These adolescents also are at increased risk for negative consequences related to risky behavior, suicidality, functional impairments, and school problems.[29,42–45] Nonetheless, few youth receive SUD treatment; many do not consider their substance use as problematic, and many of those who are interested in SUD treatment have difficulty accessing services, further underscoring the need to address substance use in mental health treatment settings.[46–48] The brief intervention model, which incorporates components of motivational interviewing and is described in more detail below, may be suitable for addressing substance use even among adolescents that are not seeking treatment for substance use problems.

Notably, adolescents who are identified in mental health care settings as having co-occurring disorders may be more likely to initiate treatment than those in primary care settings, possibly because they are already receiving psychosocial interventions or have a greater therapeutic alliance with the providers.[49] One study that examined the feasibility of SBIRT implementation in a college mental health setting found multiple advantages. Clinicians reported that the structured screening helped them start a discussion regarding substance use and helped them explore, together with the client, whether substance use was a contributing factor to the presenting mental health issue.[50] Once repercussions from substance use are identified, a clinician can use them as a fulcrum to shift the conversation toward an exploration of behavior change to prevent similar problems in the future.

Another advantage to SBIRT in mental health settings is the potential to address adolescents that fall short of an SUD diagnosis (eg, infrequent cannabis users, occasional binge drinkers) and those with mild or moderate SUDs.[27] These individuals are at particular risk of future psychopathology and impairment compared with nonsubstance users.[2,51–53] Although these adolescents are in need of treatment to address substance use, they may be inappropriate candidates for intensive SUD treatment settings. Brief intervention within the existing mental health setting in which the patient is comfortable (as specified below) may be a practical approach to reducing substance use and associated risk in this group (**Fig. 1**).

Here we review the evidence for effective screening methods and brief intervention models and address approaches to matching the severity of substance use with an appropriate intervention. We also discuss successes and challenges in SBIRT implementation, both in primary care pediatrics, where most research has been done, and in mental health treatment.

SCREENING

Asking the right questions to identify adolescent substance use and assign level of associated risk is critical to implementing early interventions that reduce the burden of morbidity and mortality. Clinical impressions, which typically rely on recognition of advanced symptoms for discerning SUDs, have very poor sensitivity for identifying regular use, early problems, or even a mild-to-moderate disorder.[54,55] A structured approach to screening may be even more important in mental health settings, as symptoms of SUDs may mimic typical psychiatric disorders (eg, substance-induced anxiety, psychotic, or bipolar disorders). Furthermore, newer adolescent SBIRT models conceptualize screen results as placing a patient on a spectrum of substance use experience, from "none" to "severe substance use disorder" and suggest an appropriate intervention for every level of experience, rather than simply categorizing an SUD as present or absent.[56] Examples are shown in **Table 1**.

SCREENING TOOLS

The ideal screening tool is easy to administer, easy to interpret, quick, accurate, and categorizes substance use in a way that guides intervention. Several screening tools have been validated for use with adolescents (**Table 2**). These tools fall into 2 broad categories: problem-based and frequency-based screens. Most of the first tools developed were problem-based screens that categorized adolescents into "low" versus "high" risk for meeting criteria for an SUD based on the number of substance use–related problems endorsed. The CRAFFT is a well-validated instrument that has screenlike properties; a score of 2 or greater indicates high risk for an SUD.[57,58] The CRAFFT has been widely disseminated and can be used as a screen, although it is longer than newer tools, does not include questions about tobacco, and mixes all psychoactive substances together for an overall score rather than giving a risk level for each individual substance.

Frequency-based screens determine risk for an SUD based on the reported frequency of past-year substance use. Three recently validated tools (National Institute on Alcohol Abuse and Alcoholism [NIAAA] Youth Alcohol Screen, Brief Screener for Tobacco, Alcohol, and other Drugs [BSTAD], and Screening to Brief Intervention tool [S2BI]) have established that frequency of use can be used to determine SUD risk for commonly used substances by adolescents.[20,59,60]

The BSTAD tool is an open-ended past-year frequency questionnaire for alcohol, tobacco, and drugs. Like the NIAAA tool, the question is posed differently depending on the age of the adolescent. This tool was validated in a primary care setting, and the authors determined the optimal cut points for identifying a SUD were ≥6 days of

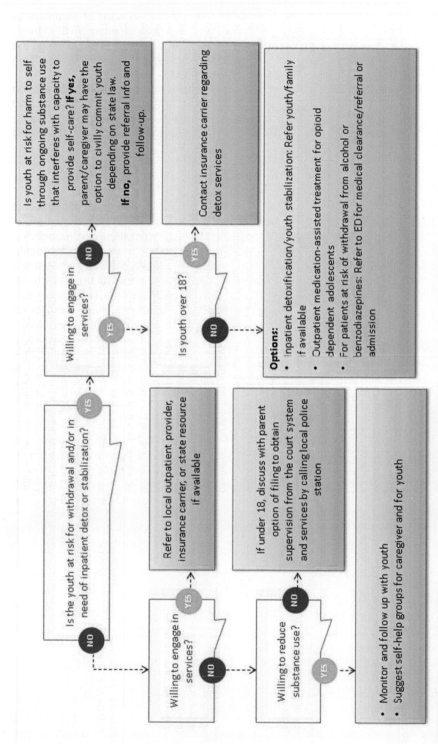

Fig. 1. Decision support for substance use disorder treatment. (*Adapted from* Levy S, Shrier LA, The Massachusetts Department of Public Health Bureau of Substance Abuse Services, et al. Adolescent SBIRT toolkit for providers. 2015. Available at: http://massclearinghouse.ehs.state.ma.us/BSASSBIRTPROG/SA3541.html. Accessed February 15, 2016; with permission.)

Table 1
Sample intervention conversations

Screening Result	Indicated Intervention	Example
No substance use	Prevention Positive reinforcement	"I think you're making a great choice to stay away from drinking and smoking. From our conversations I know getting good grades and doing your best on the track team are important to you and avoiding substances makes those things easier. The truth is, most kids your age aren't drinking or smoking and I'm glad you've made that decision too. If that changes and you decide to experiment with alcohol, marijuana or tobacco, please talk with me so I can help answer any questions you might have and make sure you have the facts you need to make an educated decision."
Limited substance use (eg, once or twice in the past year)	Brief advice	"Thanks for answering the substance use screening questions honestly. I see that you used marijuana once or twice last year. As your doctor, my hope is you will stop using it completely for the sake of your health. If it's okay, I'd like to give you a little information about marijuana. Over time it will interfere with your brain's development, making it harder to do well in school, as well as impact your lungs which works directly against all the training you are doing at track practice. I'm worried it's going to make it harder to do the things you say are important to you. For these reasons, I recommend that you quit. You may have heard lots of different things about marijuana and all of that information can be confusing. Do you have any questions about how marijuana can affect your body, mood or brain?"
Progression to more regular substance use (monthly) or meets diagnostic criteria for mild-moderate	Brief intervention	"It seems that you depend on marijuana to help you manage stress and is a way that you feel connected to your friends. At the same time, marijuana use is causing tension between you and your mother and has gotten you into trouble at school. As your physician, I recommend that you quit. Marijuana does not reduce stress in the long term. I can understand that the tension between you and your mother has been hard to manage. Would you be willing to quit for a couple of months to see how that goes? That would give you the opportunity to see how you feel when you are not using marijuana, and it may also be a great first step in rebuilding trust with your parents."
Moderate to severe SUD (weekly or more)	Treatment referral	"Thank you for being so open about your use of marijuana and alcohol. It sounds like there are some benefits to your use—it helps you relax and deal with your life—and also some major costs—you aren't doing as well as you want in school, your girlfriend thinks it is a problem and you've stopped playing football. Because I am so worried about you, I'd like to speak with your parents about this and I think it's important to get more expert help. I strongly suggest getting connected with a program that works with people in your situation—thinking about cutting down or cutting out their use but conflicted—so you can get back to doing the things you said were important to you. I'd still like to work with you and will be available while you participate in the program and afterward. How does that sound?"

Table 2	
Substance use screening and assessment tools used with adolescents	
Brief screens	
S2BI[60]	Screening to Brief Intervention • Single frequency of use question per substance • Identifies the likelihood of a DSM-5 SUD • Includes tobacco, alcohol, marijuana, and other/illicit drug use • Discriminates among no use, no SUD, moderate SUD, and severe SUD • Electronic medical record compatible • Self- or interview administered
BSTAD[59]	Brief Screener for Tobacco, Alcohol, and Other Drugs • Identifies problematic tobacco, alcohol, and marijuana use • Built on the NIAAA screening tool with added tobacco and drug questions • Electronic medical record compatible • Self- or interview administered

NIAAA
  Youth
  Alcohol Screen[68]
	Youth Guide
	• 2-question alcohol screen
	• Screens for friends' use and for personal use of 9 y and older
	• Free resource material and Web-based CME training course: http://pubs.niaaa.nih.gov/publications/Practitioner/YouthGuide/YouthGuide.pdf
	• http://www.medscape.org/viewarticle/806556

Brief assessment guides	
CRAFFT[64]	Car, Relax, Alone, Friends/Family, Forget, Trouble • Quickly assesses for problems associated with substance use • Not a diagnostic tool
AUDIT[108]	Alcohol Use Disorders Identification Test • Assesses for risky drinking • Not a diagnostic tool

Abbreviations: CME, continuing medical education; DSM-5, Diagnostic and Statistical Manual of Mental Disorders, Fifth Edition.

tobacco use (sensitivity, 0.95; specificity, 0.97); ≥2 days of alcohol use (sensitivity, 0.96; specificity, 0.85); and ≥2 days of marijuana use (sensitivity, 0.80; specificity, 0.93).[59]

The S2BI tool uses a comprehensive stem question to assess the frequency of past-year use (none, once or twice, monthly, weekly or more) for tobacco, alcohol, marijuana, and 5 other classes of substances commonly used by adolescents (**Box 1**). In the initial validation study, which recruited adolescents from both a primary care and an outpatient program for adolescents with SUDs, the S2BI had high sensitivity and specificity for discriminating between risk categories. These were no use, substance use without an SUD, which correlated to a response of "once or twice," mild or moderate SUD, which correlated to a response of "monthly," and severe SUD, which correlated to a response of "weekly or more."[61] Particularly unique is the ability to detect adolescents with severe substance use disorder, as medical settings have been notably poor in connecting this vulnerable group with treatment. SAMHSA estimates that less than 10% of teens in need of specialty substance use treatment receive it and most of those who do are referred from the justice system.[62,63]

A problem-based tool, such as the CRAFFT questions, can be used to guide further assessment if the S2BI questions generate the need for further exploration.[64] Previously used as a stand-alone screen, the CRAFFT questions can quickly guide the clinician to topics to be used later in motivational interviewing. For example, a patient who

Box 1
Screening to brief intervention

The following questions will ask about your use, if any, of alcohol, tobacco, and other drugs. Please answer every question by clicking on the box next to your choice.

In the past year, how many times have you used…

Tobacco?
- Never
- Once or twice
- Monthly
- Weekly or more

Alcohol?
- Never
- Once or twice
- Monthly
- Weekly or more

Marijuana?
- Never
- Once or twice
- Monthly
- Weekly or more

STOP if answers to all previous questions are "never." Otherwise, continue with questions on the right.

In the past year, how many times have you used…

Prescription drugs that were not prescribed for you (such as pain medication or Adderall)?
- Never
- Once or twice
- Monthly
- Weekly or more

Illegal drugs (such as cocaine or Ecstasy)?
- Never
- Once or twice
- Monthly
- Weekly or more

Inhalants (such as nitrous oxide)?
- Never
- Once or twice
- Monthly
- Weekly or more

Herbs or synthetic drugs (such as salvia, K2, or bath salts)?
- Never
- Once or twice
- Monthly
- Weekly or more

responds "yes" to the TROUBLE question can be asked for more details. This may show tension with parents, problems at school, legal problems, accidents, medical, or other problems.

Both S2BI and BSTAD are available in an electronic format and are available through the NIDAMED website (http://www.drugabuse.gov/nidamed-medical-health-professionals). Regardless of which screening tool is used, each risk category has an associated brief intervention. The next section reviews the recommended interventions for each risk category.

BRIEF INTERVENTION

Response to a substance use screen is intended to prevent, delay, or reduce substance use and associated risky behaviors and, if indicated, encourage an adolescent to accept a referral to treatment. Interventions encompass a spectrum of responses that include "positive reinforcement" for no substance use, "brief advice" to quit for occasional use and use that does not reach the level of a substance use disorder, "brief intervention" for moderate risk use, and "brief intervention" and referral for adolescents with severe SUDs. The AAP has proposed an intervention strategy that aligns with **Fig. 2**. Although designed for pediatric primary care, similar strategies have also been taught in a SAMHSA-funded, child and adolescent psychiatry SBIRT training program.[65]

No Use: Positive Reinforcement

An asynchronous, quasi-experimental trial by Harris and colleagues[66] found that adolescents that reviewed brief, electronically administered education on the medical impacts of substance use and then received 2 to 3 minutes of reinforcement were significantly less likely to start drinking alcohol 3 months after the intervention with the effect still statistically significant at 12 months. Based on this finding, the AAP recommends positive reinforcement and brief prevention messages for all adolescents that report no past-year substance use.

Reinforcement should build on a strength or interest expressed by the patient so it feels personalized. When appropriate, particularly with older adolescents who have likely had the opportunity to try substances, the report of no substance use can be framed as an active decision, which may be empowering.[67] For younger teens, the NIAAA recommends providing a "norms correction" to offset the possible implicit

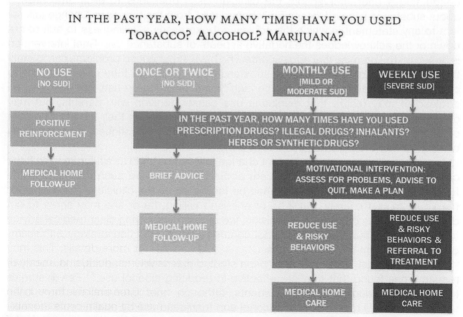

Fig. 2. S2BI algorithm. (© Copyright, Children's Hospital Boston, Center for Adolescent Substance Abuse Research, 2009. All Rights Reserved. © Copyright Boston Children's Hospital 2014. All rights reserved.)

message that screening implies an expectation that peers have already begun to use substances.[68] Delivering reinforcement in a nonjudgmental fashion may help "leave the door open" for further discussion if behavior changes in the future.

Lower Risk: Brief Advice

As noted above, the 2012 study by Harris and colleagues[66] found that adolescents in the intervention group (reviewed brief, electronically administered education on the medical impacts of substance use and then received 2–3 minutes of reinforcement) who reported past-year alcohol use at baseline were more likely to report cessation at 3- and 12-month follow-up.[66] In addition, Colby and colleagues[69] compared brief advice with motivational interviewing in daily cigarette smokers. Although there were initially differences in nicotine levels in the group who had received motivational interviewing, this difference was not sustained 6 months after the intervention, suggesting brief advice was as efficacious as motivational interviewing in this population.

As with positive reinforcement, the recommendation for brief advice is to focus on health effects and connect patient strengths. Recognizing that the adolescent took a risk in reporting honestly and delivering brief advice nonjudgmentally may help maintain the relationship between clinician and patient.

Moderate Risk: Brief Intervention

In the adolescent SBIRT framework described in this article, brief interventions are short, structured conversations, typically lasting 5 to 15 minutes that can be incorporated into a health care appointment. The goal of the intervention is to encourage an adolescent to attempt to stop or reduce substance use and associated risky behaviors.

Brief interventions are based on the principles of motivational interviewing.[70] When conducting a brief intervention, the clinician asks questions to elicit ambivalence about substance use and listens for "change talk" from the teenager. Change talk refers to any statement in which the adolescent expresses a willingness to quit or cut down or the acknowledges the negative aspects of substance use. Brief intervention is based on the premise that adolescents who have experienced problems can identify the potential benefits of reducing substance use, although they may not want to change their behavior because of the high "cost" of giving up use. For example, an adolescent may realize that marijuana use causes tension with parents, but may continue to use because smoking is a way of socializing with their friends. The core of a brief intervention involves exploring the benefits of continued substance use compared with the potential benefits of behavior change.

A summary that repeats adolescent change talk can be used as a fulcrum to shift the conversation to asking the adolescent about plans to avoid such problems in the future. Making a change plan can then be facilitated by the clinician. The goal is for the youth to quit entirely, but if he or she isn't willing, he or she may agree to cut down. Regardless of the teen's decision, we recommend giving clear medical advice to quit, ensuring that the teen does not confuse a harm reduction strategy with an implicit endorsement of continued use.

This type of brief intervention has been studied extensively in adults, and a body of research has found that they are effective in reducing alcohol use.[71] Fewer studies have been conducted with adolescents, although brief interventions have been used successfully to reduce both alcohol and marijuana use by adolescents in emergency care settings.[72–76] These studies all used multicomponent interventions delivered by peer health educators. Formative work in pediatric primary care has found that brief interventions are acceptable to both teens and clinicians.[77] A study of a structured brief motivational intervention called *The 5 A's* (Ask, Advise, Assess, Assist, Arrange) delivered by adolescent medicine specialists found reductions in both intervention and control groups with no statistically significant difference between them.[76,78] However, this study was done without a validated screening tool, and many patients were mistriaged, reducing the power of the study.[79]

Research in mental health settings has focused on using allied mental health providers such as counselors, therapists, and psychologists to administer brief interventions that are usually 1 to 5 sessions.[13,14,80] For example, a recent randomized, controlled study found that psychiatrically hospitalized adolescents with co-occurring disorders who received 2 sessions of brief interventions for SUD by master's level clinicians reported less substance use 6 months after discharge.[81] Other evidence has shown brief interventions to be effective for adolescents with comorbid tobacco use in psychiatric hospitalizations (2 sessions), adolescents with co-occurring disorders in the juvenile justice system (1 to 3 sessions), adolescents in school settings with substance-related disorders (2 sessions), and homeless youth with co-occurring disorders (2 sessions).[82–84]

Severe Risk: Referral to Treatment

Referral to treatment describes the facilitative process that provides patients identified as needing more extensive evaluation and treatment with access to appropriate services. This step comprises 2 separate, overlapping clinical activities: working with the adolescent to accept a referral and engage in treatment (see Severe substance use disorder section above) and facilitating referral to an appropriate professional or program.

Adolescents that report weekly or more use of a substance using the S2BI screen are likely to meet Diagnostic and Statistical Manual of Mental Disorders, Fifth Edition criteria for severe SUD, and referral to treatment should be considered. Often these adolescents do not consider substance use a problem and refuse treatment. Brief intervention efforts with these patients may be best targeted at accepting specialized SUD treatment. Recognizing that severe SUD (addiction) is a medical condition more akin to a chronic neurologic issue than character weakness helps frame the issue and solidifies the importance of moving the patient toward specialized treatment for SUD. If patients present acute risk to themselves or others, confidentiality may need to be broken for safety, and the limits of confidentiality need to be discussed with patients at each visit.

Deciding where to refer an adolescent in need of treatment is often complicated by limited treatment availability, insurance coverage complexities, and preferences of the adolescent and family. In mental health settings, child psychiatrists may be able to conduct a comprehensive biopsychosocial assessment and determine the appropriate level of care on the treatment spectrum, ranging from outpatient substance abuse counseling to long-term residential treatment programs (**Table 3**). Adolescents should always be treated in the least restrictive environment that can support their needs. A less restrictive setting such as a partial hospital program may be acceptable even if an adolescent meets criteria for a higher level of care such as residential treatment if the adolescent voluntarily accepts placement.

Addiction is a chronic, recurring medical condition. Although patients can recover, there is a lifelong potential to re-experience related symptoms. Wherever treatment begins, it should continue over the lifespan at a level appropriate to the activity of the disorder. Adolescents who have completed treatment in a residential or partial hospital program may continue treatment and monitoring with a psychiatrist, similar to how a psychiatrist follows up with an adolescent recovering from an acute episode

Table 3
Synopsis of the ASAM levels of care for treatment of substance use disorders

Outpatient	
Individual counseling	Adolescents with SUDs should receive specific treatment for their substance use; general supportive counseling may be a useful adjunct but should not be a substitute.[9] Several therapeutic modalities (eg, motivational interviewing, cognitive behavioral therapy, contingency management) have all shown promise in treating adolescents with SUDs.[109]
Group therapy	Group therapy is a mainstay of substance abuse treatment for adolescents with SUDs. It is a particularly attractive option because it is cost effective and takes advantage of the developmental preference for congregating with peers. However, group therapy has not been extensively evaluated as a therapeutic modality for this age group, and existing research has produced mixed results.[9,110]
Family therapy	Family-directed therapies are the best validated approach for treating adolescent substance abuse. Several modalities have been demonstrated effective. Family counseling typically targets domains that figure prominently in the etiology of substance use disorders in adolescents—family conflict, communication, parental monitoring, discipline, child abuse/neglect, and parental substance use disorders.[9]
Intensive outpatient program	IOPs serve as an intermediate level of care for patients who have needs that are too complex for outpatient treatment but do not require inpatient services. These programs allow individuals to continue with their daily routine and practice newly acquired recovery skills both at home and at work. IOPs generally comprise a combination of supportive group therapy, educational groups, family therapy, individual therapy, relapse prevention and life skills, 12- step recovery, case management, and aftercare planning. The programs range from 2–9 h/d, 2–5 times a week and last 1–3 mo. These programs are appealing because they provide a plethora of services in a relatively short period.[111]
Partial hospital program	Partial hospitalization is a short-term, comprehensive outpatient program in affiliation with a hospital that is designed to provide support and treatment for patients with SUDs. The services offered at these programs are more concentrated and intensive than regular outpatient treatment, as they are structured throughout the entire day and offer medical monitoring in addition to individual and group therapy. Participants typically attend sessions for 7 or 8 h/d at least 5 d/wk for 1–3 wk. As with IOPs, patients return home in the evenings and have a chance to practice newly acquired recovery skills.[112]

Inpatient/residential	
Detoxification	Detoxification refers to the medical management of symptoms of withdrawal. Medically supervised detoxification is indicated for any adolescent who is at risk of withdrawing from alcohol or benzodiazepines and may also be helpful for adolescents withdrawing from opioids, cocaine, or other substances. Detoxification may be an important first step but is not considered definitive treatment. Patients who are discharged from a detoxification program should then begin either an outpatient or residential substance abuse treatment program.[109,110]
Acute residential treatment	ART is a short-term (days–weeks) residential placement designed to stabilize patients in crisis, often before entering a longer-term residential treatment program.[109] ART programs typically target adolescents with co-occurring mental health disorders.
Residential treatment	Residential treatment programs are highly structured live-in environments that provide therapy for those with severe substance abuse, mental illness, or behavioral problems that require 24-h care. The goal of residential treatment is to promote the achievement and subsequent maintenance of long-term abstinence and equip each patient with both the social and coping skills necessary for a successful transition back into society. Residential programs are short term, which is a stay of <30 d, or long-term, which is longer than 30 d.
	Residential programs generally comprise individual and group therapy sessions, plus medical, psychological, clinical, nutritional, and educational components. Residential facilities aim to simulate real living environments with added structure and routine to prepare individuals with the framework necessary for their lives to continue drug and alcohol free upon completion of the program.[113]
Therapeutic boarding school	Therapeutic boarding schools are educational institutions that provide constant supervision for their students by a professional staff. These schools offer a highly structured environment with set times for all activities, smaller more specialized classes, and social and emotional support. In addition to the regular services offered at traditional boarding schools, therapeutic schools also provide individual and group therapy for adolescents with mental health or substance use disorders.[114]

Abbreviations: ART, Acute residential treatment; IOP, Intense outpatient program.

from a non–substance use–related psychiatric disorder. Relapse is common and should be identified as early as possible so that the adolescent can be referred back to a higher level of care as needed. Again, similar to the management of other psychiatric disorders, psychiatrists can also play a supportive role by working with the school, family, and third-party payers to support the youth in long-term recovery.

CHALLENGES TO SCREENING, BRIEF INTERVENTION, AND REFERRAL TO TREATMENT IMPLEMENTATION

Professionals that care for adolescents and young adults have been slow to systematically address substance use, although there is evidence that this is changing. Barriers to adoption of screening found in the literature include concerns about time, how to manage positive screens, and unfamiliarity with available standardized tools.[85–87] Despite these barriers, self-reported rates of substance use screening by primary care physicians appear to be increasing. Data from a national survey conducted by the AAP found that although screening rates for substance use among pediatricians were only 45% in 1997, they increased markedly to 89% by 2013.[88] However, the 2013 AAP needs assessment found pediatricians using a validated tool only 30% of the time. This finding was mirrored by findings in a study of Massachusetts primary care providers in which 86% reported screening for substance use, but only 34% were using a validated tool.[87] In contrast, Gordon and colleagues[89] found that a population of providers in rural Pennsylvania was much less likely to screen annually (34%) although almost all providers (92%) felt it was important.

Advances in technology, adoption of electronic medical records, and a general societal trend toward increased comfort with screen-based technologies also increase opportunities for use of screening tools.[90] Shorter, more efficient, frequency-based screens and self-administered implementation may help increase efficiency and reduce the use of clinical instincts in lieu of a formal tool. One study found that adolescents prefer self-administered screens to an interview format and said that they were more likely to be honest with self-administered questions.[86] Self-administered screens also require significantly less time to administer.[91]

The cultural shift toward use of text, phone, and computer for administering or augmenting interventions has been an area of much interest. This field is quickly evolving as technology and attitudes change rapidly and research efforts struggle to keep up.[92,93] Data so far appear to be mixed; systematic reviews of efforts to target tobacco smoking with online interventions showed no benefit, and Web-based alcohol interventions were not robust enough to show definitive benefits.[94,95]

Implementing brief interventions may be an even bigger challenge. Declining appointment lengths creates a challenge across medical settings, including child and adolescent psychiatry. Short trainings that show efficient brief interventions can impact physician practice in research settings, but recent findings show the challenges of influencing uptake in real-world settings.[96,97] Sterling and colleagues[97] offered three 1-hour trainings and access to video of these trainings for general pediatricians at a large integrated health care practice and then monitored SBIRT implementation data at quarterly meetings. Although less than 50% of physicians attended 2 or more meetings, there was a significant increase in assessment and brief interventions offered patients compared with the usual care group. This work was done in primary care pediatrics, although mental health settings likely face similar challenges.

There are also external forces aligning to promote the development and implementation of brief interventions and provider training. The Affordable Care Act requires screening in general medical settings, and while the impact of the legislation in this

Table 4	
Online resources for learning SBIRT	
Organization/Description	**Web Site**
Substance Abuse and Mental Health Services Administration	http://www.integration.samhsa.gov/clinical-practice/SBIRT
Massachusetts Department of Public Health – SBIRT toolkit for providers who see adolescents[67]	http://massclearinghouse.ehs.state.ma.us/BSASSBIRTPROG/SA1099.html
Institute for Research, Education, and Training in Addictions (IRETA) – Toolkit for providers and organizations using SBIRT in a variety of settings[115]	http://ireta.org/improve-practice/toolkitforsbirt/

area has not yet been captured, the requirement continues to focus attention on this area. Recently, there have been efforts to disseminate SBIRT training to general practitioners during residency, behavioral health counselors working with adolescents, nurses, social workers, pediatric residents, and an umbrella of residency programs including psychiatry and child and adolescent psychiatry residents.[98–106] In a recent project with pediatric residents, brief online training resulted in improved SBIRT understanding (**Table 4**).[107]

SUMMARY

SBIRT may be ideally suited for mental health clinicians to identify at-risk youth before development of SUD and apply evidence-based prevention and appropriate intervention to prevent onset or delay progression of SUD. Child and adolescent psychiatrists and other mental health clinicians may spend more time with patients, are more versed in psychosocial interventions such as motivational interviewing and cognitive behavioral therapy, and are readily able to identify and treat the common co-occurring psychopathology than their primary care peers; therefore, they are well positioned to implement these practices. Providing brief interventions for this population in mental health settings may be especially effective for preventing the progression of both substance use and mental health disorders.

REFERENCES

1. DuRant RH, Smith JA, Kreiter SR, et al. The relationship between early age of onset of initial substance use and engaging in multiple health risk behaviors among young adolescents. Arch Pediatr Adolesc Med 1999;153(3):286–91. Available at: http://www-ncbi-nlm-nih-gov.ezp-prod1.hul.harvard.edu/pubmed/10086407. Accessed June 20, 2014.
2. Hingson RW, Heeren T, Winter MR. Age at drinking onset and alcohol dependence: age at onset, duration, and severity. Arch Pediatr Adolesc Med 2006; 160(7):739–46. Available at: http://www.ncbi.nlm.nih.gov/entrez/query.fcgi?cmd=Retrieve&db=PubMed&dopt=Citation&list_uids=16818840.
3. The Partnership for a Drug Free America. 2012 Parents and Teens Full Report. Partnersh Attitude Track Study. 2013.
4. Rubino T, Zamberletti E, Parolaro D. Adolescent exposure to cannabis as a risk factor for psychiatric disorders. J Psychopharmacol 2012;26(1):177–88.
5. Meier MH, Caspi A, Ambler A, et al. Persistent cannabis users show neuropsychological decline from childhood to midlife. Proc Natl Acad Sci U S A 2012; 109(40):E2657–64.

6. Lynskey MT, Heath AC, Bucholz KK, et al. Escalation of drug use in early-onset cannabis users vs co-twin controls. JAMA 2003;289(4):427–33. Available at: http://www-ncbi-nlm-nih-gov.ezp-prod1.hul.harvard.edu/pubmed/?term=escalation+of+drug+use+in+early-onset+cannabis+users. Accessed March 4, 2016.
7. Center for Behavioral Health Statistics and Quality (CBHSQ), Substance Abuse and Mental Health Services Administration (SAMHSA), U.S. Department of Health and Human Services (HHS) and by RI. Results from the 2014 National Survey on Drug Use and Health: Mental Health Detailed Tables. Available at: http://www.samhsa.gov/data/sites/default/files/NSDUH-MHDetTabs2014/NSDUH-MHDetTabs2014.htm#tab2-9a. Accessed February 15, 2016.
8. American Psychiatric Association. The American Psychiatric Association practice guidelines for the psychiatric evaluation of adults.
9. Bukstein OG, Bernet W, Arnold V, et al. Practice parameter for the assessment and treatment of children and adolescents with substance use disorders. J Am Acad Child Adolesc Psychiatry 2005;44(6):609–21.
10. Bukstein OG, Horner MS. Management of the adolescent with substance use disorders and comorbid psychopathology. Child Adolesc Psychiatr Clin N Am 2010;19(3):609–23.
11. Hammond CJ, Upadhyaya H. Adolescent substance use disorders: principles for assessment and management. Child Adolesc Psychopharmacol News 2015;20(1):1–7, 10.
12. Hoagwood K, Burns BJ, Kiser L, et al. Evidence-based practice in child and adolescent mental health services. Psychiatr Serv 2001;52(9):1179–89.
13. Cushing CC, Jensen CD, Miller MB, et al. Meta-analysis of motivational interviewing for adolescent health behavior: efficacy beyond substance use. J Consult Clin Psychol 2014;82(6):1212–8.
14. Jensen CD, Cushing CC, Aylward BS, et al. Effectiveness of motivational interviewing interventions for adolescent substance use behavior change: a meta-analytic review. J Consult Clin Psychol 2011;79(4):433–40. Available at: http://www-ncbi-nlm-nih-gov.ezp-prod1.hul.harvard.edu/pubmed/21728400. Accessed December 7, 2015.
15. Substance Abuse and Mental Health Services Administration. About Screening, Brief Intervention, and Referral to Treatment (SBIRT). 2015. Available at: http://www.samhsa.gov/sbirt/about. Accessed February 15, 2016.
16. Patient Protection and Affordable Care Act. Patient Protection and Affordable Care Act. U.S.C.; 2010.
17. Committee on Substance Abuse, Levy SJ, Kokotailo PK. Substance use screening, brief intervention, and referral to treatment for pediatricians. Pediatrics 2011;128(5):e1330–40.
18. Hagan JF, Shaw JS, Duncan P. Bright futures guidelines for health supervision of infants, children, and adolescents. 3rd edition. Elk Grove Village, IL: American Academy of Pediatrics; 2008.
19. Elster AB, Kuznets NJ. AMA guidelines for adolescent preventive services (GAPS): recommendations and rationale. Baltimore, MD: Williams & Wilkins; 1994.
20. National Institute on Alcohol Abuse and Alcoholism. Alcohol screening and brief intervention for youth: a practitioner's guide; excerpt for MedScape CME course. 2011. Available at: http://pubs.niaaa.nih.gov/publications/Practitioner/YouthGuide/YouthGuideAlgorithm.pdf. Accessed February 15, 2016.
21. Belamarich PF, Gandica R, Stein REK, et al. Drowning in a sea of advice: pediatricians and American Academy of Pediatrics policy statements. Pediatrics 2006;118(4):e964–78.

22. Yarnall KSH, Pollak KI, Østbye T, et al. Primary care: is there enough time for prevention? Am J Public Health 2003;93(4):635–41. Available at: http://www-ncbi-nlm-nih-gov.ezp-prod1.hul.harvard.edu/pubmed/12660210. Accessed January 26, 2016.

23. Yuma-Guerrero PJ, Lawson KA, Velasquez MM, et al. Screening, brief intervention, and referral for alcohol use in adolescents: a systematic review. Pediatrics 2012;130(1):115–22.

24. Patnode CD, O'Connor E, Rowland M, et al. Primary care behavioral interventions to prevent or reduce illicit drug use and nonmedical pharmaceutical use in children and adolescents: a systematic evidence review for the U.S. Preventive Services Task Force. Ann Intern Med 2014;160(9):612–20.

25. Levy S, Williams J. Substance use screening, brief intervention, and referral to treatment. (policy statement). Pediatrics 2016. [Epub ahead of print].

26. Agerwala SM, McCance-Katz EF. Integrating screening, brief intervention, and referral to treatment (SBIRT) into clinical practice settings: a brief review. J Psychoactive Drugs 2012;44(4):307–17.

27. Mitchell SG, Gryczynski J, O'Grady KE, et al. SBIRT for adolescent drug and alcohol use: current status and future directions. J Subst Abuse Treat 2013; 44(5):463–72.

28. Center for Behavioral Health Statistics and Quality. Behavioral health trends in the United States: results from the 2014 National Survey on Drug Use and Health (HHS Publication). 2015.

29. Boys A, Farrell M, Taylor C, et al. Psychiatric morbidity and substance use in young people aged 13-15 years: results from the Child and Adolescent Survey of Mental Health. Br J Psychiatry 2003;182:509–17. Available at: http://www-ncbi-nlm-nih-gov.ezp-prod1.hul.harvard.edu/pubmed/12777342. Accessed January 25, 2016.

30. Roberts RE, Roberts CR, Xing Y. Comorbidity of substance use disorders and other psychiatric disorders among adolescents: evidence from an epidemiologic survey. Drug Alcohol Depend 2007;88(Suppl 1):S4–13.

31. Szobot CM, Rohde LA, Bukstein O, et al. Is attention-deficit/hyperactivity disorder associated with illicit substance use disorders in male adolescents? A community-based case-control study. Addiction 2007;102(7):1122–30.

32. Goldstein BI, Bukstein OG. Comorbid substance use disorders among youth with bipolar disorder: opportunities for early identification and prevention. J Clin Psychiatry 2010;71(3):348–58.

33. Wolitzky-Taylor K, Bobova L, Zinbarg RE, et al. Longitudinal investigation of the impact of anxiety and mood disorders in adolescence on subsequent substance use disorder onset and vice versa. Addict Behav 2012;37(8):982–5.

34. Conway KP, Swendsen J, Husky MM, et al. Association of lifetime mental disorders and subsequent alcohol and illicit drug use: results from the National Comorbidity Survey–adolescent supplement. J Am Acad Child Adolesc Psychiatry 2016;55(4):280–8.

35. Hollen V, Ortiz G. Mental health and substance use comorbidity among adolescents in psychiatric inpatient hospitals: prevalence and covariates. J Child Adolesc Subst Abuse 2015;24(2):102–12.

36. Holzer L, Pihet S, Passini CM, et al. Substance use in adolescent psychiatric outpatients: self-report, health care providers' clinical impressions, and urine screening. J Child Adolesc Subst Abuse 2013;23(1):1–8.

37. Storr CL, Pacek LR, Martins SS. Substance use disorders and adolescent psychopathology. Public Health Rev 2013;34(2):1–42. Available at: http://academiccommons.columbia.edu/item/ac:168536. Accessed January 26, 2016.

38. Center for Mental Health Services. Mental health care for youth: a national assessment, annual/final progress report. Rockville (MD): Center for Mental Health Services; 2001.

39. Anderson RL. Use of community-based services by rural adolescents with mental health and substance use disorders. Psychiatr Serv 2003;54(10): 1339–41.

40. Esposito-Smythers C, Spirito A, Kahler CW, et al. Treatment of co-occurring substance abuse and suicidality among adolescents: a randomized trial. J Consult Clin Psychol 2011;79(6):728–39.

41. Hawkins EH. A tale of two systems: co-occurring mental health and substance abuse disorders treatment for adolescents. Annu Rev Psychol 2009;60: 197–227.

42. Breslau J, Miller E, Joanie Chung WJ, et al. Childhood and adolescent onset psychiatric disorders, substance use, and failure to graduate high school on time. J Psychiatr Res 2011;45(3):295–301.

43. Teplin LA, Elkington KS, McClelland GM, et al. Major mental disorders, substance use disorders, comorbidity, and HIV-AIDS risk behaviors in juvenile detainees. Psychiatr Serv 2005;56(7):823–8.

44. Sarver DE, McCart MR, Sheidow AJ, et al. ADHD and risky sexual behavior in adolescents: conduct problems and substance use as mediators of risk. J Child Psychol Psychiatry 2014;55(12):1345–53.

45. Nock MK, Green JG, Hwang I, et al. Prevalence, correlates, and treatment of lifetime suicidal behavior among adolescents: results from the National Comorbidity Survey Replication Adolescent Supplement. JAMA Psychiatry 2013;70(3):300–10.

46. Johnson SD, Stiffman A, Hadley-Ives E, et al. An analysis of stressors and co-morbid mental health problems that contribute to youth's paths to substance-specific services. J Behav Health Serv Res 2001;28(4):412–26. Available at: http://www-ncbi-nlm-nih-gov.ezp-prod1.hul.harvard.edu/pubmed/?term=an+analysis+of+stressors+and+co-morbid+mental+health+problems+that+contribute. Accessed January 26, 2016.

47. Klein JD, McNulty M, Flatau CN. Adolescents' access to care: teenagers' self-reported use of services and perceived access to confidential care. Arch Pediatr Adolesc Med 1998;152(7):676–82. Available at: http://www-ncbi-nlm-nih-gov.ezp-prod1.hul.harvard.edu/pubmed/9667540. Accessed January 26, 2016.

48. Mclennan J, Shaw E, Shema S, et al. Adolescents' insight in heavy drinking. J Adolesc Health 1998;22(5):409–16.

49. Sterling S, Kline-Simon A, Wong A, et al. PS1-20: integrating alcohol and drug use screening for adolescents into mental health settings: rationale, missed opportunities and outcomes. Clin Med Res 2013;11(3):167.

50. Spear S, Tillman S, Moss C, et al. Another way of talking about substance abuse: substance abuse screening and brief intervention in a Mental Health Clinic. J Hum Behav Soc Environ 2009;19(8):959–77.

51. Englund MM, Egeland B, Oliva EM, et al. Childhood and adolescent predictors of heavy drinking and alcohol use disorders in early adulthood: a longitudinal developmental analysis. Addiction 2008;103(Suppl 1):23–35.

52. Irons DE, Iacono WG, McGue M. Tests of the effects of adolescent early alcohol exposures on adult outcomes. Addiction 2015;110(2):269–78.

53. Swift W, Coffey C, Carlin JB, et al. Adolescent cannabis users at 24 years: trajectories to regular weekly use and dependence in young adulthood. Addiction 2008;103(8):1361–70.
54. Wilson CR, Sherritt L, Gates E, et al. Are clinical impressions of adolescent substance use accurate? Pediatrics 2004;114(5):e536–40.
55. Hassan A, Harris SK, Sherritt L, et al. Primary care follow-up plans for adolescents with substance use problems. Pediatrics 2009;124(1):144–50.
56. Massachusetts Department of Public Health Bureau of Substance Abuse Services. Provider guide: adolescent screening, brief intervention, and referral to treatment—using the CRAFFT screening tool. Boston: Massachusetts Department of Public Health; 2009.
57. Knight JR, Sherritt L, Shrier LA, et al. Validity of the CRAFFT substance abuse screening test among adolescent clinic patients. Arch Pediatr Adolesc Med 2002;156(6):607–14.
58. Knight JR, Sherritt L, Harris SK, et al. Validity of brief alcohol screening tests among adolescents: a comparison of the AUDIT, POSIT, CAGE and CRAFFT. Washington, DC: Association for Medical Education and Research in Substance Abuse; 2002.
59. Kelly SM, Gryczynski J, Mitchell SG, et al. Validity of brief screening instrument for adolescent tobacco, alcohol, and drug use. Pediatrics 2014;133(5):819–26. Available at: http://pediatrics.aappublications.org/content/133/5/819.short. Accessed November 24, 2014.
60. Levy S, Weiss R, Sherritt L, et al. An electronic screen for triaging adolescent substance use by risk levels. JAMA Pediatr 2014;168(9):822–8.
61. American Psychiatric Association. Diagnostic and statistical manual of mental disorders. 5th edition. Arlington (VA): American Psychiatric Association; 2013.
62. Substance Abuse and Mental Health Services Administration. Results from the 2012 National Survey on drug use and health: summary of national findings. Rockville (MD): Substance Abuse and Mental Health Services Administration; 2013.
63. Substance Abuse and Mental Health Services Administration (SAMHSA). The TEDS Report: substance abuse treatment admissions referred by the criminal justice system. Rockville (MD): Substance Abuse and Mental Health Services Administration (SAMHSA); 2009. Available at: http://www.samhsa.gov/data/2k9/211/211CJadmits2k9.pdf.
64. Knight JR, Shrier LA, Bravender TD, et al. A new brief screen for adolescent substance abuse. Arch Pediatr Adolesc Med 1999;153(6):591–6.
65. Schram P, Harris SK, Van Hook S, et al. Implementing adolescent screening, brief intervention, and referral to treatment (SBIRT) education in a pediatric residency curriculum. Subst Abus 2015;36(3):332–8. Available at: http://www-ncbi-nlm-nih-gov.ezp-prod1.hul.harvard.edu/pubmed/25036267. Accessed November 21, 2015.
66. Harris SK, Csemy L, Sherritt L, et al. Computer-facilitated substance use screening and brief advice for teens in primary care: an international trial. Pediatrics 2012;129(6):1072–82.
67. Levy S, Shrier LA, The Massachusetts Department of Public Health Bureau of Substance Abuse Services, et al. Adolescent SBIRT toolkit for providers. 2015. Available at: http://massclearinghouse.ehs.state.ma.us/BSASSBIRTPROG/SA3541.html. Accessed February 15, 2016.
68. National Institute on Alcohol Abuse and Alcoholism. Alcohol screening and brief intervention for youth: a practitioner's guide. 2011. NIH Publication No. 11–7805.

Available at: http://pubs.niaaa.nih.gov/publications/Practitioner/YouthGuide/YouthGuide.pdf. Accessed February 15, 2016.

69. Colby SM, Monti PM, O'Leary Tevyaw T, et al. Brief motivational intervention for adolescent smokers in medical settings. Addict Behav 2005;30(5):865–74.

70. Miller WR, Rollnick S. Motivational interviewing: helping people change. 3rd edition. Spring Street (NY): Guilford Press; 2013. Available at: http://books.google.com/books?hl=en&lr=&id=o1-ZpM7QqVQC&pgis=1. Accessed June 23, 2014.

71. Vasilaki EI, Hosier SG, Cox WM. The efficacy of motivational interviewing as a brief intervention for excessive drinking: a meta-analytic review. Alcohol Alcohol 2006;41(3):328–35. Available at: http://alcalc.oxfordjournals.org.ezp-prod1.hul.harvard.edu/content/41/3/328. Accessed January 11, 2016.

72. Spirito A, Monti PM, Barnett NP, et al. A randomized clinical trial of a brief motivational intervention for alcohol-positive adolescents treated in an emergency department. J Pediatr 2004;145(3):396–402.

73. Monti PM, Barnett NP, Colby SM, et al. Motivational interviewing versus feedback only in emergency care for young adult problem drinking. Addiction 2007;102(8):1234–43.

74. Monti PM, Colby SM, Barnett NP, et al. Brief intervention for harm reduction with alcohol-positive older adolescents in a hospital emergency department. J Consult Clin Psychol 1999;67(6):989–94.

75. Stern SA, Meredith LS, Gholson J, et al. Project CHAT: a brief motivational substance abuse intervention for teens in primary care. J Subst Abuse Treat 2007;32(2):153–65. Available at: http://www-ncbi-nlm-nih-gov.ezp-prod1.hul.harvard.edu/pubmed/17306724. Accessed June 20, 2014.

76. Pbert L, Flint AJ, Fletcher KE, et al. Effect of a pediatric practice-based smoking prevention and cessation intervention for adolescents: a randomized, controlled trial. Pediatrics 2008;121(4):e738–47.

77. Haller DM, Meynard A, Lefebvre D, et al. Brief intervention addressing excessive cannabis use in young people consulting their GP: a pilot study. Br J Gen Pract 2009;59(560):166–72.

78. Haller DM, Meynard A, Lefebvre D, et al. Effectiveness of training family physicians to deliver a brief intervention to address excessive substance use among young patients: a cluster randomized controlled trial. CMAJ 2014;186(8):E263–72. Available at: http://www-ncbi-nlm-nih-gov.ezp-prod1.hul.harvard.edu/pubmed/?term=effectiveness+of+training+family+physicians+to+deliver+a+brief+intervention+to+address+excessive+substance+use+among+young+patients. Accessed April 16, 2014.

79. Levy S. Brief interventions for substance use in adolescents: still promising, still unproven. CMAJ 2014;186(8):565–6. Available at: http://www.cmaj.ca/content/186/8/565.extract. Accessed June 7, 2014.

80. Yule AM, Wilens TE. Substance use disorders in adolescents with psychiatric comorbidity: when to screen and how to treat: consider pharmacotherapy, psychotherapy when treating substance use disorders. Curr Psychiatr 2015;14(4):36. Available at: https://www.questia.com/library/journal/1G1-412981388/substance-use-disorders-in-adolescents-with-psychiatric. Accessed January 26, 2016.

81. Brown RA, Abrantes AM, Minami H, et al. Motivational interviewing to reduce substance use in adolescents with psychiatric comorbidity. J Subst Abuse Treat 2015;59:20–9.

82. Slesnick N, Guo X, Brakenhoff B, et al. A comparison of three interventions for homeless youth evidencing substance use disorders: results of a randomized clinical trial. J Subst Abuse Treat 2015;54:1–13.

83. Feldstein SW, Ginsburg JID. Motivational interviewing with dually diagnosed adolescents in juvenile justice settings. Br Treat Cris Interv 2006;6(3):218–33.

84. Winters KC, Fahnhorst T, Botzet A, et al. Brief intervention for drug-abusing adolescents in a school setting: outcomes and mediating factors. J Subst Abuse Treat 2012;42(3):279–88.

85. Baldwin JA, Johnson RM, Gotz NK, et al. Perspectives of college students and their primary health care providers on substance abuse screening and intervention. J Am Coll Health 2006;55(2):115–9.

86. Knight JR, Harris SK, Sherritt L, et al. Adolescents' preference for substance abuse screening in primary care practice. Subst Abus 2007;28(4):107–17. Available at: http://www-ncbi-nlm-nih-gov.ezp-prod1.hul.harvard.edu/pubmed?term= adolescents%20preference%20for%20substance%20abuse%20screening%20 in%20primary%20care%20practice&cmd=correctspelling. Accessed November 23, 2015.

87. Harris SK, Herr-Zaya K, Weinstein Z, et al. Results of a statewide survey of adolescent substance use screening rates and practices in primary care. Subst Abus 2012;33(4):321–6.

88. Ziemnik RE, Harris SK, Leon-Chi L, et al. Pediatrician Screening, Brief Intervention and Referral to Treatment (SBIRT) practices: Results of a National Survey. Presented at the Association for Medical Education and Research in Substance Abuse (AMERSA) 39th Annual National Conference. Washington DC, November 5-7, 2015.

89. Gordon AJ, Ettaro L, Rodriguez KL, et al. Provider, patient, and family perspectives of adolescent alcohol use and treatment in rural settings. J Rural Health 2011;27(1):81–90.

90. Borus J, Weas S, Fleegler E, et al. Email isn't just for old people: teen acceptability of internet communication with medical providers. Clin Pediatr (Phila) 2015. [Epub ahead of print].

91. Harris SK, Knight JR, Van Hook S, et al. Adolescent substance use screening in primary care: validity of computer self-administered vs. clinician-administered screening. Subst Abus 2016;37(1):197–203. Available at: http://www-ncbi-nlm-nih-gov.ezp-prod1.hul.harvard.edu/pubmed/25774878. Accessed November 23, 2015.

92. Shrier LA, Rhoads A, Burke P, et al. Real-time, contextual intervention using mobile technology to reduce marijuana use among youth: a pilot study. Addict Behav 2014;39(1):173–80.

93. Shrier LA, Rhoads AM, Fredette ME, et al. "Counselor in Your Pocket": youth and provider perspectives on a mobile motivational intervention for marijuana use. Subst Use Misuse 2013. [Epub ahead of print].

94. Hutton HE, Wilson LM, Apelberg BJ, et al. A systematic review of randomized controlled trials: web-based interventions for smoking cessation among adolescents, college students, and adults. Nicotine Tob Res 2011;13(4):227–38.

95. White A, Kavanagh D, Stallman H, et al. Online alcohol interventions: a systematic review. J Med Internet Res 2010;12(5):e62.

96. Buckelew SM, Adams SH, Irwin CE Jr, et al. Increasing clinician self-efficacy for screening and counseling adolescents for risky health behaviors: results of an intervention. J Adolesc Health 2008;43(2):198–200.

97. Sterling S, Kline-Simon AH, Satre DD, et al. Implementation of screening, brief intervention, and referral to treatment for adolescents in pediatric primary care. JAMA Pediatr 2015;169(11):e153145. Available at: http://archpedi.jamanetwork.com. ezp-prod1.hul.harvard.edu/article.aspx?articleid=2467333. Accessed January 11, 2016.

98. Wamsley MA, Steiger S, Julian KA, et al. Teaching residents screening, brief intervention, and referral to treatment (SBIRT) skills for alcohol use: Using chart-stimulated recall to assesscurricular impact. Subst Abus 2015. [Epub ahead of print].

99. Clemence AJ, Balkoski VI, Lee M, et al. Residents' experience of SBIRT as a clinical tool following practical application: a mixed methods study. Subst Abus 2016;37(2):306–14.

100. Kalu N, Cain G, McLaurin-Jones T, et al. Impact of a multicomponent screening, brief intervention, and referral to treatment (SBIRT) training curriculum on a medical residency program. Subst Abus 2016;37(1):242–7.

101. Mitchell SG, Schwartz RP, Kirk AS, et al. SBIRT implementation for adolescents in urban federally qualified health centers. J Subst Abuse Treat 2016;60:81–90.

102. McNelis A, Agley J, Carlson J, et al. One size doesn't fit all: screening, brief intervention, and referral to treatment (SBIRT) education for medical professionals. Eur Psychiatry 2015;30:512.

103. Bray JH, Kowalchuk A, Waters V, et al. Baylor Pediatric SBIRT Medical Residency Training Program: model description and evaluation. Subst Abus 2014; 35(4):442–9.

104. Whittle AE, Buckelew SM, Satterfield JM, et al. Addressing adolescent substance use: teaching screening, brief intervention, and referral to treatment (SBIRT) and motivational interviewing (MI) to residents. Subst Abus 2015; 36(3):325–31.

105. Ryan SA, Martel S, Pantalon M, et al. Screening, brief intervention, and referral to treatment (SBIRT) for alcohol and other drug use among adolescents: evaluation of a pediatric residency curriculum. Subst Abus 2012;33(3):251–60. Available at: http://www.tandfonline.com/doi/abs/10.1080/08897077.2011. 640182?journalCode=wsub20. Accessed April 17, 2014.

106. Tetrault JM, Green ML, Martino S, et al. Developing and implementing a multispecialty graduate medical education curriculum on screening, brief intervention, and referral to treatment (SBIRT). Subst Abus 2012;33(2):168–81.

107. Giudice EL, Lewin LO, Welsh C, et al. Online versus in-person screening, brief intervention, and referral to treatment training in pediatrics residents. J Grad Med Educ 2015;7(1):53–8. Available at: http://www-ncbi-nlm-nih-gov.ezp-prod1.hul.harvard.edu/pubmed/26217423. Accessed January 28, 2016.

108. Saunders JB, Aasland OG, Babor TF, et al. Development of the alcohol use disorders identification test (AUDIT): WHO Collaborative Project on early detection of persons with harmful alcohol consumption–II. Addiction 1993;88(6):791–804. Available at: http://www-ncbi-nlm-nih-gov.ezp-prod1.hul.harvard.edu/pubmed/ 8329970. Accessed November 21, 2014.

109. Fournier ME, Levy S. Recent trends in adolescent substance use, primary care screening, and updates in treatment options. Curr Opin Pediatr 2006;18(4): 352–8.

110. Vaughan BL, Knight JR. Intensive drug treatment. In: Neinstein LS, Gordon C, Katzman D, et al, editors. Adolescent healthcare: a practical guide. 5th edition. Philadelphia: Lippincott Williams & Wilkins; 2009. p. 671–5.

111. Center for Substance Abuse Treatment. Services in intensive outpatient treatment programs. In: Substance abuse: clinical issues in intensive outpatient treatment. Rockville (MD): Substance Abuse and Mental Health Services Administration (US); 2006. Available at: http://www.ncbi.nlm.nih.gov/books/NBK64094/. Accessed February 26, 2014.

112. Nemeck D, Lopez W, editors. CIGNA level of care guidelines for: behavioral health & substance abuse. Wilmington, DE: CIGNA; 2010. Available at: http://www.cignabehavioral.com/web/basicsite/provider/pdf/levelOfCareGuidelines.pdf.

113. Center for Substance Abuse Treatment. 3 Triage and Placement in Treatment Services. In: Substance abuse treatment for adults in the criminal justice system. Rockville (MD): Substance Abuse and Mental Health Services Administration (US); 2005. Available at: http://www.ncbi.nlm.nih.gov/books/NBK64131/. Accessed February 26, 2014.

114. Center for Substance Abuse Treatment. Therapeutic communities. Chapter 5. In: SAMHSA/CSAT treatment improvement protocols. Rockville (MD): Substance Abuse and Mental Health Services Administration (US); 1999. Available at: http://www.ncbi.nlm.nih.gov/books/NBK64342/.

115. Institute for Research Education and Training in Addictions. SBIRT Toolkit. Available at: http://ireta.org/improve-practice/toolkitforsbirt/. Accessed February 15, 2016.

Family-Based Treatments for Adolescent Substance Use

Viviana E. Horigian, MD[a],*, Austen R. Anderson, BS[b],
José Szapocznik, PhD[c]

KEYWORDS

- Substance use • Family therapy • Externalizing problems • Behavioral interventions
- Evidence-based treatment

KEY POINTS

- Family is a central system in adolescent's development.
- Ecologically based family therapy has been proven the most effective of approaches for adolescent substance use disorder.
- Several family-based treatments have been widely studied and have robust evidence of efficacy, effectiveness, and are being implemented in community settings. Others are promising and at earlier stages of testing.

INTRODUCTION

Adolescent substance use is a major risk factor for negative outcomes, including substance dependence later in life, criminal behavior, school problems, mental health disorders, injury, and death.[1-8] Substance use is often comorbid with various psychiatric disorders, especially in clinical samples.[9] Although there is some evidence for the effectiveness of various interventions for child and adolescent substance use prevention[10] and treatment,[11-17] continuing to develop, evaluate, and disseminate the most

Disclosures: J. Szapocznik is the developer of the BSFT model and has copyrighted the intervention. He is also the director for the BSFT training institute. This work was supported by grant UG1DA013720 awarded by the National Institute on Drug Abuse, and UL1TR000460 awarded by the Clinical and Translational Science Institute.
a Department of Public Health Sciences, Miller School of Medicine, University of Miami, 1120 Northwest 14th Street, CRB Room 910, Miami, FL 33136, USA; b Department of Public Health Sciences, Miller School of Medicine, University of Miami, 1120 Northwest 14th Street, CRB Room 1069A, Miami, FL 33136, USA; c Department of Public Health Sciences, Miller School of Medicine, University of Miami, 1120 Northwest 14th Street, CRB Room 1020, Miami, FL 33136, USA
* Corresponding author.
E-mail address: vhorigian@med.miami.edu

effective interventions will be essential to the welfare of adolescents. As it stands, there is a variety of available treatment approaches for adolescent substance use. Some focus on the treatment of individual adolescents through cognitive behavior therapy, motivation enhancement therapy, and supportive drug counseling. Others are structured to treat an adolescent peer group using group therapy. Family therapies have a long history in the treatment of adolescent substance abuse and, as a group, family-based treatments have been found to be highly effective at reducing substance use.[13,18]

This article provides a user-friendly, clinically focused, and pragmatic review of currently used and evidence-based family treatments. More in-depth comparisons of the evidence for each family-based treatment are available.[11,16–18] The theoretic background and empirical support for each family therapy are briefly reviewed, with descriptions of therapeutic techniques that illustrate how the treatment works in day-to-day treatment. Various aspects of each treatment, such as targeted population demographics, severity of population, location of service delivery, and the extent to which the various family-based treatments are ready for dissemination and implementation are also reviewed. The authors hope that readers will be able to assess which treatments would be effective for adolescents in their care or their agency's care. Emphasis will be placed on treatments that have the best empirical evidence and are most ready to be used in community settings. However, other promising treatments that are less well researched are also described.

WHY FAMILY-BASED APPROACHES?

Evidence and theory support a focus on family-based approaches to adolescent substance use treatment. A recent meta-analysis by Tanner-Smith and colleagues[13] revealed that family therapy programs were more effective than several other approaches, including behavioral therapy, cognitive behavioral therapy, motivation enhancement therapy or motivational interviewing psychoeducational therapy, group counseling, and practice as usual. In this meta-analysis, the statistical significant mean effect size reported for these comparisons is .26, which could be equated to a reduction from 10 days of use in the past month to 6 days of use, almost a 40% reduction of days of drug use. However, there are limitations to this meta-analysis. Specifically, it did not compare family therapy against all treatment types; it did not distinguish effects between family therapy and specific nonfamily-focused, empirically validated interventions; and it did not address sustained post-treatment effects.

Theoretically, adolescents lie at the confluence of several social systems (eg, school, community, peers), of which the family is central. As in our previous work, the authors propose an ecodevelopmental-systems theoretic approach that allows for more thorough description of the risk and protective factors predicting (ie, creating risk or protection against) adolescent substance use (**Fig. 1**).[19,20] This theoretic approach, based on Bronfenbrenner's integration of social ecological and life-span human development theories, assumes that children's development is influenced by several interacting systems across time. It places the child first and most centrally in the developmental ecology of the family because of the foundational role that families play across child and adolescent development. Although individual genetic, personality, and cognitive factors are important in understanding adolescent behavior, the ecodevelopmental approach knowingly emphasizes contextual factors more than individual factors because of their well-established role as central risk and protective factors.[21] Years of research have empirically shown that substance use and

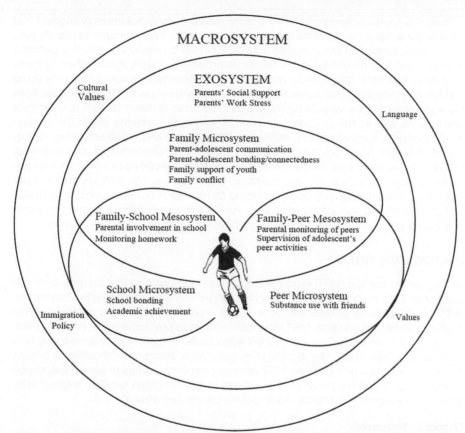

Fig. 1. Ecodevelopmental systems. (*From* Pantin H, Schwartz SJ, Sullivan S, et al. Preventing substance abuse in Hispanic immigrant adolescents: an ecodevelopmental, parent-centered approach. Hispanic Journal of Behavioral Sciences 2003;25(4):477; with permission.)

related problem behaviors are predicted by a large number of family-based risk and protective factors:

Risks
- Familial conflict[22,23]
- Abuse as children[24]
- Exposure to parents that use or used substances[25,26]

Protective
- Positive parenting[27–29]
- Parental monitoring and knowledge[30]
- Positive parent–teen affective quality[31]
- Parent–teen communication[32]
- Attachment to the family[33]
- Opportunities for prosocial behaviors[33]
- Antidrug rules and norms[34]

Research has also indicated that family involvement in treatment more generally is a key factor in obtaining successful outcomes in the treatment of adolescent substance use.[35]

Thus, the ecodevelopmental theory and the research evidence strongly suggest that adolescent substance use is inextricably linked with the functioning of the family system. This indicates that family-based approaches may be especially effective because of their emphasis on changing the family environment. Family approaches typically directly or indirectly target each of the risk and protective factors previously listed and focus on the relational interactions among family members. This article describes the ways in which the various family-based treatments attempt to alter how families function, as well as the families' interactions with other systems within the adolescent's ecology, such as friends, school, neighborhood, and extended family. Treatments that are more advanced in the phases of implementation are reviewed, followed by newer or less tested interventions. Information on each treatment was obtained through published articles, chapters, and manuals, and through online registries of evidence-based practices, including Blueprints Programs, Substance Abuse and Mental Health Administration's National Registry of Evidence-based Programs and Practices, and the National Institute of Justice's Crime Solutions database.

MULTISYSTEMIC THERAPY

Multisystemic therapy (MST) is an evidence-based intervention that focuses on family and community engagement. Based in Bronfenbrenner's social ecological framework, MST conceptualizes adolescent behavior as multidetermined and centered within multiple interacting systems. MST attempts to address problems within systems (family conflict, negative peer groups) and between systems (parent involvement in school work, peer group school attendance) to reduce the adolescent's difficulties in school, the family, and peer groups.[36] An MST therapist applies a variety of behavioral, cognitive behavioral, and family systems approaches to strengthen families; support adolescents; and, most importantly, to empower caregivers (**Box 1**).

Phases of Treatment

The sequence of therapy begins with the therapist's efforts to align with the family to gain a clear understanding of the overarching goals. Then they work to understand how the adolescent's drug use fits within the social context. This is accomplished by getting background information on the multiple systems, including a genogram, a strength and needs assessment, and a fit circle that visually displays what contextual factors are supporting the adolescent's drug use. The therapist and family collaborate to prioritize which targets of change are most important and what interventions would be most effective. Central to these efforts are the use of a weekly supervision form that contains primary goals, previous intermediary goals, barriers, gains in treatment, an updated fit circle and new intermediary goals for the coming week. The interventions are implemented and obstacles to implementation are collaboratively overcome as they arise. Interventions might include helping parents implement rewards and punishments, asking families to communicate with each other in session, blocking harmful communication patterns, discussing marital conflict and providing alternatives, and assisting caregivers in increasing monitoring. Finally, outcomes are assessed and, if more work is needed, the therapist takes the new information and creates additional working hypotheses.[36]

MST has been modified into different adaptations that attempt to address specific problems such as child abuse, problem adolescent sexual behaviors, and substance use. Although the original MST showed effectiveness in reducing substance use,[37] in an effort to focus on substance use when it is the primary difficulty, MST for substance abuse (MST-SA) was developed. This treatment integrates contingency management

---

Box 1
Multisystemic therapy core treatment principles

MST is founded on 9 core treatment principles which are:

1. Finding the fit: Proper assessment allows the therapist to understand how the adolescent's drug use fits within the context of multiple systems.

2. Focusing on positives and strengths: The positive attributes and strengths of the family, community, and the adolescent are leveraged to bring about change.

3. Increasing responsibility: Therapy should be directed toward helping individuals engage in responsible behavior such as attending school, stopping drug use, and increasing caregivers' patience.

4. Present focused, action oriented, and well-defined: Therapy emphasizes taking action to solve specific problems that are occurring now rather than past problems.

5. Targeting sequences: Interventions are targeted at changing multiple interactions that are working together to support problematic drug use.

6. Developmentally appropriate: Interventions are formulated to match the developmental stage of the adolescent.

7. Continuous effort: Interventions are meant to be applied throughout the week, requiring effort from various family members.

8. Evaluation and accountability: The efficacy of therapy is assessed according to various indicators of progress across the adolescent's life (ie, report cards, drug screens, parent reports).

9. Generalization: Although targeting specific problems, interventions should empower caregivers to handle other problems in other domains.

---

by offering vouchers and other incentives to youth who avoid drugs. In a randomized trial of MST and MST-SA in drug court setting, adolescents treated with MST-SA showed decreased drug use compared with traditional MST and drug court alone. As it stands, MST-SA is the version of MST that seems to best treat adolescent substance use problems.[38]

A primary difference from other evidence-based treatments in that it is delivered in a time-intensive manner, leading to an average of 60 direct service hours per family over 4 to 6 months.[38]

FUNCTIONAL FAMILY THERAPY

Functional family therapy (FFT)[39] is used for treating adolescent behavioral and psychological problems by improving communication between family members, increasing support, decreasing negativity, and altering dysfunctional family patterns. Through 3 phases of FFT treatment, a therapist helps the family to increase their motivation, bring about changes in behavior, and help the family maintain changes (**Box 2**).

Phases of Treatment

There are 3 phases of FFT treatment:

- Phase 1: The therapist engages the family and enhances their motivation to change through reducing negativity and by emphasizing the problem behaviors as a family issue. Reframing is a common technique whereby negative attitudes or blame are validated by the therapist and then reinterpreted in a more positive way. Thus, when a mother is angry with her daughter for using substances and

> **Box 2**
> **Functional family therapy guiding principles for bringing about change**
>
> Principle 1: Understanding clients
> - This principle includes understanding the broader community and cultural contexts within which the client and family are situated. It emphasizes the importance of identifying and working with clients' strengths as well as their risk factors.
>
> Principle 2: Understanding client problems systemically
> - Presenting problems are understood as relational problems that are the result of problematic patterns of relating within families. They are seen as functional in that they are engaged in for obtaining outcomes within an already problematic system.
>
> Principle 3: Understanding therapy and the role of the therapist as fundamentally a relational process
> - The relational engagement between therapist and family is viewed as cooperation between experts. By respecting the families, identifying meaningful change for them, and adjusting therapy to match each unique situation, therapists can guide families through the phases of treatment.
>
> *Data from* Sexton TL, Alexander JF. Functional family therapy clinical training manual. Baltimore, MD: Annie E. Casey Foundation; 2004.

blames her for their family's misfortunes, the therapist recognizes the anger and explains that those harsh feelings are likely stemming from the mothers love and concern for her daughter and the other family members.

- Phase 2: The therapist makes efforts to bring about behavior change so that families can better perform tasks related to parenting, communication, and supervision. This is accomplished by assessing risk factors, evaluating relational patterns, encouraging active listening, promoting clear communication, and helping parents implement rules and consequences for negative behavior. One example is that parents are taught to offer alternatives rather than ultimatums in their discussions with their adolescents, which will in turn reduce conflict.
- Phase 3: The therapist focuses on helping the family to maintain changes accomplished during therapy and to generalize those changes to new issues. This occurs as families are taught how to take new communication, problem-solving, and parenting skills used to target specific behaviors into new situations. The therapist helps by linking new situations to successful navigation of previous situations. As the therapist reframes continued struggles as normal, the client families will be motivated to continue acting in adaptive ways rather than resorting to past behavior patterns.

The techniques in FFT are not based on step-by-step, 1 size fits all procedures but, instead, allow for flexible, individualized treatment of families based on their unique relational and contextual factors. The theoretic foundation of FFT is systemic, behavioral, and cognitive in nature.[39] It is described as protocol driven but also involving an essential level of creativity at the hand of the therapist. Originally developed for treating externalizing behaviors more broadly, FFT has shown reductions in adolescent substance use in various clinical trials. FFT is also being tested for treating rural adolescents' substance use problems through a video teleconference version.

MULTIDIMENSIONAL FAMILY THERAPY

Multidimensional family therapy (MDFT) is a family-based treatment that makes use of individual therapy and multiple-systems approaches to treat adolescent substance use and other problematic behaviors.[9] MDFT techniques target intrapersonal (ie, feeling and thinking processes) and interpersonal factors that are leading the adolescent to act out in problematic ways. MDFT addresses problematic conditions and processes in the various domains of adolescent development, including the individual, the parents, the family environment, and extrafamilial systems.[40] The family is the central context of adolescent development healthy functioning and is theorized to be based on interdependent relations between parents and adolescents rather than emotional distance.[41] Importantly, MDFT is understood not as a universally applied procedural approach but rather as a flexible system of treatment that can adapt to individual circumstances (**Box 3**).

Phases of Treatment

The MDFT treatment course moves through 3 stages: (1) build the foundation, (2) prompt action and change by working the themes, and (3) seal the changes and exit.

The first stage begins with an assessment of various risk and protective factors that the individual, parents, family, and extrafamily systems exhibit. The therapist uses crises and stress to increase motivation, collects information from various sources to set personally relevant goals, talks to all members of the family, and explains the MDFT process. The second phase involves therapeutic interventions that are designed to address risk factors and other impediments to healthy family functioning. The therapist actively listens and empathizes with the adolescent to increase their hope and encourages them to share their inner experience. Therapists also work with parents through psychoeducation and behavioral coaching with the aim to help them improve their

---

Box 3
Multidimensional family therapy assumptions underlying treatment

1. Adolescent drug abuse is a multidimensional phenomenon; it is based on an ecological and developmental perspective that takes into account various social contexts.

2. Family functioning is instrumental in creating new, developmentally adaptive lifestyle alternatives for adolescents.

3. Problem situations provide information and opportunity; these are often the target of interventions.

4. Change is multifaceted, multideterminded, and stage oriented. Although complex, the coordination of treatment across systems and domains in a sequential way.

5. Motivation is malleable but it is not assumed. Clients are not always going to be motivated to engage in treatment and increasing motivation is central to MDFT.

6. Multiple therapeutic alliances are required and they create a foundation for change. Relationships with each family member and others are important.

7. Individualized interventions foster developmental competencies. Treatment must fit the family's historical and cultural contexts to be successful.

8. Treatment occurs in stages. Continuity is stressed as treatment proceeds; finding the continuity in themes across the stages is important for change to occur.

9. Therapist responsibility is emphasized. Therapists are responsible for many aspects of MDFT treatment and must adjust their approach relevant to feedback.

10. Therapist attitude is fundamental to success. They are optimistic and realistic in advocating for adolescent and parent improvement.

parenting by strengthening their abilities to set limits, monitor, and support their child. New skills and perceptions are taught by the therapist, who helps the family deal with problematic patterns of interaction that occur in-session. The extrafamily systems are also engaged by the therapist so that parents and adolescents can have the additional support offered by community agencies.[42]

Multiple randomized clinical trials have shown the effectiveness of MDFT for reducing adolescent substance use in controlled, and community-based settings. There is also evidence that therapist adherence to the MDFT model improves substance use outcomes.[43]

BRIEF STRATEGIC FAMILY THERAPY

Brief strategic family therapy (BSFT)[44,45] is an evidence-based integrative model, that combines structural and strategic family therapy theory and intervention techniques to address systemic or relational (primarily family) interactions that are associated with adolescent substance use and related behavior problems. BSFT considers adolescent symptoms to be rooted in maladaptive family interactions such as inappropriate family alliances, overly rigid or overly permeable family boundaries, and parents' tendency to believe that a single individual (usually the adolescent) is responsible for the family's problems. These maladaptive patterns of family interactions may result in the symptoms or merely prevent the family from effectively correcting the symptoms. Key characteristics of the intervention are that it is problem-focused, directive, practical, and follows a prescribed format (**Box 4**).

Interventions are organized into 4 domains, and are delivered in treatment phases to achieve specific goals at different times during treatment.[46,47]

Box 4
Brief strategic family therapy foundational concepts

- Systems: A social system assumes that a group of people (in the case of BSFT it is the family) is better understood as a whole organism rather than as individual independent actors. Every action that a member of the system undertakes can be understood as affecting the whole system, thus positive changes in the adolescent or the parent may bring changes to the whole family.

- Structure: Patterns of social interaction are habitual and repetitive interactions that can be understood as structure. As family members interact with each other, structure, sometimes maladaptive, can be formed that promote adolescents to behave poorly.

- Strategy: The strategic aspects of treatment refer to the practical (whatever interventions that will help bring about change), problem-focused (limiting the scope of treatment to interactions related to the presenting problem), and planned nature of BSFT treatment (based on the therapist's assessment of problematic interactions).

- Content versus process: More important than what is said in BSFT therapy, the quality of the listening, sharing, and interacting between the family members helps the therapist diagnose and work on problematic repetitive patterns.

- Context: Relying on Bronfenbrenner's (1979) theory, BSFT assumes that individuals are affected by the various social contexts within which they exist. The family is the most important of these contexts; however, peers, neighborhoods, wider culture, and counseling can also be understood as contributing contexts to adolescent development and behavior.

Data from Szapocznik J, Hervis O, Schwartz S. Brief strategic family therapy for adolescent drug abuse. Bethesda (MD): National Institute on Drug Abuse; 2003.

Table 1
Treatment characteristics: target population, treatment parameters, dissemination and research evidence

Treatment	Population	Therapist Qualifications or Fidelity	Treatment Parameters	Dissemination	Stage of Research
Multisystemic Therapy	Demographics: • Age: 12–18 y • Race: all races and ethnicities	Qualifications: • Masters level clinician (License not required) Fidelity: • Weekly group supervision • Therapist, supervisor and consultant adherence measures. Review of audio-taped treatment sessions	Families per therapist: 4–6 families per therapist (Therapist available 24 h/d, 7 d/wk) # of sessions: Minimum session 1/wk (as often as 1/d in the first weeks) Length of treatment: 3–5 mo # of treatment hours: 60 h of client contact Treatment locations: Home; juvenile justice setting; mental health center; school; juvenile drug court	Manual: Available for purchase Training: 5-d initial training. Quarterly booster training. Ongoing support for the agency and treatment team. # of countries: 15 # of implementing sites: >500 (teams) Certification: By site (3–4 therapists per team) Website: www.mstservices.com	• Blueprints Programs–Model Plus program • SAMHSA–NREPP • NIJ–Effective 48 published outcomes, independent and benchmarking studies. Space restrictions limit our coverage to the substance abuse adaptation of MST and a comprehensive meta-analysis. MST-SA Effectiveness: *1999[37,58] 2002[59]* MST-SA vs UCS *EOT* ↓ Drug use *6 mo* ↑ School attendance ↓ Out of home placements *4 y* ↓ Violent crime ↓ Drug use *2006[60] 2008[61]* MST-SA vs family court *12 mo* ↓ Substance use ↓ Delinquency *18 mo* ↓ Sibling substance use *2014[62]* 22 study meta-analysis — ↓ Delinquency ↓ Psychopathology ↓ Substance use ↓ Family problems ↓ Out of home placement ↓ Peer problems

(continued on next page)

Table 1
(continued)

Treatment	Population	Therapist Qualifications or Fidelity	Treatment Parameters	Dissemination	Stage of Research
Multidimensional Family Therapy	Demographics: • Age: 11–18 y • Race: white (US and European), African American, Hispanic	Qualifications: • Usually licensed masters level clinicians Fidelity: • Weekly supervision of cases. Monthly DVD or live supervision	Families per therapist: no more than 6 # of sessions: About 2 45–90-min sessions/wk. 40% youth, 20% parent, and 40% family. Telephone calls between sessions. Some sessions with community organizations Length of treatment: 3–6 mo depending on severity # of treatment hours: — Treatment locations: Clinic; Home; School; Family Court	Manual: Publicly available Training: 6 mo for therapists with 3 onsite trainings, weekly telephone consultations and access to the online program. Supervisor training takes an additional 4 mo. # of countries: 8 # of implementing sites: >110 (53 international sites) Certification: by site (2+ therapists per team) Website: www.mdft.org	• SAMHSA–NREPP • NIJ–Effective Efficacy: *2001*[63] MDFT vs GT vs multifamily education *2008*[64] MDFT vs CBT Effectiveness: *2004*[65] MDFT & MET or CBT & CRA *2004*[66] MDFT vs GT *2009*[67] MDFT vs GT *12 mo* ↓ Substance use ↓ Externalizing ↑ Family competence ↑ GPA *6 mo* ↓ Marijuana use *12 mo* ↑ Abstinence ↑ Recovery *EOT* ↓ Substance use ↓ Externalizing ↓ Internalizing ↑ Family functioning *12 mo* ↓ Substance use ↓ Externalizing

		↓ Internalizing
		↓ Family problems
		↓ School problems
		↓ Peer problems
2011[68]	MDFT & CBT	*12 mo*
		↓ Substance use
		↓ Externalizing
	MDFT vs CBT	↓ Substance use for high severity
2013[69]	MDFT vs IT	*12 mo*
		↓ Cannabis dependence
		↑ Treatment retention
		↓ Drug use for severe subgroup
2014[70]	MDFT vs IT	*12 mo*
	MDFT & IT	↓ Externalizing
		↓ Internalizing
		↑ Family functioning
2015[71]	MDFT & GT	*EOT*
		↓ Externalizing
		↓ Substance use
		↓ Delinquency
	MDFT vs GT	*24 mo*
		↓ Externalizing
		↓ Felony arrests
		↓ Serious crimes

(continued on next page)

Table 1
(continued)

Treatment	Population	Therapist Qualifications or Fidelity	Treatment Parameters	Dissemination	Stage of Research
Functional Family Therapy	Demographics • Age: 11–19 y • Race: white, African American, Hispanic • Runaway adolescents	Qualifications: • Developer recommends master's level except in extraordinary circumstances Fidelity: • Weekly supervision (by FFT consultant for year 1, by FFT-trained on-site supervisor from year 2 onward) • Biweekly call with site supervisor • Review of outcome and adherence data from FFT database	Families per therapist: 10–12 # of sessions: 12–14 1 h family sessions for mild cases. Up to 30 sessions for difficult cases. Length of treatment: 3–5 mo # of treatment hours: 12–30 Location of treatment: Home, clinic	Manual: Publically available Training: 1 1-d introductory training, 2 2 d clinical trainings, 3 2-d implementation trainings, 2 2-d supervisor trainings # of countries: 10 # of sites: >180 Certification: By site (3–8 therapists per team) Website: www.fftllc.com	• Blueprints Programs–Model program • SAMHSA–NREPP • NIJ–Effective Efficacy: 1973[72] FFT vs FT & NTC *EOT* ↑ Family communication 1973[73] FFT vs FT & NTC *EOT* ↑ Family communication 18 mo ↓ Recidivism 1977[74] FFT vs FT & NTC *EOT* ↑ Family communication 18 mo ↓ Recidivism 2.5–3.5 y ↓ Sibling court referrals

1989[75]	FFT vs Parenting group	*15+ mo* ↓ Substance use ↑ Retention ↑ Parent involvement ↑ Mental health ↑ Family functioning
2001[76]	FFT vs CBT vs GT	*7 mo* ↓ Substance use
2009[77]	FFT & UCS & EBFT	*15 mo* ↓ Substance use
2011[78]	FFT & CBT FFT vs CBT	*18 mo* ↓ HIV risk behaviors ↑ HIV risk behaviors relative to CBT
2014[79]	FFT or CWD & CWD or FFT & CT Effectiveness:	*18 mo* ↓ Depression ↓ Substance use
2010[80]	FFT vs UCS	*12 mo* ↓ Recidivism for high-adherence therapists
2015[81]	FFT vs NTC	*EOT* ↓ Psychosocial problems ↑ Family functioning

(continued on next page)

Table 1
(continued)

Treatment	Population	Therapist Qualifications or Fidelity	Treatment Parameters	Dissemination	Stage of Research
Brief Strategic Family Therapy	Demographics • Age: 6–17 y • Race: white, African American, Hispanic	Qualifications: Master's level Fidelity: • Weekly on-site supervision • Monthly phone supervision from BSFT institute • Weekly video review	Families per therapist: 10–12 # of sessions: 12–16 90 min family sessions Length of treatment: 4 mo # of treatment hours: 12–24 Location of treatment: Home, clinic	Manual: Publicly available Training: 3 3-d trainings # of countries: 2 # of sites: 10 Certification: By site (4 therapists per team) Website: www.bsft.org	• SAMHSA–NREPP • NIJ–Promising Efficacy: *1988[82] 1996[83] 2001[84]* BSFT vs UCS *EOT* ↑ Engagement ↑ Retention *EOT* ↓ Behavior problems ↓ Emotional problems ↑ Family functioning 12 mo ↑ Family functioning *EOT* *1989[85]* BSFT vs IT *2003[86]* BSFT vs GT ↓ Marijuana use ↓ Behavior problems ↑ Family functioning *EOT* *2006[87]* BSFT vs Supportive questioning or listening ↓ Bullying ↓ State or trait anger ↓ Cortisol levels ↑ Mental health ↑ Social functioning

2006[88]	BSFT vs Supportive questioning or listening	1 y ↓ Substance use ↓ Bullying ↓ Risky sex behavior ↓ Anger ↓ Interpersonal problems ↑ Mental health ↑ Social functioning
2013[89]	BSFT vs Referrals to treatment	6 mo ↓ Alcohol use ↓ Conduct problems
Effectiveness: 2011[46,48] 2013[90] 2015[49]	BSFT vs UCS	EOT ↑ Engagement ↑ Retention
	BSFT vs UCS BSFT & UCS	12 mo ↑ Family functioning ↓ Depression or anxiety ↓ Drug use for high-adherence therapists
	BSFT vs UCS	3-7 y ↓ Lifetime or last year arrests ↓ Lifetime or last year incarcerations ↓ Externalizing

(continued on next page)

Table 1
(continued)

Treatment	Population	Therapist Qualifications or Fidelity	Treatment Parameters	Dissemination	Stage of Research
Ecologically Based Family Therapy	Demographics • Age: 12–17 y • Race: African American, Hispanic, white • Runaway youth	Qualifications: Not listed Fidelity: • Ongoing audiotape review is standard	Families per therapist: — # of sessions: 12 1 h family sessions, 2–4 1 h individual sessions (HIV prevention) Length of treatment: 3–6 mo # of treatment hours: 14–16 Location of treatment: Home, clinic	Manual: Available from developer Training: Available from developer. 2-d training followed by weekly role-play training. # of countries: 0 # of sites: 0 Certification: NA Website: NA	• NIJ–Promising Efficacy: 2005[91] EBFT vs UCS EBFT & UCS 2009[77] EBFT vs UCS EBFT & UCS 2013[92] EBFT & CRA & MI	*12 mo* ↓ Substance use ↓ psychological functioning ↑ Family functioning ↑ HIV knowledge *15 mo* ↓ Substance use ↓ Psychological diagnoses ↓ Externalizing ↓ Delinquency ↑ Family functioning *24 mo* ↓ Substance use

	Demographics	Qualifications / Fidelity	Treatment Details	Manual / Training / Certification	Efficacy	Outcomes
Family Behavior Therapy	Demographics • Age: 12–21 y • Race: white, African American, Hispanic or Latino (Minorities are somewhat underrepresented)	Qualifications: • State licensed mental health professionals Fidelity: • Review of audio tapes with feedback • Weekly supervision • Client reported rating form available	Families per therapist: maximum of 13 # of sessions: 12–19 1-h sessions Length of treatment: 4–12 mo # of treatment hours: About 14–15 Location of treatment: Home, clinic	Manual: Available for purchase. Online videos Training: Available from treatment developer. 3 d workshop and 2 3 d booster workshops. Ongoing phone training # of countries: — # of sites: 19 have been trained Certification: Agency Website: https://web.unlv.edu/labs/frs/fbt.htm	• SAMHSA–NREPP Efficacy: 1994[51] FBT vs GT 2001[50] FBT & IT FBT vs IT	12 mo ↓ Substance use ↓ Institutionalization ↓ Depression ↑ Employment ↑ School attendance ↑ Family functioning 6 mo ↓ Substance use ↓ Hard drug use
Culturally Informed & Flexible Family Treatment for Adolescents	Demographics • Age: 14–17 y • Race: Hispanic	Qualifications: • No baselines defined Fidelity: • Not described	Families per therapist: — # of sessions: up to 32 2/wk family, parents, and adolescent sessions Length of treatment: 4 mo # of treatment hours: 32 Location of treatment: —	Manual: Not publically available Training: Not currently available # of countries: — Certification: NA Website: NA	Efficacy: 2011[54] CIFFTA vs FT	8 mo ↓ Drug use ↑ Parenting practices

(continued on next page)

Table 1
(continued)

Treatment	Population	Therapist Qualifications or Fidelity	Treatment Parameters	Dissemination	Stage of Research
Strengths-Oriented Family Therapy	Demographics • Age: 12–18 y • Race: mostly white (76%)	Qualifications: • Bachelors level (Masters recommended) Fidelity: • Audio recording with feedback • Weekly group and individual supervision using a set of theoretically related questions. • Client-rated treatment integrity	Families per therapist: Not known # of sessions: 5 biweekly family sessions; 10 multifamily group sessions; 1 booster session Length of treatment: 3 mo # of treatment hours: About 25 h total Treatment locations: Home, clinic	Manual: Publically available Training: 5 d training # of countries: — # of sites: — Certification: Therapist Website: NA	Efficacy: 2006[57] SOFT & 7C *6 mo* ↓ Substance use ↓ Substance-related problems

Abbreviations: 7C, the 7 challenges; CBT, cognitive behavioral therapy; CRA, community reinforcement approach; CT, combined treatment (FFT and CWD); CWD, coping with depression; EOT, end of treatment; FT, family therapy; GT, group therapy; IT, individual therapy; MET, motivational enhancement therapy; MI, motivational interviewing; NIJ, National Institute of Justice; NREPP, National Registry of Evidence-based Programs and Practices; NTC, no treatment control; SAMHSA, Substance Abuse and Mental Health Services Administration; UCS, usual community services.

Phases of Treatment

Early sessions are characterized by joining interventions that are intended to establish a therapeutic alliance with each family member and with the family as a whole. The therapist joins the family by demonstrating acceptance of and respect toward each individual family member, as well as the way in which the family as a whole is organized. Early sessions also include tracking and diagnostic enactment interventions. These interventions are designed to systematically identify family strengths and weaknesses and develop a treatment plan. The therapist encourages the family to behave as they would usually behave if the counselor were not present by, for example, asking them to speak with each other about the concerns that bring them to therapy rather than directing comments to the therapist. From these observations, the therapist is able to diagnose both family strengths and problematic relations. Reframing interventions are used to reduce family conflict and create a sense of hope or possibility for positive change. Over the course of treatment, therapists are expected to continue to maintain an effective working relationship with family members (joining), facilitate within-family interactions (tracking and diagnostic enactment), and to directly address negative affect or beliefs and family interactions. As treatment progresses, the focus of treatment shifts to implementing restructuring strategies to transform family relations from problematic to effective and mutually supportive. Restructuring strategies include redirecting or blocking communication, assisting in the development of behavior management, helping families develop conflict resolution skills, shifting family alliances, and promoting parental leadership.

BSFT has been evaluated in several randomized clinical trials. Adherence to the BSFT intervention strategies by therapists has been linked to improved adolescent outcomes.[48] A recent study demonstrated long-term effects of the intervention on arrests, incarcerations, and externalizing behaviors.[49]

OTHER FAMILY THERAPY TREATMENTS

Ecologically based family therapy (EBFT) is a treatment that has been investigated in a few efficacy studies with runaway adolescents who use substances. It is based on the Homebuilders Family Preservation model, which is an intervention created to keep youth in their own homes. EBFT is based on the assumption that most children are better off with their own families than in outside placements. Treatment begins by meeting with the adolescent and the family members individually so that they can be prepared to talk about the factors behind the runaway episode in a family session. At that point, the therapist assists the family in addressing these problems together, with the goal of changing dysfunctional interactions. During treatment, the therapist uses an intrapersonal to interpersonal perspective in interpreting the adolescent's problems by making use of questions and reframes that focus on the family relationships.

Unlike some of the previous therapies, there is no underlying assumption in EBFT treatment that adolescent substance use stems directly from family dysfunction and conflict. As a result, the treatment occurs in both individual and family sessions, allowing the therapist to help the youth make individual changes. This is accomplished through the use of cognitive behavioral techniques that teach the adolescent new skills for coping with intrapersonal and interpersonal problems.

Family behavior therapy (FBT) is a family-based treatment with some initial efficacy in the treatment of adolescent substance use.[50,51] The treatment involves the youth and at least 1 caregiver. The focus of the treatment is teaching families how to use behavioral techniques to improve family functioning. FBT is composed of 4 main components: behavioral contracting, stimulus control (identifying risky associations), urge control (coping skills), and communication skills training. The treatment argues that a strong relationship between the adolescent and their caregiver is central to dealing with the problem behaviors.[52] As families successfully implement these strategies, it is expected that negative behaviors, such as substance use and externalizing, will decrease, while positive outcomes, such as success in school and work, will increase.

Culturally informed and flexible family treatment for adolescents (CIFFTA)[53] was originally developed to cater to Hispanic families. It recognizes that there are commonalities across ethnicities, such as family conflict and clinical diagnoses, but that there are differences due to immigration, acculturation, and cultural experiences. CIFFTA emphasizes the interaction between the family context and the wider cultural context because these create circumstances that lead to adolescent substance use. The flexible aspect of the treatment is based in a modular design that can be adjusted depending on adolescent, family, and community characteristics. It also incorporates individual interventions such as motivational interviewing and other psychoeducational topics. There is some initial evidence of the efficacy of CIFFTA, including improvement compared with weekly traditional structural family therapy.[54]

Strengths-oriented family therapy (SOFT)[55,56] has some initial efficacy evidence in the treatment of adolescent substance use.[57] Adolescents are seen in family and multifamily groups for about 2 hours each session. The treatment also includes some case management when deemed necessary. SOFT was specifically developed in an effort to build on previous family therapy treatments by adding motivational components, solution-focused terminology, and a strengths assessment. The emphasis on both youth and parent motivation shows the importance of the family context in adolescent substance use, while the strengths assessment attempts to leverage protective factors for the benefit of the youth. The initial efficacy trial found that SOFT and a group therapy treatment reduced adolescent substance use at a 6-month follow-up.

SELECTING A TREATMENT

Table 1 presents information on the various family-based treatments for adolescent substance use. It includes information on the populations treated, the location of the service, therapist qualifications, treatment parameters, and the stage of research. The goal is that this summary together with the narrative of each mode previously described, will inform the reader in the selection of an appropriate treatment of adolescent substance users.

SUMMARY

The increasing evidence for the impact of these family interventions compared with individual and group intervention adds to prior evidence on the importance of family protective and risk factors, which supports the importance of the family in adolescent development and drug use. Several EBFT treatments have been evaluated for efficacy and effectiveness, and are now widely implemented in the United States and abroad. Fidelity to these manualized interventions is key for sustained outcomes. Some new models are accruing evidence for specific populations and will be tested for effectiveness in community settings. Continued research into the implementation and dissemination, as well as formal cost-benefit analyses, are needed to further document the effectiveness of FBT.

REFERENCES

1. Brook JS, Cohen P, Brook DW. Longitudinal study of co-occurring psychiatric disorders and substance use. J Am Acad Child Adolesc Psychiatry 1998;37(3): 322–30.
2. Degenhardt L, Coffey C, Carlin JB, et al. Outcomes of occasional cannabis use in adolescence: 10-year follow-up study in Victoria, Australia. Br J Psychiatry 2010; 196(4):290–5.
3. Degenhardt L, Hall W. Extent of illicit drug use and dependence, and their contribution to the global burden of disease. Lancet 2012;379(9810):55–70.
4. Fergusson DM, Horwood LJ, Swain-Campbell N. Cannabis use and psychosocial adjustment in adolescence and young adulthood. Addiction 2002;97(9):1123–35.
5. McCambridge J, McAlaney J, Rowe R. Adult consequences of late adolescent alcohol consumption: a systematic review of cohort studies. PLoS Med 2011; 8(2):e1000413.
6. Miller JW, Naimi TS, Brewer RD, et al. Binge drinking and associated health risk behaviors among high school students. Pediatrics 2007;119(1):76–85.
7. Moore TH, Zammit S, Lingford-Hughes A, et al. Cannabis use and risk of psychotic or affective mental health outcomes: a systematic review. Lancet 2007; 370(9584):319–28.
8. Squeglia LM, Jacobus J, Tapert SF. The influence of substance use on adolescent brain development. Clin EEG Neurosci 2009;40(1):31–8.
9. Rowe CL. Multidimensional family therapy: addressing co-occurring substance abuse and other problems among adolescents with comprehensive family-based treatment. Child Adolesc Psychiatr Clin N Am 2010;19(3):563–76.
10. Vermeulen-Smit E, Verdurmen JE, Engels RC. The effectiveness of family interventions in preventing adolescent illicit drug use: a systematic review and meta-analysis of randomized controlled trials. Clin Child Fam Psychol Rev 2015;18(3):218–39.
11. Hogue A, Henderson CE, Ozechowski TJ, et al. Evidence base on outpatient behavioral treatments for adolescent substance use: updates and recommendations 2007–2013. J Clin Child Adolesc Psychol 2014;43(5):695–720.
12. Belendiuk KA, Riggs P. Treatment of adolescent substance use disorders. Curr Treat Options Psychiatry 2014;1(2):175–88.
13. Tanner-Smith EE, Wilson SJ, Lipsey MW. The comparative effectiveness of outpatient treatment for adolescent substance abuse: a meta-analysis. J Subst Abuse Treat 2013;44(2):145–58.
14. Calabria B, Shakeshaft AP, Havard A. A systematic and methodological review of interventions for young people experiencing alcohol-related harm. Addiction 2011;106(8):1406–18.
15. Macgowan MJ, Engle B. Evidence for optimism: behavior therapies and motivational interviewing in adolescent substance abuse treatment. Child Adolesc Psychiatr Clin N Am 2010;19(3):527–45.
16. Waldron HB, Turner CW. Evidence-based psychosocial treatments for adolescent substance abuse. J Clin Child Adolesc Psychol 2008;37(1):238–61.
17. Becker SJ, Curry JF. Outpatient interventions for adolescent substance abuse: a quality of evidence review. J Consult Clin Psychol 2008;76(4):531–43.
18. Baldwin SA, Christian S, Berkeljon A, et al. The effects of family therapies for adolescent delinquency and substance abuse: a meta-analysis. J Marital Fam Ther 2012;38(1):281–304.

19. Szapocznik J, Douglas J. An ecodevelopmental framework for organizing the influences on drug abuse: a developmental model of risk and protection. In: Glantz MD, Hartel CR, editors. Drug abuse: origins & interventions. Washington, DC: American Psychological Association; 1999. p. 331–66.
20. Pantin H, Schwartz SJ, Sullivan S, et al. Preventing substance abuse in Hispanic immigrant adolescents: an ecodevelopmental, parent-centered approach. Hisp J Behav Sci 2003;25(4):469–500.
21. Hawkins JD, Catalano RF, Miller JY. Risk and protective factors for alcohol and other drug problems in adolescence and early adulthood: implications for substance abuse prevention. Psychol Bull 1992;112(1):64–105.
22. Burnette ML, Oshri A, Lax R, et al. Pathways from harsh parenting to adolescent antisocial behavior: a multidomain test of gender moderation. Dev Psychopathol 2012;24(3):857–70.
23. Skeer M, McCormick MC, Normand SL, et al. A prospective study of familial conflict, psychological stress, and the development of substance use disorders in adolescence. Drug Alcohol Depend 2009;104(1–2):65–72.
24. Oshri A, Rogosch FA, Burnette ML, et al. Developmental pathways to adolescent cannabis abuse and dependence: child maltreatment, emerging personality, and internalizing versus externalizing psychopathology. Psychol Addict Behav 2011; 25(4):634–44.
25. Kaplow JB, Curran PJ, Dodge KA. Child, parent, and peer predictors of early-onset substance use: a multisite longitudinal study. J Abnorm Child Psychol 2002;30(3):199–216.
26. Biederman J, Faraone SV, Monuteaux MC, et al. Patterns of alcohol and drug use in adolescents can be predicted by parental substance use disorders. Pediatrics 2000;106(4):792–7.
27. Capaldi DM, Stoolmiller M, Kim HK, et al. Growth in alcohol use in at-risk adolescent boys: two-part random effects prediction models. Drug Alcohol Depend 2009;105(1–2):109–17.
28. Soloski KL, Kale Monk J, Durtschi JA. Trajectories of early binge drinking: a function of family cohesion and peer use. J Marital Fam Ther 2016;42(1):76–90.
29. Henderson CE, Rowe CL, Dakof GA, et al. Parenting practices as mediators of treatment effects in an early-intervention trial of multidimensional family therapy. Am J Drug Alcohol Abuse 2009;35(4):220–6.
30. Barnes GM, Hoffman JH, Welte JW, et al. Effects of parental monitoring and peer deviance on substance use and delinquency. J Marriage Fam 2006;68(4): 1084–104.
31. Montgomery C, Fisk JE, Craig L. The effects of perceived parenting style on the propensity for illicit drug use: the importance of parental warmth and control. Drug Alcohol Rev 2008;27(6):640–9.
32. Caughlin JP, Malis RS. Demand/Withdraw communication between parents and adolescents: connections with self-esteem and substance use. J Soc Pers Relat 2004;21(1):125–48.
33. Beyers JM, Toumbourou JW, Catalano RF, et al. A cross-national comparison of risk and protective factors for adolescent substance use: the United States and Australia. J Adolesc Health 2004;35(1):3–16.
34. Schinke SP, Fang L, Cole KC. Substance use among early adolescent girls: risk and protective factors. J Adolesc Health 2008;43(2):191–4.
35. Bukstein OG. Practice parameter for the assessment and treatment of children and adolescents with substance use disorders. J Am Acad Child Adolesc Psychiatry 2005;44(6):609–21.

36. Henggeler SW, Schoenwald SK, Borduin CM, et al. Multisystemic therapy for anti-social behavior in children and adolescents. 2nd edition. New York: Guilford Press; 2009.
37. Henggeler SW, Pickrel SG, Brondino MJ. Multisystemic treatment of substance-abusing and -dependent delinquents: outcomes, treatment fidelity, and trans-portability. Ment Health Serv Res 1999;1(3):171–84.
38. Zajac K, Randall J, Swenson CC. Multisystemic therapy for externalizing youth. Child Adolesc Psychiatr Clin N Am 2015;24(3):601–16.
39. Sexton TL, Alexander JF. Functional family therapy clinical training manual. Balti-more, MD: Annie E. Casey Foundation; 2004.
40. Liddle HA, Rodriguez RA, Dakof GA, et al. Multidimensional family therapy: a science-based treatment for adolescent drug abuse. In: Lebow J, editor. Hand-book of clinical family therapy. New York: John Wiley and Sons; 2005. p. 128–63.
41. Liddle HA. Multidimensional family therapy treatment (MDFT) for the adolescent cannabis users; cannabis youth treatment (CYT) manual series, vol. 5. Rockville (MD): US Department of Health and Human Services; 2001.
42. Liddle HA. Treating adolescent substance abuse using multidimensional family therapy. In: Weisz JR, Kazdin AE, editors. Evidence-based psychotherapies for children and adolescents. 2nd edition. New York: Guilford Press; 2010. p. 416–32.
43. Rowe C, Rigter H, Henderson C, et al. Implementation fidelity of multidimensional family therapy in an international trial. J Subst Abuse Treat 2013;44(4):391–9.
44. Szapocznik J, Hervis O, Schwartz S. Brief strategic family therapy for adolescent drug abuse. Bethesda (MD): National Institute on Drug Abuse; 2003. NIH Publi-cation 03–4751.
45. Horigian VE, Szapocznik J. Brief strategic family therapy: thirty-five years of inter-play among theory, research, and practice in adolescent behavior problems. In: Scheier LM, editor. Handbook of adolescent drug use prevention: research, inter-vention strategies, and practice. Washington, DC: American Psychological Asso-ciation; 2015. p. 249–65.
46. Robbins MS, Feaster DJ, Horigian VE, et al. Brief strategic family therapy versus treatment as usual: results of a multisite randomized trial for substance using ad-olescents. J Consult Clin Psychol 2011;79(6):713–27.
47. Szapocznik J, Kurtines WM. Breakthroughs in family therapy with drug-abusing problem youth. New York: Springer; 1989.
48. Robbins MS, Feaster DJ, Horigian VE, et al. Therapist adherence in brief strategic family therapy for adolescent drug abusers. J Consult Clin Psychol 2011;79(1): 43–53.
49. Horigian VE, Feaster DJ, Robbins MS, et al. A cross-sectional assessment of the long term effects of brief strategic family therapy for adolescent substance use. Am J Addict 2015;24(7):637–45.
50. Azrin NH, Donohue B, Teichner GA, et al. A controlled evaluation and description of individual-cognitive problem solving and family-behavior therapies in dually-diagnosed conduct-disordered and substance-dependent youth. J Child Ado-lesc Subst Abuse 2001;11(1):1–43.
51. Azrin NH, McMahon PT, Donohue B, et al. Behavior therapy for drug abuse: a controlled treatment outcome study. Behav Res Ther 1994;32(8):857–66.
52. Donohue B, Azrin N, Allen DN, et al. Family behavior therapy for substance abuse and other associated problems a review of its intervention components and appli-cability. Behav Modif 2009;33(5):495–519.

53. Santisteban DA, Mena MP. Culturally informed and flexible family-based treatment for adolescents: a tailored and integrative treatment for Hispanic youth. Fam Process 2009;48(2):253–68.

54. Santisteban DA, Mena MP, McCabe BE. Preliminary results for an adaptive family treatment for drug abuse in Hispanic youth. J Fam Psychol 2011;25(4):610–4.

55. Smith DC, Hall JA. Strengths-oriented family therapy for adolescents with substance abuse problems. Soc Work 2008;53(2):185–8.

56. Hall JA, Smith DC, Williams JK. Strengths-oriented family therapy (SOFT): a manual guided treatment for substance-involved teens and their families. In: Lecroy CW, editor. Handbook of evidence-based treatment manuals for children and adolescents. New York: Oxford Press; 2008. p. 491–545.

57. Smith DC, Hall JA, Williams JK, et al. Comparative efficacy of family and group treatment for adolescent substance abuse. Am J Addict 2006;15:131–6.

58. Brown TL, Henggeler SW, Schoenwald SK, et al. Multisystemic treatment of substance abusing and dependent juvenile delinquents: effects on school attendance at posttreatment and 6-month follow-up. Child Serv Soc Pol Res Pract 1999;2(2):81–93.

59. Henggeler SW, Clingempeel WG, Brondino MJ, et al. Four-year follow-up of multisystemic therapy with substance-abusing and substance-dependent juvenile offenders. J Am Acad Child Adolesc Psychiatry 2002;41(7):868–74.

60. Henggeler SW, Halliday-Boykins CA, Cunningham PB, et al. Juvenile drug court: enhancing outcomes by integrating evidence-based treatments. J Consult Clin Psychol 2006;74(1):42–54.

61. Rowland M, Chapman JE, Henggeler SW. Sibling outcomes from a randomized trial of evidence-based treatments with substance abusing juvenile offenders. J Child Adolesc Subst Abuse 2008;17(3):11–26.

62. van der Stouwe T, Asscher JJ, Stams GJ, et al. The effectiveness of multisystemic therapy (MST): a meta-analysis. Clin Psychol Rev 2014;34(6):468–81.

63. Liddle HA, Dakof GA, Parker K, et al. Multidimensional family therapy for adolescent drug abuse: results of a randomized clinical trial. Am J Drug Alcohol Abuse 2001;27(4):651–88.

64. Liddle HA, Dakof GA, Turner RM, et al. Treating adolescent drug abuse: a randomized trial comparing multidimensional family therapy and cognitive behavior therapy. Addiction 2008;103(10):1660–70.

65. Dennis M, Godley SH, Diamond G, et al. The Cannabis Youth Treatment (CYT) Study: main findings from two randomized trials. J Subst Abuse Treat 2004; 27(3):197–213.

66. Liddle HA, Rowe CL, Dakof GA, et al. Early intervention for adolescent substance abuse: pretreatment to posttreatment outcomes of a randomized clinical trial comparing multidimensional family therapy and peer group treatment. J Psychoactive Drugs 2004;36(1):49–63.

67. Liddle HA, Rowe CL, Dakof GA, et al. Multidimensional family therapy for young adolescent substance abuse: twelve-month outcomes of a randomized controlled trial. J Consult Clin Psychol 2009;77(1):12–25.

68. Hendriks V, van der Schee E, Blanken P. Treatment of adolescents with a cannabis use disorder: main findings of a randomized controlled trial comparing multidimensional family therapy and cognitive behavioral therapy in The Netherlands. Drug Alcohol Depend 2011;119(1–2):64–71.

69. Rigter H, Henderson CE, Pelc I, et al. Multidimensional family therapy lowers the rate of cannabis dependence in adolescents: a randomised controlled trial in

Western European outpatient settings. Drug Alcohol Depend 2013;130(1–3): 85–93.

70. Schaub MP, Henderson CE, Pelc I, et al. Multidimensional family therapy decreases the rate of externalising behavioural disorder symptoms in cannabis abusing adolescents: outcomes of the INCANT trial. BMC Psychiatry 2014;14:26.

71. Dakof GA, Henderson CE, Rowe CL, et al. A randomized clinical trial of family therapy in juvenile drug court. J Fam Psychol 2015;29(2):232–41.

72. Parsons B, Alexander J. Short-term family intervention: a therapy outcome study. J Consult Clin Psychol 1973;41(2):195–201 [serial online].

73. Alexander J, Parsons B. Short-term behavioral intervention with delinquent families: impact on family process and recidivism. J Abnorm Psychol 1973;81(3): 219–25.

74. Klein N, Alexander J, Parsons B. Impact of family systems intervention on recidivism and sibling delinquency: a model of primary prevention and program evaluation. J Consult Clin Psychol 1977;45(3):469–74.

75. Friedman AS. Family therapy vs. parent groups: effects on adolescent drug abusers. Am J Fam Ther 1989;17:335–47.

76. Waldron HB, Slesnick N, Brody JL, et al. Treatment outcomes for adolescent substance abuse at 4- and 7-month assessments. J Consult Clin Psychol 2001;69(5): 802–13.

77. Slesnick N, Prestopnik JL. Comparison of family therapy outcome with alcohol-abusing, runaway adolescents. J Marital Fam Ther 2009;35:255–77.

78. Hops H, Ozechowski TJ, Waldron HB, et al. Adolescent health-risk sexual behaviors: effects of a drug abuse intervention. AIDS Behav 2011;15:1664–76.

79. Rohde P, Waldron HB, Turner CW, et al. Sequenced versus coordinated treatment for adolescents with comorbid depressive and substance use disorders. J Consult Clin Psychol 2014;82(2):342–8.

80. Sexton T, Turner CW. The effectiveness of functional family therapy for youth with behavioral problems in a community practice setting. J Fam Psychol 2010;24(3): 339–48.

81. Hartnett D, Carr A, Sexton T. The effectiveness of functional family therapy in reducing adolescent mental health risk and family adjustment difficulties in an Irish context. Fam Process 2015;55(2):287–304.

82. Szapocznik J, Perez-Vidal A, Brickman AL, et al. Engaging adolescent drug abusers and their families in treatment: a strategic structural systems approach. J Consult Clin Psychol 1988;56(4):552–7.

83. Santisteban DA, Szapocznik J, Perez-Vidal A, et al. Efficacy of intervention for engaging youth and families into treatment and some variables that may contribute to differential effectiveness. J Fam Psychol 1996;10(1):35–44.

84. Coatsworth JD, Santisteban DA, McBride CK, et al. Brief strategic family therapy versus community control: engagement, retention, and an exploration of the moderating role of adolescent symptom severity. Fam Process 2001;40(3): 313–32.

85. Szapocznik J, Rio A, Murray E, et al. Structural family versus psychodynamic child therapy for problematic Hispanic boys. J Consult Clin Psychol 1989;57(5): 571–8.

86. Santisteban DA, Perez-Vidal A, Coatsworth JD, et al. Efficacy of brief strategic family therapy in modifying Hispanic adolescent behavior problems and substance use. J Fam Psychol 2003;17(1):121–33.

87. Nickel MK, Muehlbacher M, Kaplan P, et al. Influence of family therapy on bullying behaviour, cortisol secretion, anger, and quality of life in bullying male

     adolescents: a randomized, prospective, controlled study. Can J Psychiatry 2006;51(6):355–62.

88. Nickel M, Luley J, Krawczyk J, et al. Bullying girls - changes after brief strategic family therapy: a randomized, prospective, controlled trial with one-year follow-up. Psychother Psychosom 2006;75(1):47–55.

89. Valdez A, Cepeda A, Parrish D, et al. An adapted brief strategic family therapy for gang-affiliated Mexican American adolescents. Res Soc Work Pract 2013;23(4): 383–96.

90. Horigian VE, Weems CF, Robbins MS, et al. Reductions in anxiety and depression symptoms in youth receiving substance use treatment. Am J Addict 2013;22(4): 329–37.

91. Slesnick N, Prestopnik JL. Ecologically based family therapy outcome with substance abusing runaway adolescents. J Adolesc 2005;28(2):277–98.

92. Slesnick N, Erdem G, Bartle-Haring S, et al. Intervention with substance-abusing runaway adolescents and their families: results of a randomized clinical trial. J Consult Clin Psychol 2013;81(4):600–14.

Cognitive Behavioral Therapy and Motivational Enhancement Therapy

Sarah S. Wu, PhD[a], Erin Schoenfelder, PhD[a],
Ray Chih-Jui Hsiao, MD[b,c],*

KEYWORDS

- Cognitive behavioral therapy • Treatment • Adolescent substance abuse
- Motivational enhancement therapy • Motivational interviewing

KEY POINTS

- Although cognitive behavioral therapy (CBT) is widely recognized as the preferred treatment of psychiatric disorders, such as depression or anxiety, less is known about the application of CBT to substance use disorders (SUDs), particularly in adolescence.
- This article discusses how CBT conceptualizes substance use and how it is implemented as a treatment of adolescent substance abuse.
- To achieve this goal, we draw on several manuals for CBT that implement it as a standalone treatment or in combination with motivational enhancement therapies, such as motivational interviewing.
- This article also reviews several studies that examined the efficacy of CBT, to get a better sense of its appropriateness as a treatment.
- Numerous starting resources are provided to help a clinician implement CBT with clients.

OVERVIEW OF COGNITIVE BEHAVIORAL THERAPY

Cognitive behavioral therapy (CBT)[1–3] is psychotherapeutic treatment approach based on the theory that psychiatric symptoms and distress are caused and maintained by maladaptive cognitions and behaviors. A CBT framework posits that beliefs that one holds about oneself, the world, and the future are formed by previous experiences and shape an individual's perceptions and reactions to future experiences. For example, from a CBT perspective, an individual who has negative patterns of

[a] Psychiatry and Behavioral Health, Seattle Children's Hospital, 4800 Sand Point Way, OA.5.154, PO Box 5371, Seattle, Washington 98145-5005, USA; [b] Child and Adolescent Psychiatry Residency Training Program, Washington State Medical Association, University of Washington School of Medicine, 4800 Sand Point Way Northeast, Mailstop OA.5.154, PO Box 5371, Seattle, WA 98105-0371, USA; [c] Adolescent Substance Abuse Program, Seattle Children's Hospital, 4800 Sand Point Way Northeast, Mailstop OA.5.154, PO Box 5371, Seattle, WA 98105-0371, USA
* Corresponding author. Adolescent Substance Abuse Program, Seattle Children's Hospital, 4800 Sand Point Way Northeast, Mailstop OA.5.154, PO Box 5371, Seattle, WA 98105-0371.
E-mail address: ray.hsiao@seattlechildrens.org

Child Adolesc Psychiatric Clin N Am 25 (2016) 629–643
http://dx.doi.org/10.1016/j.chc.2016.06.002
1056-4993/16/$ – see front matter © 2016 Elsevier Inc. All rights reserved.

thinking will interpret an event more harshly and therefore feel and act more negatively than a person with more positive schemas. In the case of substance use, abusing behaviors can engender certain beliefs and emotions (eg, "I drink because it's the only way I can enjoy social events") that then in turn reinforce the substance use. CBT aims to mitigate psychological distress by targeting and changing maladaptive thoughts and behaviors, and consequently the beliefs and emotions that ensue as a result.

CBT is implemented in the context of a collaborative relationship between therapist and client where the therapist systematically guides the client in linking events, beliefs, and actions, and identifying maladaptive beliefs. Through self-monitoring, Socratic questioning (ie, systematically questioning the validity of one's belief), and reality-testing (ie, testing out a belief to see if the feared consequences transpire), the client learns to evaluate situations in a more adaptive and realistic manner. Therapy also focuses on encouraging behaviors that support the client reaching his or her goals. For example, a client may create a plan to try using behavioral relaxation strategies when feeling overwhelmed, rather than avoiding the situation. Eventually, with repeated practice, the client is able to anticipate triggering situations, and the maladaptive thoughts and behaviors that typically ensue, and instead respond with more adaptive thoughts and behaviors.

To date, the efficacy of CBT has been studied across a multitude of psychiatric disorders, including depression, anxiety, eating disorders, schizophrenia and other psychotic disorders, and chronic pain, although it is most classically identified with depression[2] and anxiety.[4] More recently, clinicians and researchers have applied CBT to the treatment of substance abuse disorders (SUDs) as a standalone treatment,[5] and as adjunct to motivational interviewing (MI) or motivational enhancement techniques (MET). This article reviews how CBT can be applied to SUDs and explores evidence for the efficacy of this treatment in adults, children, and adolescents. Also examined are issues related to implementation. Practical information for clinicians who wish to implement CBT to treat SUDs is provided.

COGNITIVE BEHAVIORAL THERAPY AND SUBSTANCE ABUSE DISORDERS

CBT for substance use is predicated on the belief that strategies for helping one change their use of substances should be based on an understanding of how the patient originally learned to use substances. CBT relies heavily on the principles of social learning, modeling, and classical and operant conditioning.[6,7] With modeling, for example, a child may learn that drinking is a coping mechanism by watching a frustrated parent deal with a stressful day by having several drinks each night. Through repeated exposure, the child learns that drinking may be an "appropriate" way to deal with stress.

Kadden[8] conceptualizes operant conditioning as learning by consequences, whereas classical conditioning is described as "learning by association." Both are key ideas in how CBT frames and conceptualizes substance abuse. With respect to operant conditioning, there are many reasons why an individual may be reinforced for using a substance. The primary motivation is often the immediate physiologic effect of using the substance, such as the feeling of being "high," euphoria, or relaxation. Secondary motivations include thoughts and behaviors that are shaped over time with repeated use. For example, Carroll[6] describes how cocaine can directly change one's mood (eg, reducing feelings of depression), thoughts (eg, "I feel really good"), or behavior (eg, feeling emboldened, increasing social interaction). These secondary effects may become the primary motivations for use over time, and are therefore important to elucidate during treatment. Such components serve as excellent targets for CBT intervention.

With respect to classical conditioning, it is the pairing of cues and substance use that becomes reinforced over time. For example, an adolescent who drinks with a group of friends every day after school on the bleachers may begin to crave alcohol whenever he sees bleachers or is in the presence of those friends.

One treatment approach that considers classical conditioning is to try to reduce the occurrence of triggers (eg, reducing exposures to friends who drink), but CBT does not specifically try to reduce the impact of the triggers themselves. Instead, according to Kadden,[9] CBT accepts the consequences of use as a given (eg, excessive drinking will inevitably lead to a loss of control that cannot be mitigated) and instead tries to teach the client to develop more effective coping skills and responses.

Based on this theoretic framework, CBT treatment consists of two major components: functional analysis and skills training. Although there are many manuals for CBT for substance abuse, for brevity's sake, we focus on a few flagship manuals (**Box 1**) to explain how CBT might be implemented with substance abuse disorders. During functional analysis, the therapist's goal is to help clients determine why they began to use substances, the effects of their usage, with the goal of helping them identify ways to more effectively manage their behavior in response to the cues that triggers their use. Another approach, as suggested in the manual produced by the Addiction Technology Transfer Centers,[10] is to use a recent substance-using episode to help a client think through the antecedents and consequences of their usage. Although the questions were specifically written for treating cocaine, they are easily adapted to other substances. Examples include the following:

1. Where were you and what were you doing?
2. What happened before?
3. How were you feeling?
4. When was the first time you were aware of wanting to use?
5. What was the high like at the beginning?
6. What was it like later?
7. Can you think of anything that happened as a result?

Box 1
Treatment manuals

The following manuals may be useful for learning CBT for substance use:

1. Cognitive Behavioral Approach: Treating Cocaine Addiction: https://archives.drugabuse.gov/TXManuals/CBT/CBT1.html

2. CBT and MET for adolescent cannabis users: http://store.samhsa.gov/shin/content//SMA05-4010/SMA05-4010.pdf

3. CBT and MET for adolescent cannabis users supplement: https://store.samhsa.gov/shin/content/SMA08-3954/SMA08-3954.pdf

4. Cognitive behavioral coping skills therapy manual: http://pubs.niaaa.nih.gov/publications/ProjectMatch/match03.pdf

5. Cognitive Behavioral Therapy for Substance Use: Coping Skills Training: http://www.bhrm.org/guidelines/CBT-Kadden.pdf

6. SAMHSA Brief Interventions for Substance Use: http://www.integration.samhsa.gov/clinical-practice/sbirt/brief-interventions

8. What about negative consequences?

More advanced and in-depth questions for conducting functional analysis are provided by Carroll,[6] who suggests that therapists may want to pay particular attention to five domains within the client's life that may involve substance use: (1) social, (2) environmental, (3) emotional, (4) cognitive, and (5) physical. In the previous example, the therapist could also explore such factors as who the patient was with before the use (social), what they were thinking before they began to use (cognitive), and if they were feeling any particular physical symptoms (physical) that led to use. Alternatively, Kadden[8] and Carroll[6] suggest that standardized assessment measures may also be useful in helping to elucidate the factors contributing to substance use (**Table 1**). Such measures can be administered repeatedly throughout treatment to evaluate improvement.

McHugh and colleagues[5] also suggest that, during the functional analysis stage of CBT, the therapist should also be building a broader case conceptualization that accounts for other factors and difficulties that may perpetuate the substance use. For

Table 1
Assessment measures for SUDs that can be used during functional analysis and to track progress

Assessment Measure	Authors	Description
Inventory of Drug-Taking Situations	Annis & Martin,[11] 1985	50-item self-report questionnaire to assess for situations where the patient has consumed alcohol or other drugs over the past year
The Drinker Inventory of Consequences	Miller et al,[12] 1995	45-item scale to assess for the range of lifetime and recent consequences of drinking-related behavior in the patient
The Global Appraisal of Individual Needs	Dennis et al,[13] 2003	1.5–2.5 h interview intended to be conducted on first day of treatment that assesses for several areas of the patient's background history, and the patient's current problems, services being received, attitudes and beliefs, and desire for treatment and recovery
Addiction Severity Index	McLellan et al,[14] 1992	Semistructured interview to assess the problems that a patient may be experiencing as a result of substance abuse in seven life domains: medical, employment/support status, alcohol, drug, legal, family/social, and psychiatric
University of Rhode Island Change Assessment Scale	DiClemente & Hughes,[15] 1990	Assesses patients on where they stand with respect to the four stages of change: precontemplation, contemplation, action, and maintenance
The Treatment Attitudes and Expectation Form	Elkin et al,[16] 1985	A self-report instrument of treatment attitudes and a patient's beliefs regarding the causes of substance abuse adapted from the National Institute of Mental Health Treatment of Depression Collaborative Research Program
Revised Drinking Motives Questionnaire	Kuntsche et al,[17] 2006	Assesses an individual's reasons and motivations for drinking along four dimensions: social, coping, enhancement, and social pressure and conformity

example, co-occurring psychiatric conditions may add additional barriers or result in skill deficits that contribute to use (eg, a patient with severe social anxiety who drinks to participate socially). Although these difficulties necessarily vary between patients, they need to be discussed and incorporated into the treatment plan.

Once the patterns underlying substance use are clarified, the therapist moves onto skills training. The goal of skills training is to teach clients new and more adaptive behaviors and ways of thinking in response to triggers. Therapists should first introduce the rationale behind each skill, how it relates conceptually to the client's specific concerns, and why it is a useful step to achieving sobriety.[8] Therapists may choose to start with easier skills (eg, behavioral skills, such as diaphragmatic breathing and relaxation techniques), and work upward in difficulty. Skills should be summarized at the end of each session, and homework should be assigned to help the client practice the relevant skill.

According to Kadden,[8] skills can be categorized as involving the client only, or for managing substance use situations in which other individuals (in addition to the client) are involved (**Box 2**). For coping with one's own urges and thoughts, for example,

---

Box 2
Sample list of coping skills and skills training that may be implemented in CBT

Client-Centered Skills

- Distress tolerance
- Distraction
- Seeking social support
- Urge surfing
- Challenging and restructuring one's thoughts and cognitive distortions
- Anger management
- Relaxation
- Problem solving and decision making
- Finding new activities that can be enjoyed without substance use
- Reduce negative thinking

Interpersonal-Focused Skills

- Skills to refuse substance use
- Learning how to handle criticisms
- Learning how to refuse requests
- General social skills
- Encouraging healthy relationships
- Planning for relapse
- Helping clients identify how small, seemingly insignificant decisions may contribute to substance use behaviors
- Cognitive restructuring with respect to interpersonal interactions and beliefs
- Working with partners and families to support treatment goals

Data from Kadden RM. Cognitive-behavioral therapy for substance dependence: coping skills training. 2002. Available at: ccgt.nl/teksten/CBT-Kadden.pdf.

some relevant skills may include distress tolerance (ie, skills to help an individual manage the experience of intense motions, such as diaphragmatic breathing, holding a cold ice cube); distraction; talking with friends and family; and urge surfing, which is the skill of using mindfulness to observe and experience an urge as it peaks and diminishes (see Ref.[18]). A key skill in CBT for any presenting concern involves cognitive restructuring, or challenging and changing one's thoughts. Cognitive restructuring begins with identifying cognitive distortions, or ways in which thoughts may be inaccurate or skewed. Clients are coached to evaluate the supposed benefits or merits of thoughts versus ways in which the thoughts are detrimental or lead to negative consequences.[5,19] In restructuring thoughts, therapists help clients create more adaptive appraisals about the function and benefit of substance use. In addition to cognitive restructuring, other relevant skills also include anger management, reducing negative thinking, relaxation, guided problem solving, and decision making.[8] Additionally, clients may need help in finding new activities that can be enjoyed without substance use[5] and need support to schedule positive, productive, and healthy activities to create a new lifestyle.

With respect to interpersonal interactions, CBT skills include teaching clients how to firmly refuse invitations for substance use, handle criticisms, set personal boundaries with others, general social skills, and build healthy communication and relationships. For the longer term, the therapist also helps the client plan for relapse and identify how small, seemingly insignificant decisions, such choosing to walk home on a route that takes one by an old drinking spot, may contribute to substance use behaviors.[19] McHugh and colleagues[5] suggest that cognitive restructuring also helps improve interpersonal interactions, because clients often have maladaptive beliefs that substance use improves their relationships or sense of belonging when the opposite is often true.

As is the case with all cognitive behavioral approaches, CBT with substance use is guided by a few overarching principles: therapy is structured, brief, and time limited; present-centered; thought focused; based in practice and homework; and based in a sound therapeutic relationship (ATTC [Addiction Technology Transfer Centers]).

Kadden and colleagues[19] note that practice and homework are particularly important components of treatment for generalizing skills outside of the therapy session. Homework can include thought records that ask clients to track events that triggered maladaptive beliefs and feelings related to their substance abuse. Many CBT for substance abuse treatment manuals include worksheets for clients to complete as homework (see **Box 1**). In addition, although clients may be reluctant to participate in rehearsal role playing, Carroll[6] and Kadden and colleagues[19] note that it is highly effective in helping clients to directly experience the benefit and outcome of their skills.[8]

Kadden[8] also notes that therapists should be flexible in their treatment approach and may also want to include partners and family members in treatment. For example, a partner may be able to support the client in removing substances from the house, and can benefit from learning skills to reinforce the client as he or she learns to change. If the relationship is a trigger, teaching the partner more effective coping skills may have secondary benefits that extends to the client. The therapist should continually review previously taught skills and concepts, so as to further generalization. Finally, it is important for clients to reward themselves when they have successfully practiced a new skill. The therapist should engage in contingency management[5] and shape the client's behaviors by providing rewards and praise for efforts that are proximal to the intended goal.[6] Initially, rewards may take the form of more concrete rewards, such as prizes, money, or treatment "privileges" to engage the client. Once abstinence is achieved, however, rewards may be more naturally occurring, taking the form, for example, of healthier relationships or success at work.

McHugh and colleagues[5] also suggest that exposures may want to be incorporated as part of the CBT regiment wherein cues that usually lead to substance abuse are gradually decoupled from the act of use. For example, therapists can include exposures to external cues for use, such as showing patients drug paraphernalia or the drugs themselves and teaching them skills to manage the desire to use. For individuals for whom the cues are internal (eg, an individual who smokes whenever he or she is anxious), exposures can also be conducted for internal affective cues using interoceptive exposures wherein the symptoms of those internal cues are recreated (eg, by having the patient hyperventilate or by elevating the heart rate) without allowing for the usual ensuing substance use. One study, for example, found that interoceptive exposures successfully used the emotional arousal that an individual experienced during his panic attack.[20,21] By reducing the arousal and increasing coping skills, social support, and supporting goal setting, the treatment team was able to reduce the patients substance use.

Some research has also suggested that third-wave therapies based in mindfulness, such as acceptance commitment therapy or dialectical behavioral therapy, are useful in treating SUDs. Hayes and colleagues,[22] for example, found that adding an ACT (Acceptance and Commitment Therapy) component to therapy was associated with lower opiate and total drug use during follow-up than with methadone treatment alone. Research has also suggested that dialectical behavioral therapy, which also focuses heavily on coping skills and mindfulness, has had some efficacy in the substance abuse area.[23,24]

COGNITIVE BEHAVIORAL THERAPY WITH MOTIVATIONAL ENHANCEMENT THERAPY

Although CBT has been proposed as a standalone treatment of substance abuse disorders, it is often used in conjunction with MI/MET, a therapeutic approach that focuses on evoking the desire for change in patients.[25] The Cannabis Youth Treatment (CYT) series[26] is an example of a manualized treatment that incorporates cognitive behavioral and motivational techniques. The CYT currently exists in several formats: (1) two individual MET sessions coupled with group CBT sessions, (2) MET plus CBT and family support, or (3) a family- or family-specific treatment approach.[26]

In the case of CYT, the motivational component first emphasizes using the client's reasons for change to engage him or her in treatment. This is done in an individual setting so that the client can contemplate their ambivalence alone, without added peer pressure or fear of social evaluation. Indeed, as part of the MI/MET component, some of the treatment manuals[19] even incorporate a contract, asking the client to commit to certain parameters regarding attendance, promptness, alcohol and drug use, and completion of homework.

Next, we review the current literature available on the efficacy of CBT-based treatments to address substance abuse. We first focus on a several meta-analyses that have been conducted in adults, and then review the literature currently available regarding the efficacy of CBT for use with substance using and abusing adolescents and children.

COGNITIVE BEHAVIORAL THERAPY EFFICACY IN ADULTS WITH SUBSTANCE USE

Hofmann and colleagues[4] conducted a review of 106 meta-analytic studies examining the efficacy of CBT across several psychiatric conditions that included SUDs. As was found by McHugh and colleagues[5] and Magill and Ray,[27] the review found support for the efficacy of CBT with cannabis dependence, and efficacy increased with more sessions (as opposed to a single session). There was also a lower dropout rate with CBT than with control conditions. Most notably, Hofmann and colleagues did not find a significant advantage in CBT over other interventions, such as contingency management, relapse prevention, or MI and medication treatments (ie, agonists). However, one meta-analysis identified better outcomes for addressing nicotine dependence when CBT was implemented, either alone or in conjunction with nicotine-replacement therapy, than when nicotine-replacement therapy was used alone.[28,29] Similarly, another meta-analysis found that CBT was effective when used in conjunction with other nonpharmacologic treatments (eg, MI) as compared with the pharmacologic treatments alone.[30] However, CBT did not seem to be more effective than the other nonpharmacologic treatments when they were implemented alone.

In a meta-analytical review of 34 randomized control trials (which included 2340 patients), McHugh and colleagues[5] found an average effect size of d = .45 for CBT treatment compared with treatment-as-usual or general drug counseling. Effect sizes across the included studies ranged in size, with the largest treatment effects found for cannabis, and the smallest for the treatment of polysubstance abuse, and cocaine and opiates falling in the middle. Several of the studies have found evidence for sustained treatment effects over time. For example, in one study of the treatment of cocaine dependence, 60% of patients who received CBT provided clean toxicology screens at the 52 weeks posttreatment.[31]

Magill and Ray[27] also conducted a meta-analytic review of 52 studies that used CBT to treat adult alcohol and drug users. The studies included 9308 patients, 80% of which were diagnosed as substance dependent. The meta-analysis indicated that 29% of the patients who received CBT had better outcomes than the typical person who did not receive any treatment at all. About 8% of the patients who received CBT had better outcomes than the typical person who received a treatment without CBT. The effects were strongest for women and for cannabis users. However, in contrast to the findings of McHugh and colleagues,[5] the results did not suggest that treatment benefits were maintained across time.

Taken together, the currently available literature seems to suggest that CBT is particularly effective for treating cannabis and nicotine use and somewhat effective for treating alcohol and other noncannabis substances relative to control and treatment-as-usual conditions, or no treatment at all. However, CBT does not seem to be particularly effective for treating polysubstance use disorders. The preponderance of the evidence seems to suggest that CBT confers its biggest advantage when used in conjunction with other psychosocial treatments, such as MI or with pharmacologic treatments versus alone.

COGNITIVE BEHAVIORAL THERAPY EFFICACY IN ADOLESCENTS WITH SUBSTANCE USE DISORDERS

Tanner-Smith and colleagues[32] conducted a meta-analysis to compare the effects of family therapy, MET, psychoeducational therapy, and CBT on adolescent substance abusers. The results indicated that CBT, behavioral therapy, family therapy, and MET yielded the largest decreases in substance use. Moreover, CBT resulted in better treatment outcomes than psychoeducational therapy and no treatment or placebo control conditions. CBT, MET/CBT, and behavioral treatments were difficult to distinguish in terms of efficacy.

Vaughn and Howard[33] also conducted a meta-analytic review of adolescent substance abuse treatments, and evaluated studies based on their methodologic characteristics. Overall, the results indicated that group CBT and multidimensional family therapy (MDFT) had the highest levels of support in the research findings. CBT combined with functional family support received a "B" rating, along with psychoeducational therapy and behavioral therapy. Individual CBT received a "D" rating, suggesting that perhaps CBT is most effective for SUDs when presented in a group or family setting.

Macgowan and Engle[34] reviewed 34 studies that examined the efficacy of behavior therapies (N = 12), MI, or combined behavioral-psychosocial therapies in treating youth with alcohol or other drug use. Although the format of CBT varied greatly across the reviewed studies, the authors concluded that CBT effectively reduced alcohol and other drug use over time, and in some cases, relative to the comparative treatment condition. Becker and Curry[35] evaluated 31 randomized studies of treatment efficacy for adolescent substance abuse on 14 study characteristics. The results indicated that although it was not the most commonly used intervention, CBT was supported by the most methodologically sound studies. Moreover, the studies suggested that CBT was superior to group interactional therapy to treatment as usual but similar in treatment outcome to group psychoeducation or family behavior therapy.

Waldron and Kaminer[36] also conducted a review of controlled trials of CBT for adolescent substance use. They note that CBT may be an effective mechanism of change in part because of the skills that are taught. In one study they cite, researchers found that adolescents treated for SUDs, abstinence, and minor relapse used more problem-solving coping strategies than adolescents who had major relapses.[37,38] In addition, coping skills were found in another study to be predictive of treatment outcome.[39] In reviewing numerous studies, Waldron and Kaminer conclude that the evidence did support CBT to treat drug use, but that CBT was not necessarily more efficacious than family therapy at reducing drug use. These findings mirror those of a meta-analysis conducted by Waldron and Turner,[40] in which MDFT, functional family therapy, and group CBT were found to be the most "well-established" for adolescent substance abuse treatment, without significant between-treatment differences.

In a review of their own work, Waldron and Kaminer[36] discuss that individual CBT was found to be particularly effective in encouraging abstinence in a study of adolescent marijuana use, but that this effect decreased in significance by 7 months, and no longer existed at 19 months posttreatment. In another study to address adolescent drinking, Waldron and colleagues[41] found that group and individual CBT resulted in significantly smaller percentage of days of alcohol use 5 months posttreatment as compared with pretreatment, and in a reduction in percentage of days of any substance use 8 months posttreatment as compared with pretreatment. Interestingly, Waldron also found that, in both comparisons, the significant results were driven by the adolescents who received individual CBT.

Finally, Deas[9] conducted a review of studies that examined treatment efficacy of evidence-based practices for alcohol and other drug disorders in adolescents. Studies included were conducted between 1990 and 2005, and all used random assignment to different treatment conditions. The treatments that were compared were family-based interventions, MET therapies, behavioral therapy, CBT, and pharmacotherapy. Although the evidence seemed to suggest that evidence-based therapies, such as CBT, seem to be validated for adolescent use, Deas also cautioned that the studies included a broad range of ages and did not account for developmental variables, such as cognitive development in their findings. Additionally, outcome variables varied greatly across the studies and targeted the treatment of multiple substance abuses, because adolescents frequently coabuse. Deas cautions that future studies need to come to a consensus as to how to address developmental factors and outcome variables to provide a more complete picture of whether CBT and other evidence-based practices are indeed effective for treating adolescent substance abuse.

ISSUES RELATED TO IMPLEMENTATION

As discussed by Waldron and Turner,[40] there are moderators of treatment effects that should be considered when using CBT. Briefly, moderators of treatment are pretreatment characteristics that influence the relationship between treatment type (or any other independent variable) and treatment outcome.[42] Although moderator variables such as these are often not measured in treatment outcome studies, they are important to incorporate when making treatment decisions and in the interpretation of research outcomes. Some prime moderators may include, but are not limited to, sex of the patients, comorbidities, ethnicity, motivation for change, parenting and family factors, and baseline levels of coping skills and functioning.

With respect to ethnicity, for example, Waldron and Turner[40] review several studies in which treatment efficacy varied as a function of patient ethnicity. One study suggested that patient-therapist ethnicity matching was particularly effective when treating Hispanic adolescents with substance abuse, but less so for Anglo adolescents. Another study found that Hispanic adolescents seemed to benefit more from family-based interventions than CBT.

Hendriks and colleagues[43] conducted a study to determine whether individual characteristics in adolescent cannabis users affected the outcomes of treatment. In general, their review of adult substance abusers suggested no improved efficacy when matching patients to treatment type. Patients were assigned to either MDFT or the CYT 5-session format of CBT. Significant patient characteristics included demographic background (eg, age, gender), characteristics related to substance use and severity, substance-use related problems, delinquency, treatment history, comorbid psychopathology, family functioning, or school- or work-related problems. Although there were no between treatment-group differences on outcome, MDFT did prove to be more effective than CBT depending on age, conduct disorder (CD)/ODD comorbidity, and level of internalizing problems. For example, younger adolescents with comorbid CD/ODD or internalizing problems had greater reductions in their cannabis use with MDFT than CBT. These findings are consistent with those of Deas,[9] who suggested that CBT treatment outcomes may vary as a function of age, in part because of developmental differences, such as cognitive understanding or emotional readiness, which interact with how different therapies work.

Comorbid Diagnoses

Similar to the study conducted by Hendricks and colleagues,[43] several other studies have explicitly examined the treatment outcomes in adolescents with comorbid psychiatric conditions. Cornelius and colleagues[44] examined the efficacy of combined CBT/MET compared with treatment as usual for adolescents with comorbid major depressive disorder and alcohol use disorder. The biggest treatment gains, in terms of reduction in severity of MDD (Major Depressive Disorder) symptoms and alcohol-related behaviors, were found in the group that received CBT/MET. These results are similar to those found by Hides and colleagues[45] who examined the treatment outcomes of CBT/antidepressants on alcohol- and substance-abusing adolescents and adults with comorbid depression. At the end of treatment, the CBT/antidepressants yielded reductions in levels of self-rated depression and anxiety, whereas self-ratings of social and occupational functioning increased. Additionally, there was a significant decrease in the number of those meeting criteria for SUDs, substance use, and an increase in the number of days of abstinence. Although these results were found at Week 20 posttreatment, they were also maintained at Week 40.

Riggs and colleagues[46] compared the efficacy of CBT plus fluoxetine hydrochloride, versus placebo on adolescents who were diagnosed with nontobacco substance use, major depression, and CD. The results indicated that the CBT plus fluoxetine and CBT plus placebo groups had an overall decrease in self-reported substance use and in overall levels of CD symptoms but the difference in reduction between the two groups was nonsignificant. In addition, there were more substance-free weekly urine analyses in the CBT-placebo group, than in the CBT-fluoxetine group. Again, these results suggest that CBT can confer benefits to substance abuse treatment when used in conjunction with pharmacotherapy. In addition, these results suggest that CBT can have greater beneficial effects that may generalize to other comorbid conditions that adolescents with substance abuse disorders may also be experiencing.

Esposito-Smythers and colleagues[47] compared the efficacy of CBT for adolescents with co-occurring suicidality and alcohol use disorder. Although the sample size was small (five families), the results indicated that the CBT yielded reductions in suicidality and alcohol use over the course of treatment. The authors suggest that CBT can be effectively used with alcohol-using adolescents who are also suicidal in an outpatient setting.

Taken together, these results suggest that CBT seems to be effective for addressing several substance use concerns in adolescents ranging from 13 to 18 years in age, and adolescents with comorbid mental health problems. Although the evidence is strongest for CBT to treat cannabis use, alcohol can also be successfully treated with CBT in outpatient and community settings. Interestingly, no significant differences were found between CBT and family therapies, although the evidence suggests that the greatest benefits of CBT are seen in the short term. Moreover, these results indicate that CBT can be used effectively in adolescent substance users with comorbid conditions (at least with respect to depression, anxiety, and suicidality) and that delivery is effective in individual and group formats. Finally, when implementing CBT, it is important to account for developmental variables and moderators, such as age and cognitive skill level.

LIMITATIONS IN TREATMENT

Many of these manuals, namely Project MATCH and CYT, were designed as protocols for research studies and consequently have strict implementation criteria. The Project MATCH manual, for example, is intended only for outpatient settings and deviations from the protocol is strongly discouraged. With the CYT manual, Sampl and Kadden[26] note that the therapy is only appropriate as an early treatment or outpatient treatment for children between the ages of 12 and 18 who are abusing or dependent on marijuana. In addition, the authors caution that CBT is not appropriate for polysubstance dependence or those who are using other substances heavily in addition to marijuana. Children with severe social anxiety, CD, or another acute psychological condition may also not be appropriate for CYT.

Additionally, as discussed by Moyers and Houck,[48] there may be some limitations in using CBT along with MI. Practitioners have traditionally emphasized complete abstinence as the ultimate treatment goal in CBT. However, MI supports the client's right to make decisions in therapy and choose their treatment goal. This may result in conflicting goals for the therapist; on one hand, the therapist will want to support the client's autonomy, and on the other, encourage a goal the client is ambivalent about. Moyers and Houck[48] emphasize that, whereas MI brings value added to other treatments, such as CBT, conflicts such as these needs to be considered and addressed when combining the two treatments.

IMPLICATIONS FOR CLINICIANS

With the help of training manuals, such as those described in this review, CBT can be successfully implemented for the treatment of substance use problems in adults and adolescents in a variety of settings. When determining if CBT is the appropriate treatment modality for a given client, it is helpful to consider the client's level of motivation, their ability to commit to participating in homework outside of therapy, a client's level of insight into his or her own metacognition, and whether the client might benefit from additional skills and tools that can be offered by other therapeutic approaches. The current research to date suggests that CBT, as a standalone and complementary therapy, can benefit adolescents who use a wide range of substances across several treatment settings.

Medical and mental health clinicians can also support a patient's referral to a CBT program by providing psychoeducation about this treatment modality and outcomes and supporting the client in overcoming barriers to treatment initiation and continuation. Although many of the essential treatment components of CBT are not specific to the treatment only, it is useful in that it provides a structured, client-driven, time-limited, and active form of treatment through which therapists can engage clients. Most importantly, it seems that individual and group formats of CBT can have efficacy, which suggests that the treatment is scalable and appropriate in resource-limited settings.

REFERENCES

1. Beck AT. Depression: clinical, experimental, and theoretical aspects. Philadelphia: University of Pennsylvania Press; 1967.
2. Beck JS. Cognitive therapy. John Wiley & Sons, Inc; 1979.
3. Ellis A. Reason and emotion in psychotherapy. Oxford (United Kingdom): Lyle Stuart; 1962.
4. Hofmann SG, Asnaani A, Vonk IJ, et al. The efficacy of cognitive behavioral therapy: a review of meta-analyses. Cognit Ther Res 2012;36(5):427–40.
5. McHugh RK, Hearon BA, Otto MW. Cognitive behavioral therapy for substance use disorders. Psychiatr Clin North Am 2010;33(3):511–25.
6. Carroll KM. Therapy manuals for drug addiction, manual 1: a cognitive-behavioral approach: treating cocaine addiction. Rockville (MD): National Institute on Drug Abuse; 1998.
7. Kaminer Y, Spirito A, Lewander W. Brief motivational interventions, cognitive-behavioral therapy, and contingency management for youth substance use disorders. In: Kaminer Y, Winters K, editors. Clinical manual of adolescent substance abuse treatment. Arlington (TX): American Psychiatric Association; 2011. p. 213–38.
8. Kadden, R. Cognitive-behavioral therapy for substance dependence: coping skills training. 2002. Available at: http://www.ci2i.research.va.gov/CI2IRESEARCH/docs/Cogbehtrpguidelines.pdf. Accessed February 19, 2016.
9. Deas D. Evidence-based treatments for alcohol use disorders in adolescents. Pediatrics 2008;121(Suppl 4):S348–54.
10. Addiction Technology Transfer Center Network. Cognitive behavioral therapy training manual. 2013. Available at: http://www.nattc.org/regcenters/productDocs/10/CBT%20Manual%20%20Revised%20March%202013.pdf. Accessed February 19, 2016.

11. Annis HM, Martin G. Inventory of drug-taking situations. Toronto: Addiction Research Foundation; 1985.

12. Miller WR, Tonigan JS, Longabaugh R. The Drinker Inventory of Consequences (DrInC): an instrument for assessing adverse consequences of alcohol abuse: test manual (No. 95). Rockville (MD): US Department of Health and Human Services; Public Health Service; National Institutes of Health; National Institute on Alcohol Abuse and Alcoholism; 1995.

13. Dennis ML, Titus JC, White MK, et al. Global appraisal of individual needs: administration guide for the GAIN and related measures. Bloomington (IL): Chestnut Health Systems; 2003.

14. McLellan AT, Kushner H, Metzger D, et al. The fifth edition of the addiction severity index. J Subst Abuse Treat 1992;9(3):199–213.

15. DiClemente CC, Hughes SO. Stages of change profiles in outpatient alcoholism treatment. Journal of Substance Abuse 1990;2(2):217–35.

16. Elkin I, Parloff MB, Hadley SW, et al. NIMH treatment of Depression Collaborative Research Program: background and research plan. Arch Gen Psychiatry 1985; 42(3):305–16.

17. Kuntsche E, Knibbe R, Gmel G, et al. Replication and validation of the drinking motive questionnaire revised (DMQ-R, Cooper, 1994) among adolescents in Switzerland. Eur Addict Res 2006;12(3):161–8.

18. Bowen S, Marlatt A. Surfing the urge: brief mindfulness-based intervention for college student smokers. Psychol Addict Behav 2009;23(4):666.

19. Kadden, R, Carroll, K, Donovan, D, et al. Cognitive-behavioral coping skill therapy manual: a clinical research guide for therapists treating individuals with alcohol abuse and dependence. 2003. Available at: http://pubs.niaaa.nih.gov/publications/ProjectMatch/match03.pdf. Accessed February 19, 2016.

20. Zvolensky MJ, Lejuez CW, Kahler CW, et al. Integrating an interoceptive exposure-based smoking cessation program into the cognitive-behavioral treatment of panic disorder: theoretical relevance and case demonstration. Cogn Behav Pract 2003;10(4):347–57.

21. Zvolensky MJ, Yartz AR, Gregor K, et al. Interoceptive exposure-based cessation intervention for smokers high in anxiety sensitivity: a case series. J Cogn Psychother 2008;22(4):346–65.

22. Hayes SC, Wilson KG, Gifford EV, et al. A preliminary trial of twelve-step facilitation and acceptance and commitment therapy with polysubstance-abusing methadone-maintained opiate addicts. Behav Ther 2004;35(4):667–88.

23. Linehan MM, Dimeff LA, Reynolds SK, et al. Dialectical behavior therapy versus comprehensive validation therapy plus 12-step for the treatment of opioid dependent women meeting criteria for borderline personality disorder. Drug Alcohol Depend 2002;67(1):13–26.

24. Linehan MM, Schmidt H, Dimeff LA, et al. Dialectical behavior therapy for patients with borderline personality disorder and drug-dependence. Am J Addict 1999; 8(4):279–92.

25. Miller WR, Yahne CE, Tonigan JS. Motivational interviewing in drug abuse services: a randomized trial. J Consult Clin Psychol 2003;71(4):754.

26. Sampl, S, & Kadden, R. Motivational enhancement therapy and cognitive behavioral therapy for adolescent cannabis users: 5 sessions. Cannabis Youth Treat (cyt) Ser, Volume 1. 2001. Available at: http://store.samhsa.gov/shin/content//SMA05-4010/SMA05-4010.pdf. Accessed February 19, 2016.

27. Magill M, Ray LA. Cognitive-behavioral treatment with adult alcohol and illicit drug users: a meta-analysis of randomized controlled trials. J Stud Alcohol Drugs 2009;70(4):516–27.
28. Vera MPG, Sanz J. Análisis de la situación de los tratamientos para dejar de fumar basados en terapia cognitivo-conductual y en parches de nicotina. Psicooncología 2006;3(2/3):269–89.
29. Hasler G, Klaghofer R, Buddeberg C. The University of Rhode Island Change Assessment Scale (URICA). Psychother Psychosom Med Psychol 2002; 53(9–10):406–11 [in German].
30. Leung KS, Cottler LB. Treatment of pathological gambling. Curr Opin Psychiatry 2009;22(1):69–74.
31. Rawson RA, Huber A, McCann M, et al. A comparison of contingency management and cognitive-behavioral approaches during methadone maintenance treatment for cocaine dependence. Arch Gen Psychiatry 2002;59(9):817–24.
32. Tanner-Smith EE, Wilson SJ, Lipsey MW. The comparative effectiveness of outpatient treatment for adolescent substance abuse: a meta-analysis. J Subst Abuse Treat 2013;44(2):145–58.
33. Vaughn MG, Howard MO. Adolescent substance abuse treatment: a synthesis of controlled evaluations. Res Soc Work Pract 2004;14(5):325–35.
34. Macgowan MJ, Engle B. Evidence for optimism: behavior therapies and motivational interviewing in adolescent substance abuse treatment. Child Adolesc Psychiatr Clin N Am 2010;19(3):527–45.
35. Becker SJ, Curry JF. Outpatient interventions for adolescent substance abuse: a quality of evidence review. Journal of Consulting and Clinical Psychology 2008; 76(4):531.
36. Waldron HB, Kaminer Y. On the learning curve: the emerging evidence supporting cognitive–behavioral therapies for adolescent substance abuse. Addiction 2004;99(Suppl 2):93–105.
37. Myers MG, Brown SA. Coping responses and relapse among adolescent substance abusers. J Subst Abuse 1990;2(2):177–89.
38. Myers MG, Brown SA. Coping and appraisal in potential relapse situations among adolescent substance abusers following treatment. J Child Adolesc Subst Abuse 1990;1(2):95–115.
39. Myers MG, Brown SA, Mott MA. Coping as a predictor of adolescent substance abuse treatment outcome. J Subst Abuse 1993;5(1):15–29.
40. Waldron HB, Turner CW. Evidence-based psychosocial treatments for adolescent substance abuse. J Clin Child Adolesc Psychol 2008;37(1):238–61.
41. Waldron HB, Slesnick N, Brody JL, et al. Treatment outcomes for adolescent substance abuse at 4-and 7-month assessments. J Consult Clin Psychol 2001;69(5):802.
42. Kazdin AE. Mediators and mechanisms of change in psychotherapy research. Annu Rev Clin Psychol 2007;3:1–27.
43. Hendriks V, van der Schee E, Blanken P. Matching adolescents with a cannabis use disorder to multidimensional family therapy or cognitive behavioral therapy: treatment effect moderators in a randomized controlled trial. Drug Alcohol Depend 2012;125(1):119–26.
44. Cornelius JR, Douaihy A, Bukstein OG, et al. Evaluation of cognitive behavioral therapy/motivational enhancement therapy (CBT/MET) in a treatment trial of comorbid MDD/AUD adolescents. Addict Behav 2011;36(8):843–8.
45. Hides L, Carroll S, Catania L, et al. Outcomes of an integrated cognitive behaviour therapy (CBT) treatment program for co-occurring depression and substance misuse in young people. J Affect Disord 2010;121(1):169–74.

46. Riggs PD, Mikulich-Gilbertson SK, Davies RD, et al. A randomized controlled trial of fluoxetine and cognitive behavioral therapy in adolescents with major depression, behavior problems, and substance use disorders. Arch Pediatr Adolesc Med 2007;161(11):1026–34.

47. Esposito-Smythers C, Spirito A, Kahler CW, et al. Treatment of co-occurring substance abuse and suicidality among adolescents: a randomized trial. J Consult Clin Psychol 2011;79(6):728.

48. Moyers TB, Houck J. Combining motivational interviewing with cognitive-behavioral treatments for substance abuse: lessons from the COMBINE Research Project. Cogn Behav Pract 2011;18(1):38–45.

Advances in Research on Contingency Management for Adolescent Substance Use

Catherine Stanger, PhD*, Amy Hughes Lansing, PhD,
Alan J. Budney, PhD

KEYWORDS

- Contingency management • Adolescent • Substance use • Treatment • Review

KEY POINTS

- The literature on the use of contingency management (CM) for reducing adolescent substance use continues to grow and generally shows positive effects for enhancing outcomes during treatment.
- As with other models of treatment, obtaining enduring effects post-treatment remains a challenge, and tests of innovative CM programs targeting maintenance are lacking.
- Implementation research indicates strong interest in adoption of CM, and initial findings suggest that structured workshops can provide effective training for some types of programs.
- Parameters of CM programs, such as the frequency and magnitude of contingent incentives, context of the contingency (home vs clinic), target behavior, and selected population, should be clearly specified when evaluating and discussing the efficacy of CM interventions.

In 2010, the research base for CM applications in adolescent substance use disorder treatment settings was only just emerging; however, the overwhelming positive evidence base from the adult treatment literature provided reason for high expectations.[1] The adolescent literature in this area continues to progress at a moderate pace, with many indicators of budding interest in its application and in finding cost-effective models to enhance dissemination and implementation. Mixed findings have been reported, which are not unexpected given the struggle to find inexpensive, effective treatment models that could readily be adopted by the current health care system. Outcomes from other psychosocial interventions for adolescent substance

This work was supported by National Institutes of Health grants DA15186 and AA01691. None of the authors has any conflict of interest or other disclosures.
Department of Psychiatry, Geisel School of Medicine at Dartmouth, Lebanon, NH 03766, USA
* Corresponding author. Department of Psychiatry, Geisel School of Medicine at Dartmouth, 46 Centerra Parkway, Suite 300, HB 7255, Lebanon, NH 03766.
E-mail address: catherine.stanger@dartmouth.edu

Child Adolesc Psychiatric Clin N Am 25 (2016) 645–659
http://dx.doi.org/10.1016/j.chc.2016.05.002
1056-4993/16/© 2016 Elsevier Inc. All rights reserved.

childpsych.theclinics.com

use disorders clearly indicate that these problems are not easy to treat and that success rates have much room for improvement.[2] As discussed in the prior review of the adolescent CM literature,[1] the schedule of reinforcement (magnitude, timing, and frequency) of a CM program is likely the most important determinant of its success in changing the target behavior. For example, greater magnitude and more frequent delivery of contingent reinforcement (incentives) as soon as possible after the target behavior occurs usually engender better outcomes than lesser magnitude, delayed, and lower-frequency delivery, yet enlisting higher-magnitude and more frequent incentives has greater cost and requires more time and effort. Unfortunately, those seeking to use CM to enhance treatment outcome may err toward keeping costs down in this way, at the peril of reducing efficacy. Details are highlighted of newly reviewed CM programs to alert readers to the parameters (eg, target and schedule of reinforcement) under study to facilitate more nuanced interpretations of the findings.

This article first provides a review of recent controlled trials focused on adolescent substance use for teens referred to outpatient treatment. Second, a brief summary of the continued innovative applications of CM to tobacco cessation among youth is presented. Investigations of predictors and mechanisms of the CM outcomes from treatment studies are summarized to highlight recent efforts to better understand mechanisms and predictors of CM approaches and how these may be used to effectively guide future research endeavors. Emerging literature on dissemination and implementation of CM and the use of CM as platform or backbone treatment in experimental studies of novel interventions is discussed, which indicate growing recognition and acceptance of CM as a viable model for community treatment. A brief review is provided of a few studies that illustrate the influence of CM research occurring in the area of adolescent substance use treatment and how it is extended to or paralleled by new applications targeting other health behaviors or disorders.

CLINICAL TRIALS TESTING CONTINGENCY MANAGEMENT FOR SUBSTANCE USE DISORDERS

Six new controlled trials of adolescent CM have been published since 2010. Outcomes from each are reviewed, focusing on the intervention characteristics across the domains of inclusion/exclusion criteria, the platform intervention to which CM was added, whether the control condition included any contingent incentives, and whether parents of adolescents participated in the delivery of contingent incentives was or was not part of CM. In addition, the CM interventions are characterized along the dimensions recommended by Stanger and colleagues[1]: target of the intervention (eg, abstinence), monitoring strategy, and the incentive schedule, magnitude, and type (**Table 1**).

First, there have been 2 negative trials, reporting no significant differences for youth receiving CM versus a comparison condition. The smaller trial randomized 31 youth over 2.5 years into outpatient substance use treatment as usual versus a CM intervention.[3] Youth met *Diagnostic and Statistical Manual of Mental Disorders* (*DSM*) diagnostic criteria for a cannabis use disorder, and parents were not involved in the intervention. The usual care youth did receive attendance incentives using a fishbowl, with a maximum value of approximately $200. In the CM condition, the target behavior was abstinence from all tested substances (no attendance incentives), monitored by urine tests conducted twice a week for 10 weeks. The incentive schedule was escalating, with a reset contingency if use occurred; however, incentives were not reinstated if abstinence recurred and draws could be lost. A fishbowl prize incentive program was used, with pulls earning $5.20 on average, a maximum of 112 pulls, and estimated maximum earnings of approximately $580. There were no significant differences between CM and usual care youth in substance use outcomes, with youth in both conditions achieving a mean of approximately 5 consecutive weeks of abstinence. A potential explanation for finding no effect for CM might include the small sample size (N = approximately 15 per condition). In addition there may have been selection bias in the sample due to the very small percentage of youth treated at the agencies who elected to enroll in the study. These youth were likely not representative of treated youth generally and, based on the positive outcomes in both conditions, may have reflected a motivated, low-problem sample likely to achieve positive outcomes regardless of additional interventions. Furthermore, the CM schedule was generally more punitive than is typical in the instance of a lapse. Accumulated draws could be lost and were not reinstated back to maximum levels if abstinence was regained.

The second study with negative results enrolled 60 youth and compared 10-week group cognitive behavior therapy (CBT) with or without a CM intervention.[4] Youth were required to meet *DSM* cannabis use disorder criteria and have a positive urine sample for cannabis at intake. The requirement of a positive cannabis test at intake is not typical across studies and may have resulted in an overall sample at higher than usual risk of poor treatment outcome. Parents were not involved in the intervention, and youth in the control condition received incentives yoked to youth in the CM groups. In the CM condition, the target behavior was abstinence from all tested substances, monitored by urine tests conducted once a week for 2 weeks, then twice a week for 8 weeks. The incentive schedule was escalating, with a reset contingency if use occurred. A voucher program was used with maximum earnings of $242. Overall, neither condition showed improvement in substance use based on weekly tetrahydrocannabinol (THC)-positive urine drug tests, with 71% of youth positive for THC at the end of the intervention. Potential explanations for the lack of efficacy of CM in this trial include the low magnitude of incentives, no parental involvement, and restricting the sample to the most high-risk youth.

The first of the 4 positive trials published in the past 5 years compared juvenile drug court (JDC) with or without a family CM (FAM-CM) intervention (N = 104).[5] All youth in drug court were eligible, and the majority met cannabis use disorder criteria (80%). The usual drug court condition did not receive attendance incentives. The CM target was abstinence from all substances tested, and monitoring involved urine tests weekly plus additional random tests. The CM portion of the intervention lasted 4 months on average; however, drug court participation, including ongoing urine testing throughout the 9-month postrecruitment follow-up period. The schedule was escalating; however, earned points could not be redeemed for rewards when a urine test was positive and not until the fifth week. Points were deducted for positive tests. Incentives were negotiated with the teen and parent and were provided both by parents (monetary and nonmonetary) and staff. Incentives started at 12 points per negative urine test (1 point = $1), and escalated after the first 4 weeks of the program up to a maximum of 24 points per negative test. The total number potential earnings was not clearly defined; however, it seemed that the incentive system was designed so that the majority of incentives earned would be delivered by parents and not program staff, who had a maximum of $150 in their part of the program. Youth receiving CM had decreased odds of a THC-positive test through the 9-month intervention relative to the drug court as usual control youth. At the 9-month assessment, 20% of the FAM-CM and 34% of the control youth tested positive for THC. Differences across conditions were not observed on self-report of substance use, with 30% of youth in

Table 1
Summary of recent adolescent contingency management interventions: characteristics and outcomes

Study/N	Inclusion Criteria/Setting	Platform	Control Incentives	Parent Participation in Contingency Management	Contingency Management Target	Monitoring Schedule	Incentive Schedule	Incentive Magnitude	Incentive Type	Trial Outcome
Killeen et al,[3] 2012 (N = 31)	Cannabis use + diagnosis/outpatient	Community care, 12-step, group	Yes	No	Abstinence	2×/wk UA for 10 wk	Escalating with reset	$583[b]	Fishbowl/prize cabinet	Negative: CM = control; both conditions improved
Kaminer et al,[4] 2014 (N = 60)	THC-positive UA + cannabis diagnosis/outpatient	10 wk group CBT	Yes	No	Abstinence	1×/wk UA for 2 wk; 2×/wk for 8 wk	Escalating with reset	$242	Vouchers/gift cards	Negative: CM = control; poor outcomes in both conditions
Stanger et al,[8] 2015 (N = 153)	Cannabis use + diagnosis/outpatient	Individual Met/CBT 5 + 7	Yes	Yes + incentives for parents	Abstinence	2×/wk UA for 14 wk	Escalating with reset	$725	Vouchers/gift cards + fishbowl/gift cards	Positive: CM > control; during treatment differences; not sustained to 12-mo follow-up
Henggeler et al,[5] 2012 (N = 104)	Drug court (80% with cannabis diagnosis)/outpatient	Usual drug court services	No	Yes	Abstinence	1×/wk UA + random tests for ~4 mo	Escalating/can't redeem points if not abstinent/no reset	$150	Vouchers/gift cards	Positive: CM > control; during treatment differences to 9 mo of continued drug court involvement

Godley et al,[9] 2014 (N = 337)	Post residential treatment/ past year substance use disorder (91% with cannabis diagnosis)/ home visits	UCC/ACC	No	No[a]	Abstinence + prosocial activities	1×/wk UA for 12 wk + activity verification	Escalating with reset	$298[b]	Fishbowl/ prize cabinet	Positive: CM > control; effects sustained to 9 mo follow-up.
Stewart et al,[10] 2015 (N = 136)	Referral by school staff due to substance use/substance use in prior 3 mo (88% cannabis use disorder)/ school based	MI	No	No	Abstinence + self-reported abstinence or reduction ("change plan improvements")	1×/wk self-report + 50% chance of saliva test for 4 wk	Fixed with no reset	$15[b]	Fishbowl/ gift cards	Positive: CM > control; during treatment differences; not sustained to 2-mo follow-up

Abbreviation: UA, urinalysis.

[a] Parents participated in one of the comparison conditions (ACC).

[b] Maximum earnings not presented in article; amount extrapolated from information in article.

both conditions reporting any days of use in the past 90 days. CM youth also significantly reduced general delinquency and person and property offenses.

Stanger and colleagues compared motivational enhancement therapy MET/CBT 5 + 7 sessions[6,7] to 2 CM conditions, CM with and without comprehensive parent training (PT) (N = 153).[8] This study followed-up on an initial study comparing MET/CBT + abstinence CM + PT to MET/CBT + attendance CM to replicate the positive effects of CM on cannabis abstinence and to isolate the efficacy of PT. Youth were referred to outpatient substance use counseling, and all met *DSM* (Fourth Edition) diagnostic criteria for cannabis use disorder. The MET/CBT control condition received attendance incentives ($5 per visit and provision of urine specimens; maximum = $140), and results of urine tests were provided to parents. The CM target was abstinence from all substances tested, and monitoring involved twice-weekly urine tests for 14 weeks. There were 2 CM components: clinic based and home based. The clinic-based schedule was escalating, with a reset, and maximum earnings were $590. An additional fishbowl program provided incentives (gift cards) for early abstinence (first 4 weeks of the program: pulls earned $2.43 on average; 112 pulls maximum; and estimated maximum earnings = $135). For home-based CM, parents worked with the teen's therapist to develop a contingency contract specifying rewards and consequences to be implemented at home contingent on the results of the teen's urine test results. Parents also earned incentives for session attendance, and compliance with the youth substance contract procedure (fishbowl: pulls earned $2.43 on average; 111 pulls maximum; and estimated maximum earnings = $270). In the CM + PT condition, parents received additional PT focused on youth conduct problems more generally. Youth in either CM condition were more likely to achieve 4 weeks of continuous cannabis abstinence during treatment (48%) than were those who received MET/CBT only (30%). Between-condition differences were not maintained during 12-month follow-up.

No additional benefit was observed for the comprehensive PT, that is, no differences were observed between the 2 CM conditions. The failure of PT to improve outcomes may be due to several factors. First, therapist fidelity to the PT intervention was only moderate (although it was comparable to other studies in which the intervention showed positive effects). Second, the inclusion of some youth with low levels of conduct problems in the treatment sample may have limited the impact of PT. Third, the home-based CM delivered to those who did not receive PT is an evidence-based parenting intervention that focuses specifically on substance use. Therefore, the 2 CM conditions differ in the dose/breadth of PT, including an exclusive focus on substance use versus a broader focus on conduct problems and family communication, including substance use. Thus, these results do not suggest that parenting interventions fail to improve outcomes relative to individual interventions. The findings do suggest, however, that the addition of a broad-spectrum parenting intervention, as delivered in this study, focusing on conduct problems did not boost outcomes over and above home-based CM focusing on substance use more specifically.

A third positive trial enrolled substance-using youth leaving residential treatment (N = 337) who met criteria for a past year substance use disorder (91% for a cannabis use disorder).[9] Using a 2 × 2 design, youth were randomly assigned to usual continuing care (UCC) services versus assertive continuing care (ACC) services and to CM versus no CM. There were no incentives provided to youth who did not receive CM. CM targeted 2 behaviors: abstinence from all substances tested, monitored via weekly urine tests for 12 weeks, and documented participation in prosocial activities. The schedule was escalating, with a reset. A fishbowl system with a prize cabinet was used ($2.55 per pull; 117 pulls maximum abstinence and 117 for activities; and estimated maximum earnings = $298 each for abstinence and activities). Parents did not participate in CM; however, ACC involved parent/caregivers in 4 sessions focused on communication and problem solving. Youth receiving CM only and receiving ACC only had more days of abstinence from cannabis through the 9-month post-treatment follow-up compared with UCC. Outcomes for the CM + ACC condition were not significantly different from UCC, which the investigators suggest may have resulted from the high demands in the combined intervention.

The final positive CM trial was conducted in a school setting (N = 136) and enrolled youth referred by school personnel due to concern about substance use (88% met cannabis use disorder criteria).[10] The platform intervention was 4 sessions of motivational interviewing (MI), which was followed by either a CM condition or no additional intervention (MI only). No incentives were provided to the MI-only youth. One CM target was abstinence from all substances tested, with monitoring achieved by a 50% (random) chance of a saliva test (substances tested and window of detection not specified) for 4 weeks. CM youth also received incentives for self-reported abstinence or change plan improvements. A fishbowl system with fixed, nonescalating pulls (1 pull for each target) was used (50% chance of winning $5 gift card per pull; $2.50 per pull; 6 pulls maximum; and estimated maximum earnings seem to be $15–$25). Parents did not participate. Results indicated greater reductions in marijuana use days per month among CM than MI-only youth, with significant differences between conditions at the end of the 8-week intervention period but not at the 16-week follow-up assessment.

These diverse CM interventions for substance-using youth are challenging to summarize. They all highlight cannabis use as the primary clinical outcome, regardless of the method of recruitment or setting, likely reflecting the ubiquitous and frequent cannabis use patterns across samples of adolescents enrolled in general outpatient settings. All programs targeted abstinence using objective biological sampling measured typically once or twice per week. They also generally demonstrate short-term CM efficacy across highly diverse settings (school, clinic, juvenile justice, and continuing care), platform interventions (many were evidence based, ranging from 4-session MI to 14 weeks of MET/CBT) using varying types of incentives (fishbowl vs vouchers), schedules (although most were escalating), and magnitude (approximately $25 to $725 total/approximately $6 to $50 per week).

No trial has tested the impact of CM magnitude (ie, compared different magnitudes or schedules) for substance-using youth. Neither of the 2 trials with negative findings involved parents, and both were conducted in outpatient treatment settings, whereas 2 of the 4 positive trials directly involved parents in the administration of CM at home. To date, no trial has systematically tested the independent or combined efficacy of clinic-based versus parent-based CM. It seems possible that both negative trials may reflect some recruitment bias, with 1 trial showing generally positive outcomes in all conditions across a small and highly select sample of perhaps highly motivated youth,[3] and the other showing poor outcomes across groups where youth were required to test positive for cannabis at baseline, a unique inclusion criteria not typical of CM studies and perhaps more severe than other comparable studies.[4] The best outcomes across studies were reported for youth with the lowest rates of baseline substance use, that is, those in JDC or those entering continuing care after residential treatment.[5,9] Intermediate, less long-lasting outcomes[8,10] were reported for youth in outpatient and school-based settings. Finally, across studies, long-term reduction in use or abstinence among youth remains a serious challenge, even among those who show better post-treatment outcomes. The 1 study focused on continuing care suggests that including additional targets of CM, such as engagement in specific types of prosocial activities, together with targeting abstinence might better facilitate enduring change.[9]

Moderators and Mediators

Several recent studies have tested moderators and mediators of adolescent CM interventions. Overall, the list of tested relations that failed to reach significance is longer than positive associations. For example, with the CM-FAM intervention integrated with JDCs, no demographic characteristics (age <16 years, gender, and ethnicity) or psychiatric problems (presence of internalizing or externalizing disorder) showed main effects on treatment outcome and did not interact with CM.[5] Similarly, demographic predictors (mandated treatment, psychiatric medications, living with both parents, and receipt of additional services) did not predict outcomes or interact with CBT + CM.[4] One study has reported a moderating effect of disruptive behavior disorder diagnosis (DBD) on treatment outcome related to MET/CBT + attendance incentives versus MET/CBT plus abstinence-based CM.[11] DBD-positive adolescents generally reported a higher frequency of marijuana use across all assessment periods, but those who received abstinence-based CM showed a significantly greater reduction in frequency of marijuana use than those who received MET/CBT plus attendance incentives. Among DBD-negative adolescents who received abstinence-based CM did not have significantly better marijuana use outcomes compared with MET/CBT + attendance-based incentives. This may have been due to a ceiling effect; that is, DBD-negative compared with those who received MET/CBT + attendance incentives had good marijuana outcomes, making it more difficult to demonstrate greater outcomes with abstinence-based CM.

Several studies have tested treatment engagement, secondary targets (eg, prosocial activities) or cognitive mechanisms. For example, in the study of CM and ACC, although both were associated with greater treatment engagement (attending 4 or more sessions in the first 6 weeks) and increased prosocial activities, neither mediated relations between treatment condition and outcome.[9] The school-based CM study (discussed previously) tested engagement in external substance use treatment and self-reported use of temptation coping skills in high-risk situations at the end of the trial as mechanisms.[10] The number of temptation coping strategies endorsed mediated relations between treatment condition and end-of-treatment cannabis use frequency, after controlling for baseline marijuana use frequency. Youth receiving CM reported more use of temptation coping, which in turn predicted fewer cannabis use days, despite receiving no direct instruction in using these strategies. Although youth receiving CM were more likely to engage in outside treatment, this engagement did not mediate the intervention effects.

Overall, findings generally indicate that CM appears efficacious across broad demographic groups of adolescents. Only 1 recent study reported greater CM efficacy among a subpopulation, youth with concurrent DBDs. Research is particularly limited on moderation of CM efficacy by cognitive characteristics among adolescents, such as delay discounting or other characteristics related to executive function, including self-regulation or emotion regulation. Research on mechanisms of CM is similarly limited, but the study of the school-based intervention represents a notable exception.[10]

Applying Contingency Management to Tobacco Cessation

The earlier review[1] also highlighted the promising initial CM studies targeting tobacco cessation in a school-based setting, which found that adding CM to CBT could substantially enhance cessation rates in the short term.[12] A subsequent 4-week, randomized trial designed to dismantle the effects of CM and CBT has since been published.[13] Youth (n = 82) seeking cessation treatment in their school setting received either CM alone, CBT alone, or CM + CBT. Participants included 82 adolescent smokers seeking smoking cessation treatment. A greater percentage of CM + CBT and CM youth (36.7% and 36.3%, respectively) than CBT-alone youth (0%) were abstinent for 7 days or more immediately preceding the end of treatment. One-month and 3-month post-treatment assessment did not reveal any between-condition differences but suggested a slower increase in tobacco use over time in the CM-alone group. Secondary analyses of these data suggest that the significant main effect of CM seemed primarily accounted for by its robust positive impact on youth with higher levels of behavioral impulsivity or greater self-regulation deficit.[14] An additional analysis examined whether exposure to stressful life events or type of coping style interacted with type of treatment to predict tobacco abstinence outcomes.[15] Greater use of behavioral coping skills predicted positive smoking outcomes among those who received only CM, and the converse was observed among those in the CM + CBT condition, that is, less use of behavioral coping predicted abstinence. Last, in response to concerns about potential negative effects of providing monetary incentives in the CM conditions, this group assessed how youth spent their incentive earnings. Youth self-reports suggested that CM was not associated with increased spending on tobacco or other substances, and, generally, those who earned the most incentives tended to increase spending on more prosocial goods or services.[16]

Another tobacco cessation trial evaluated a home-based CM protocol focused on reaching a high-risk adolescent sample with little access to treatment.[17] Modeled after a similar Internet-delivered protocol developed by Dallery and colleagues[18] for adult smokers that was tested successfully in a prior study with 4 adolescents,[19] 62 youth received either contingent incentives based on carbon monoxide (CO) levels indicative of smoking abstinence (verified by video recordings from a CO monitor 3 times per day) or incentives for just submitting the videos on schedule with no contingency on CO levels. The innovative reinforcement schedule included shaping, abstinence, and thinning phases. The CO-based contingencies engendered greater decreases in CO across the 30-day trial, and those in this condition also maintained reductions during a 6-week post-treatment phase. Overall, the CM approaches to adolescent tobacco smoking have illustrated that systematically providing contingent incentives for smoking reduction and cessation has strong potential, certainly for motivating and engendering initial change. Reinforcement schedules that focus on reducing relapse, such as thinning or fading,[19] warrant more study to better achieve more enduring positive effects.

DISSEMINATION AND IMPLEMENTATION OF CONTINGENCY MANAGEMENT FOR ADOLESCENT SUBSTANCE USE

Despite strong evidence in support of the effectiveness of CM interventions in adults and the increasing literature demonstrating positive effects with adolescents, dissemination and implementation of CM programs have been limited. During the past few years, research examining methods of dissemination and implementation of CM for adolescent substance use indicates that CM is fairly straightforward to teach and implement and represents a relatively low-cost intervention that can be integrated with other treatment models and readily adopted by a variety of organization types (eg, substances use services, mental health provider services, and JDCs).[20–24]

One study examined 2 implementation models for integrating CM with multisystemic therapy (MST) for cannabis-using adolescents with 38 MST-trained providers.[21]

One model included an intensive quality assurance system (ie, manualized information, expert consolation, organizational support, and ongoing training) and a CM workshop, whereas the other model included the CM workshop only. Therapist adherence to CM was not significantly increased for providers who received the intensive quality assurance + workshop compared with those who received the workshop only, suggesting that a CM workshop alone may be sufficient for adequate integration of CM into a clinic providing MST. This study also found that across both implementation groups, higher therapist adherence to CM was associated with increased cannabis abstinence, reinforcing the importance of developing effective training models for increasing and maintaining provider adherence to CM.

Another study examined 3 implementation models for the integration of a CBT + CM intervention for adolescent substance use into community outpatient substance abuse treatment services with substance abuse and mental health practitioners.[20] Three models, a workshop and resources (WS+), WS+ with computer-assisted training (WS+/CAT), and WS+/CAT with supervisory support, were tested in 10 organizations across 161 therapists. No benefit was observed for the 2 more intensive training models compared with the less intensive WS + model in terms of CM knowledge, CM use, and CM adherence. This again suggests that a workshop with additional resources was sufficient to facilitate adequate adoption of CM into public sector outpatient substance abuse treatment services.

Finally, 1 study examined strategies for implementing CM-FAM into JDCs.[22] Six JDCs, 104 families, 51 therapists, and 74 JDC stakeholders received either training in CM-FAM or continued with providing usual services. Outcomes supported the feasibility of implementing CM-FAM in the JDCs, and CM-FAM–trained therapists and stakeholders had more favorable perceptions of incentive-based interventions for substance use. This finding is critical because nonfavorable perceptions of incentive-based interventions are a primary obstacle to the dissemination of CM into community treatment settings. Additional education about and exposure to CM interventions for providers and stakeholders might help to overcome this obstacle.[25,26]

Other Indicators of Acceptance of Contingency Management Models

One sign of the growing recognition and utilization of CM interventions for adolescent substance use comes from clinical trials that choose to use abstinence-based or attendance-based CM as treatment platforms on which to test the efficacy of other new behavioral or pharmacologic treatments. For example, 2 published trials investigating the efficacy of bupropion and N-acetylcysteine for adolescent tobacco cessation and cannabis use, respectively, used study designs that involved between-condition comparisons of CM plus medication versus CM plus placebo. Although not clearly asserted, the rationale for the design likely included the contention that before using a medication in an adolescent population, it should be determined if it increases efficacy compared with an optimal noninvasive, psychosocial intervention (ie, CM). Similarly, CM has been used as the base treatment on which to build and test a sexual risk reduction intervention for substance-using adolescents.[27,28]

Another indicator of growing interest in using CM to enhance outcome comes from pilot or demonstration trials conducted in community clinics. Most recently, a report appeared evaluating a very-low-cost CM program that targeted attending substance use treatment sessions in an urban outpatient clinic.[29] A quasiexperimental design (comparing attendance prior to vs after implementation of the CM program) showed that those in the CM program attended significantly more sessions on average (79% vs 61%), with expenditures for the CM program averaging approximately

$29 per participant or $3 per session. Such demonstrations, although not well controlled, show that clinical operations can readily modify CM to fit their programs and suggest a growing interest in how to use CM to optimize outcomes.

CONTINGENCY MANAGEMENT TARGETING OTHER HEALTH BEHAVIORS IN ADOLESCENTS

Literature on CM interventions targeting adolescent substance use behaviors continues to expand and just recently has extended its reach to other important adolescent health behaviors, such as weight loss or medication adherence. Although many health behavior theories (eg, health belief model, social learning model, and theory of planned behavior) have foundations in learning theory, supporting the relevance of immediate and long-term contingencies for adolescent health behavior decision making, the integration of CM with behavioral therapies for nonsubstance use health behaviors in adolescence has lagged behind.

Since 2010, there have been 4 pilot studies examining the use of CM for modifying adolescent health behaviors, including 3 studies targeting self-monitoring of blood glucose (SMBG) in adolescents with type 1 diabetes mellitus and 1 study targeting adolescent weight loss. The research groups who first applied CM methods to adolescent or adult substance use conducted all of these studies. Stanger and colleagues[30] reported positive findings for parent-led CM and clinic-based incentives for SMBG in conjunction with MET/CBT for increasing SMBG and improving glycemic control in youth with poorly controlled type 1 diabetes mellitus. Consistent with those findings, both Petry and colleagues[31] and Raiff and Dallery[32] conducted pilot tests of clinic-based incentives for SMBG, without any additional counseling or parent-led CM, and also found improvements in SMBG and glycemic control. Last, Hartlieb and colleagues[33] conducted a pilot test of CM combined with behavioral skills training to enhance adolescent weight loss and found that parent-involved CM, but not adolescent-only CM, enhanced the effect of behavioral skills training on youth weight loss.

Empirical support for the importance of incorporating parent-led and clinic-based CM interventions into treatments targeting the modification of adolescent health behaviors continues to grow.[34,35] Future experimental and implementation efforts should continue to examine the effectiveness of CM for targeting a wide variety of adolescent health behaviors, with the hope that findings will generalize across behaviors and inform new interventions.

FUTURE DIRECTIONS

Continued and new avenues of CM research and exploration seem to offer one promising path to the development of more effective programming for adolescents with substance use–related problems. Two possibilities not yet addressed are briefly discussed:

1. Exploration of neural mechanisms may provide alternative ways of thinking about the development and specification of CM-based interventions.[36–38] For example, exposure to CM might produce activation or connectivity changes in 1 or more neural networks involved with making behavioral choices, including executive (top-down) and motivational and emotional (bottom-up) processes. Such changes might be directly related to CM or occur indirectly through effects of abstinence from substance use, which may also affect brain structure and function. The use of experimental methods, including neuroimaging to identify intervention effects

on behavioral and motivational/emotional neural mechanisms, should provide clues as to how to improve the effectiveness of CM or how to target these important neural systems through other interventions, for example, cognitive training to improve outcomes.

2. Utilization of technology has great potential to facilitate or enhance CM approaches to substance use and other health behaviors.[39] Studies with adults have demonstrated how Web-based delivery of CBT interventions can increase access to and reduce costs of delivery of integrated CBT and CM interventions, which reflect an optimal treatment combination.[40] Similarly, the adolescent smoking cessation interventions, reviewed previously, provide models for how technology can be used to support effective monitoring of target behaviors outside the clinic, which can extend the reach and perhaps facilitate more effective CM programs.[17] Another example comes from Stanger and colleagues that used automated payments to debit cards to ease staff burden associated with providing the incentive earnings to participants.[8] The growing development and application of diverse technological devices and platforms to improve health behavior should provide a surplus of ideas and innovations for adapting and implementing CM-based programs to better address adolescent substance use problems.

SUMMARY

CM-based models of intervention continue to garner attention from clinical researchers seeking to enhance the effectiveness of treatments for adolescent substance use disorders. Studies are searching for CM models that can improve outcomes, enable more access to these interventions, or both. Findings to date generally provide positive support for the value of adding CM to established treatments or for providing a primarily CM-based approach. A few key observations from this body of work to keep in mind include the following:

1. No study has yet to provide a careful test of the efficacy of a parent-administered CM intervention that is not delivered in concert with an associated clinic-based CM program. If efficacious, such a home-based program might provide a transportable option that would be lower cost than typical clinic-based CM programs. That said, engaging regular parent participation in treatment and facilitating application of a structured home-based CM poses substantial challenges of its own.

2. The substantial variation in the parameters of CM programs under study (outcome target, magnitude of reinforcement, frequency of monitoring, and reinforcement) should hopefully remind readers that CM programs can vary greatly in many aspects, and each program must be evaluated on its own merits. Enough data have now accumulated from adult and adolescent treatment studies to indicate that the question to be asked is not whether or not CM is an efficacious intervention model but whether a particular CM program works and what specific parameters were used.

3. CM programs, even the most effective tested to date, like all other interventions for adolescent substance use disorders, have much room for improvement, particularly related to longer duration outcomes. Innovative CM models focused on maintaining treatment gains are sorely needed to address the ubiquitous problem of relapse.

4. The nascent literature on implementation of CM in new treatment settings and the integration of CM with other treatment models suggest that adoption of and adherence to CM can be accomplished via comprehensive WSs, perhaps without intensive training and supervision. That said, CM interventions can vary

substantially in complexity, so, again, the challenges for disseminating any one CM program may differ substantially from others. As with other treatment models, integrity and fidelity are essential to achieving good outcomes with CM and thus should not be taken for granted.

REFERENCES

1. Stanger C, Budney AJ. Contingency management approaches for adolescent substance use disorders. Child Adolesc Psychiatr Clin N Am 2010;19(3):547–62.
2. Hogue A, Henderson CE, Ozechowski TJ, et al. Evidence base on outpatient behavioral treatments for adolescent substance use: updates and recommendations 2007-2013. J Clin Child Adolesc Psychol 2014;43(5):695–720.
3. Killeen TK, McRae-Clark AL, Waldrop AE, et al. Contingency management in community programs treating adolescent substance abuse: a feasibility study. J Child Adolesc Psychiatr Nurs 2012;25(1):33–41.
4. Kaminer Y, Burleson JA, Burke R, et al. The efficacy of contingency management for adolescent cannabis use disorder: a controlled study. Subst Abus 2014;35(4): 391–8.
5. Henggeler SW, McCart MR, Cunningham PB, et al. Enhancing the effectiveness of juvenile drug courts by integrating evidence-based principles. J Consult Clin Psychol 2012;80(2):264–75.
6. Sampl S, Kadden R. Motivational enhancement therapy and cognitive behavioral therapy for adolescent cannabis users: 5 sessions, vol. 1. Rockville (MD): Center for Substance Abuse Treatment; Substance Abuse and Mental Health Services Administration; 2001.
7. Webb C, Scudder M, Kaminer Y, et al. The MET/CBT 5 supplement: 7 sessions of cognitive behavioral therapy (CBT 7) for adolescent cannabis users. Rockville, MD: Center for Substance Abuse Treatment; 2002.
8. Stanger C, Ryan SR, Scherer EA, et al. Clinic- and home-based contingency management plus parent training for adolescent cannabis use disorders. J Am Acad Child Adolesc Psychiatry 2015;54(6):445–53.e442.
9. Godley MD, Godley SH, Dennis ML, et al. A randomized trial of assertive continuing care and contingency management for adolescents with substance use disorders. J Consult Clin Psychol 2014;82(1):40–51.
10. Stewart DG, Felleman BI, Arger CA. Effectiveness of motivational incentives for adolescent marijuana users in a school-based intervention. J Subst Abuse Treat 2015;58:43–50.
11. Ryan SR, Stanger C, Thostenson J, et al. The impact of disruptive behavior disorder on substance use treatment outcome in adolescents. J Subst Abuse Treat 2013;44:506–14.
12. Krishnan-Sarin S, Duhig AM, McKee SA, et al. Contingency management for smoking cessation in adolescent smokers. Exp Clin Psychopharmacol 2006; 14(3):306–10.
13. Krishnan-Sarin S, Cavallo DA, Cooney JL, et al. An exploratory randomized controlled trial of a novel high school based smoking cessation intervention for adolescent smokers using abstinence-contingent incentives and cognitive behavioral therapy. Drug Alcohol Depend 2013;132:346–51.
14. Morean ME, Kong G, Camenga DR, et al. Contingency management improves smoking cessation treatment outcomes among highly impulsive adolescent smokers relative to cognitive behavioral therapy. Addict Behav 2015;42:86–90.

15. Schepis TS, Cavallo DA, Kong G, et al. Predicting initiation of smoking cessation treatment and outcome among adolescents using stressful life events and coping style. Subst Abus 2015;36(4):478–85.
16. Cavallo DA, Nich C, Schepis TS, et al. Preliminary examination of adolescent spending in a contingency management based smoking cessation program. J Child Adolesc Subst Abuse 2010;19(4):335–42.
17. Reynolds B, Harris M, Slone SA, et al. A feasibility study of home-based contingency management with adolescent smokers of rural Appalachia. Exp Clin Psychopharmacol 2015;23(6):486–93.
18. Dallery J, Glenn IM, Raiff BR. An Internet-based abstinence reinforcement treatment for cigarette smoking. Drug Alcohol Depend 2007;86(2-3):230–8.
19. Reynolds B, Dallery J, Shroff P, et al. A web-based contingency management program with adolescent smokers. J Appl Behav Anal 2008;41(4):597–601.
20. Henggeler SW, Chapman JE, Rowland MD, et al. Evaluating training methods for transporting contingency management to therapists. J Subst Abuse Treat 2013; 45(5):466–74.
21. Holth P, Torsheim T, Sheidow AJ, et al. Intensive quality assurance of therapist adherence to behavioral interventions for adolescent substance use problems. J Child Adolesc Subst Abuse 2011;20(4):289–313.
22. McCart MR, Henggeler SW, Chapman JE, et al. System-level effects of integrating a promising treatment into juvenile drug courts. J Subst Abuse Treat 2012;43(2):231–43.
23. Henggeler SW, Sheidow AJ, Cunningham PB, et al. Promoting the implementation of an evidence-based intervention for adolescent marijuana abuse in community settings: testing the use of intensive quality assurance. J Clin Child Adolesc Psychol 2008;37(3):682–9.
24. Henggeler SW, Chapman JE, Rowland MD, et al. Statewide adoption and initial implementation of contingency management for substance-abusing adolescents. J Consult Clin Psychol 2008;76(4):556–67.
25. Rash CJ, Dephilippis D, McKay JR, et al. Training workshops positively impact beliefs about contingency management in a nationwide dissemination effort. J Subst Abuse Treat 2013;45(3):306–12.
26. Kirby KC, Carpenedo CM, Stitzer ML, et al. Is exposure to an effective contingency management intervention associated with more positive provider beliefs? J Subst Abuse Treat 2012;42(4):356–65.
27. Letourneau EJ, McCart MR, Asuzu K, et al. Caregiver involvement in sexual risk reduction with substance using juvenile delinquents: overview and preliminary outcomes of a randomized trial. Adolesc Psychiatry (Hilversum) 2013;3(4): 342–51.
28. McCart MR, Sheidow AJ, Letourneau EJ. Risk reduction therapy for adolescents: targeting substance use and HIV/STI-risk behaviors. Cogn Behav Pract 2014; 21(2):161–75.
29. Branson CE, Barbuti AM, Clemmey P, et al. A pilot study of low-cost contingency management to increase attendance in an adolescent substance abuse program. Am J Addict 2012;21(2):126–9.
30. Stanger C, Ryan SR, Delhey L, et al. A multicomponent motivational intervention to improve adherence among adolescents with poorly controlled type 1 diabetes: a pilot study. J Pediatr Psychol 2013;36(6):629–37.
31. Petry NM, Cengiz E, Wagner JA, et al. Testing for rewards: a pilot study to improve type 1 diabetes management in adolescents. Diabetes Care 2015; 38(10):1952–4.

32. Raiff BR, Dallery J. Internet-based contingency management to improve adherence with blood glucose testing recommendations for teens diagnosed with type 1 diabetes. J Appl Behav Anal 2010;43(3):487–91.
33. Hartlieb KB, Naar S, Ledgerwood DM, et al. Contingency management adapted for African-American adolescents with obesity enhances youth weight loss with caregiver participation: a multiple baseline pilot study. Int J Adolesc Med Health 2015. [Epub ahead of print].
34. Boutelle KN, Bouton ME. Implications of learning theory for developing programs to decrease overeating. Appetite 2015;93:62–74.
35. Stoeckel M, Duke D. Diabetes and behavioral learning principles: often neglected yet well-known and empirically validated means of optimizing diabetes care behavior. Curr Diab Rep 2015;15(7):39.
36. Stanger C, Budney AJ, Bickel WK. A developmental perspective on neuroeconomic mechanisms of contingency management. Psychol Addict Behav 2013; 27(2):403–15.
37. Stanger C, Elton A, Ryan S, et al. Neuroeconomics and adolescent substance abuse: individual differences in neural networks and delay discounting. J Am Acad Child Adolesc Psychiatry 2013;52(7):747–55.
38. Stanger C, Garavan H. Potential neural influences in contingency management for adolescent substance use. In: Feldstein Ewing S, Witkiewitz K, Filbey F, editors. Neuroimaging and psychosocial addiction treatment. London: Palgrave Macmillan; 2015. p. 244–56.
39. Budney AJ, Marsch LA, Bickel WK. Towards an addiction treatment technology test. In: el-Guebaly N, Carra G, Galanter M, editors. Textbook of addiction treatment: international perspectives. Berlin: Springer-Verlag; 2015. p. 987–1006.
40. Budney AJ, Stanger C, Tilford JM, et al. Computer-assisted behavioral therapy and contingency management for cannabis use disorder. Psychol Addict Behav 2015;29(3):501–11.

Meeting Youth Where They Are

Substance Use Disorder Treatment in Schools

Margaret M. Benningfield, MD, MSCI

KEYWORDS

- Substance use disorder • Adolescent • School mental health

KEY POINTS

- School is an ideal setting for mental health interventions including treatment for substance use disorders.
- Substance use assessment—alone or paired with brief intervention—is associated with decreased substance use in high school students.
- More intensive intervention is required to effect sustained behavior change.
- Cognitive–behavioral therapies are effective and can be easily adapted for implementation in schools.
- Several models for school-based intervention have been studied, but additional research is needed.

SCHOOL AS AN IDEAL SETTING FOR MENTAL HEALTH INTERVENTION

Youth in the United States spend, on average, more than a thousand hours in school each year. Meeting these students where they are—in schools—offers an opportunity to bridge a significant gap in mental health treatment needs. Implementing evidenced-based substance abuse treatment schools has the potential to reach youth at earlier stages of substance severity, reduce the risk of progression to more chronic addiction with considerable cost savings to society.[1]

A significant number of high school–aged youth are in need of services for problematic substance use. The 2011 national Youth Risk Behavior Surveillance Survey[2] reports that of youth in grades 9 to 12, 21.9% reported binge drinking, 23.1% smoked marijuana, and 25.6% sold, offered, or were given illegal drugs on school property in the past month. The range of illness in these youth is wide. Based on 2011 National Survey on Drug Use and Health data, 14.4% of youth aged 12 to 18 years met *Diagnostic and Statistical Manual of Mental Disorders* (DSM)-V criteria

Department of Psychiatry, Vanderbilt University, 1601 23rd Avenue South, #3068C, Nashville, TN 37212, USA
E-mail address: meg.benningfield@Vanderbilt.edu

Child Adolesc Psychiatric Clin N Am 25 (2016) 661–668
http://dx.doi.org/10.1016/j.chc.2016.05.003
1056-4993/16/$ – see front matter © 2016 Elsevier Inc. All rights reserved.
childpsych.theclinics.com

Abbreviations	
CRAFFT	Car, Relax, Alone, Forget, Friends, Trouble
DSM	Diagnostic and Statistical Manual of Mental Disorders
SBIRT	Screening, brief, intervention, and referral to treatment
SUD	Substance use disorder

for substance use disorders (SUD), with about one third endorsing mild SUD (2-3 symptoms), about one third endorsing moderate SUD (4-5 symptoms) and about one third endorsing severe SUD (6-11 symptoms).[1,3] Unfortunately, only about one-third of the 14% to 20% of school-aged youth with a behavioral health disorder receive treatment, and SUD are among the least likely to be treated.[4] Schools provide an important venue to increase access to care, especially for families who are least likely to access care in traditional clinic settings.[5] In fact, 70% to 80% of those youth who are able to access services receive treatment in schools.[6] Currently, however, treatment services are most often funded by juvenile justice and social services and provided in community-based programs.[7]

In addition to increasing access to care, addressing mental health and substance use in schools can have a positive impact across a variety of emotional, behavioral, and educational outcomes in children and adolescents.[8] Substance use is associated with poor academic performance, greater rates of discipline referrals, and higher rates of dropout. Despite the high rate of drop out, more than 90% of the youth with SUD are still in school.[1]

SCHOOLS OFFER AN OPPORTUNITY TO ADDRESS SIGNIFICANT UNMET NEED FOR TREATMENT

Commonly reported barriers to receiving care included cost of treatment, perception that substance use is not a problem, not knowing where to access treatment, and lack of transportation.[9] Providing SUD treatment services in schools can overcome these barriers by meeting youth where they are.[6,10,11] Schools are a unique setting for increasing the availability of adolescent substance treatment and access to care, especially for minority and disadvantaged youth.[12,13] Youth who have access to school-based health centers are 10 times more likely to make a mental health or substance use visit and participate in screening for other high-risk behaviors compared with youth receiving services in community-based treatment settings.[14]

Despite the urgent need for services and call to provide services in schools, few published studies address school-based substance abuse treatment. In a review of the literature published to date, 16 studies of substance use treatment interventions delivered in schools were identified from 7 groups across the United States and 1 group in Great Britain. These reports include results from 5 randomized, controlled trials of brief interventions. The remaining reports are feasibility studies and analyses of the mechanisms of change in 5 nonexperimental implementation of school-based substance abuse treatment including one 8-week intervention. Findings from these published studies will be reviewed here. A significant gap in the literature remains in the absence of randomized studies of robust, integrated treatment for SUDs in schools.

SCREENING FOR SUBSTANCE USE DISORDERS IN SCHOOLS

Treatment for SUDs necessarily begins with identifying youth in need of services. Use of a validated screening tool significantly improves identification of youth with problematic substance use[15] and is recommended. Multiple screening instruments for adolescent substance use such as the Car, Relax, Alone, Forget, Friends, Trouble (CRAFFT),[16] Alcohol Use Disorders Identification Test,[17] Problem Oriented Screening Instrument for Teenagers,[18] and the Brief Screener for Tobacco, Alcohol, and other Drugs[19] are freely available in the public domain (see Benningfield and colleagues[20] for a list of these and other screening measures).

The CRAFFT is a 6-item tool that asks the adolescent to report on whether they have driven while intoxicated or ridden in a car (C) with an intoxicated driver, they use substances to relax (R), they use when alone (A), they forget (F) things done while intoxicated, their friends or family (F) have been concerned about their use, or they have gotten into trouble (T) as a result of substance use.[16] A positive response to more than 1 of these items is a positive screen, indicating need for further assessment and potential need for treatment. In a study of prevalence of positive substance use screens using the CRAFFT,[21] rates were highest in school-based health centers. Rates found in school-based health centers were nearly 30% compared with rates of 8% to 24% reported in community primary care settings. In another study of statewide implementation of the CRAFFT screening tool in high schools, 15% of 168,801 students screened reported use of alcohol or other drugs. Of these, 49% endorsed 0 or 1 CRAFFT question, 33% endorsed 2 to 3 questions, and 18% endorsed 4 or more of the CRAFFT questions, again indicating a significant population in schools who are in need of services.[22]

INTERVENTIONS: FROM BRIEF INTERVENTION TO INTEGRATED TREATMENT
Brief Interventions

Brief interventions show robust benefit in young adults; however, the support for these interventions in adolescents is more modest. For adolescents, brief interventions to address substance use have generally demonstrated small to medium effect sizes that decay over time.[23,24] These treatments remain popular, however, presumably because they are brief and therefore require fewer resources for implementation.[25]

Delivery of screening, brief, intervention, and referral to treatment (SBIRT) has been shown to be feasible in school settings. For example, a recent description of SBIRT delivery in 2 urban schools in New York reported that youth were more likely to report substance use when screened by a clinician than on anonymous survey (42% vs 28%) and students readily accepted feedback and brief intervention.[26] Another study reported on delivery of SBIRT in a large school-based health center in New Mexico.[27] A single session of motivational interviewing resulted in significant decrease in alcohol and marijuana use as well as greater engagement in additional services in students who endorsed 1 to 5 CRAFFT questions.

Some challenges of school-based delivery may be inferred from the description of a third study in which only 18 of 59 students who were invited to participate completed a brief intervention implemented in alternative schools in Los Angeles.[28] Students in this population were noted to have much greater use of substances than the general high school population. Students who did participate in the study rated the experience positively. Furthermore, initial assessment of the students' readiness to change predicted substance use at 3-month follow-up. The primary reason for lack of participation in the study was failure to return the consent form. The authors speculate that the severity of drug and alcohol use in the population may have contributed to lack of engagement and recommended providing incentives for returning consent regardless of whether students chose to participate. Such incentives may be more difficult to implement in school settings than in a traditional research setting.

Randomized, Controlled Trials of Brief Interventions

Several studies have examined delivery of brief interventions (1–3 sessions) in school settings using randomized controlled trials[29] and tested whether a single session of motivational interviewing session would lead to greater reduction in alcohol and other drug use compared with an "education as usual" control condition. Two hundred students completed the study. At 3 months, the intervention group showed significantly greater reduction in self-reported use of cigarettes, alcohol, and cannabis with small to moderate effect sizes (0.37, 0.34, and 0.75, respectively). At the 12-month follow-up, sustained decreases in alcohol and drug use were found in both intervention and control groups without differences between groups.[30] A second randomized, controlled trial from the same group compared a single session of motivational interviewing with a session of advice giving in 326 students.[31] This study found no difference between groups in drug use at 3 months. The authors note, however, that motivational interviewing fidelity was rather low.

Consistent with these findings, a randomized, controlled trial comparing (1) brief intervention with adolescent only, (2) brief intervention with adolescent plus a parent session, and (3) assessment only control found at 6 months that youth in both the brief intervention groups had greater decreases in substance use compared with control. Parent involvement provided added benefit in the 6-month follow-up.[32] At the 12-month follow-up, the initial gains observed from brief intervention were sustained, but the added parent session showed no additional benefit at 12 months.[33]

Another randomized, controlled trial of a brief intervention, The Teen Marijuana Check-Up,[34,35] recruited high school students through educational presentations in 349 classrooms targeting a total of more than 7000 students, of whom 619 volunteered to participate. The program was described as a "free, non-judgmental, and confidential service for teens who would like information on their use of cannabis."[35] Similar to the findings described, all participants who received assessment significantly reduced self-reported use of substances compared with a delayed assessment control group. Added brief intervention showed no significant benefit over assessment with education. The authors of this study note that selection bias may be a confounder that prevented demonstration of significant results in their studies: students who volunteered for the study were self-selected and may have been more amenable to change than youth who declined to participate.

In summary, significant progress has been made in implementing screening and brief interventions for adolescent substance use in school settings. Studies of brief interventions delivered in schools typically find that youth who volunteer for these studies and participate in assessment for alcohol or cannabis decrease their use in the short term, with some studies showing persistent decreased use of up to 1 year. However, as noted in the literature regarding brief intervention for adolescents in other settings, the benefits of screening and brief intervention are modest and the between-group differences diminish over time.[36]

THE NEED FOR MORE ROBUST TREATMENT OF SUBSTANCE USE DISORDERS IN SCHOOLS

These findings suggest that many high school students would benefit from more robust school-based substance treatment interventions. Despite this need, treatment options remain extremely limited for the estimated 10% of US high school students who would meet diagnostic criteria for SUD.[1] Considerable progress has been made in the development of efficacious substance treatment interventions predominantly found in community-based substance treatment settings that largely serve youth referred by the juvenile justice system.[7,37] There is a need to adapt and implement adolescent substance treatment interventions with proven efficacy for implementation and outcomes evaluation in school settings. Randomized, controlled trials of treatment interventions delivered in school settings are to this point lacking, however, several descriptive studies have been published and at least one randomized, controlled trial of an integrated treatment program is currently underway.

Project READY is a motivation enhancement based program implemented in several high schools in the Northwest.[38] Two hundred sixty-four high school students aged 14 to 18 years self-referred or were referred by school staff for any concern about substance use. Typical referral concerns were being intoxicated at school, frequent absences, frequent disciplinary referrals, or being found with drug paraphernalia. Students had to endorse use of alcohol or drugs at least once during the past 3 months, but a DSM diagnosis of SUD was not required. Participants received 4 sessions of motivational interviewing (assessment, feedback, decisional balance, and change planning) followed by 4 weeks of monitoring. The authors report a significant decrease in substance use over the course of the treatment that was maintained at the 16-week follow-up.[38–40]

Preliminary research addressing the need for randomized, controlled trials is underway in at least 1 clinical trial of an integrated treatment for adolescents with SUD and cooccurring disorders in a school setting. Investigators at the University of Colorado have adapted a 16-week individual motivational enhancement therapy/cognitive—behavioral therapy plus a contingency management substance treatment intervention as a brief, 8-week, school-based intervention. A recently completed pilot study of the school-based adaptation demonstrated implementation feasibility and acceptability of the intervention in a high school setting (www.ucdenver.edu/encompass).[41] A larger outcomes study of this school-based intervention is currently underway in 5 Denver-area high schools.

POTENTIAL BARRIERS TO THE IMPLEMENTATION OF SUBSTANCE ABUSE SERVICES IN SCHOOLS

Meeting youth where they are (in schools) has many potential benefits; however, significant challenges must be addressed. First, patient confidentiality must be protected. Services should be provided in a private setting and medical records should be maintained separate from the educational record. Second, clinicians who hope to build a school-based presence must address the need for staff buy-in and appreciate the unique nature of each school setting. Getting to know the school culture and identifying key stakeholders who can support services is essential to successful work in school settings. Thus, understanding the particular needs of a school community and the availability of community resources is crucial for successful partnerships in schools. Third, access to families can be a significant challenge in school settings. When parental consent is required for treatment, particular attention must be paid to not engaging students before obtaining consent. In states where youth may consent for treatment without parental consent, this challenge has less impact. The challenge of engaging families also has the potential to impact treatment. Recent evidence suggests that individual treatment can be more effective than family intervention.[42] Family engagement when possible is recommended, however, because of the potential to enhance the effectiveness of individual treatment, at least in the short term.[32] Fourth, verification of youth reports of drug use using toxicology can be more challenging in a school setting. Finally, some school administrators express concern for screening and identifying substance use in student owing to fear that their school will be viewed negatively.[32] These concerns can be addressed through careful planning and engaging school personnel with sensitivity to each school's particular needs.

Significant attention has been paid to the need for parity in treatment for mental health and SUDs.[1] Progress in the context of national health care reforms and significant expansion of school based health clinics provide a unique opportunity to significantly increase access to high quality behavioral health services for youth and families. Efforts to adapt and successfully implement evidence based interventions for SUDs will certainly make a significant impact on adolescent health.

SUMMARY

Providing school-based mental health treatment offers an opportunity to reach a greater number of affected youth by providing services in the setting where youth spend the majority of their time. In some contexts, even a single session of assessment has been linked with significant decreases in substance use; however, more robust treatments are likely needed to sustain these decreases over time. Empirically based individual and group treatments designed for delivery in clinic settings can readily be adapted for implementation in school settings. School-based delivery of substance use services offers an important opportunity to bridge a significant gap in services.

REFERENCES

1. Dennis ML, Clark HW, Huang LN. The need and opportunity to expand substance use disorder treatment in school-based settings. Adv Sch Ment Health Promot 2014;7(2):75–87.
2. Centers for Disease Control and Prevention. Youth risk behavior surveillance — United States, 2011. MMWR Surveill Summ 2012;61(4):1–162.
3. SAMHSA, Substance Abuse and Mental Health Services Administration. National survey on drug use and health, 2011 [ICPSR34481-v1]. Ann Arbor (MI): Inter-university Consortium for Political and Social Research; 2012.
4. Merikangas KR, He JP, Burstein M, et al. Service utilization for lifetime mental disorders in U.S. adolescents: results of the National Comorbidity Survey-Adolescent Supplement (NCS-A). J Am Acad Child Adolesc Psychiatry 2011; 50(1):32–45.
5. Evans SW. Mental health services in schools: utilization, effectiveness, and consent. Clin Psychol Rev 1999;19(2):165–78.
6. Rones M, Hoagwood K. School-based mental health services: a research review. Clin Child Fam Psychol Rev 2000;3(4):223–41.
7. Committee on Crossing the Quality Chasm: Adaptation to Mental Health and Addictive Disorders. Improving the quality of health care for mental and substance-use conditions: quality chasm series. Washington, DC: The National Academies Press; 2006.
8. Stephan SH, Weist M, Kataoka S, et al. Transformation of Children's Mental Health Services: the role of school mental health. Psychiatr Serv 2007;58(10):1330–8.
9. Substance Abuse and Mental Health Services Administration (SAMHSA). Results from the 2013 National Survey on Drug Use and Health: summary of national findings. NSDUH Series H-48, HHS Publication No. (SMA) 14–4863. Rockville (MD): U.S. Department of Health and Human Services; 2014.
10. New Freedom Commission on Mental Health. Achieving the promise: transforming mental health care in America, final report (DHHS Pub. No. SMA-03–3832). Rockville (MD): U.S. Department of Health and Human Services; 2003.

11. U.SDepartment of Health and Human Services. U.S. public health service, report of the Surgeon General's conference on children's MH: a national action agenda. Washington, DC: U.S. Department of Health and Human Services; 2000.
12. Mills C, Stephan SH, Moore E, et al. The President's New Freedom Commission: capitalizing on opportunities to advance school-based mental health services. Clin Child Fam Psychol Rev 2006;9(3–4):149–61.
13. American Academy of Pediatrics. Insurance coverage of mental health and substance abuse services for children and adolescents: a consensus statement. Pediatrics 2000;106(4):860–2.
14. Kaplan DW, Calonge BN, Guernsey BP, et al. Managed care and school-based health centers use of health services. Arch Pediatr Adolesc Med 1998;152(1):25–33.
15. Wilson CR, Sherritt L, Gates E, et al. Are clinical impressions of adolescent substance use accurate? Pediatrics 2004;114(5):e536–40.
16. Knight JR, Sherritt L, Shrier LA, et al. Validity of the CRAFFT substance abuse screening test among adolescent clinic patients. Arch Pediatr Adolesc Med 2002;156(6):607–14.
17. Reinert DF, Allen JP. The alcohol use disorders identification test: an update of research findings. Alcohol Clin Exp Res 2007;31(2):185–99.
18. Rahdert ER, editor. The adolescent assessment/referral system manual. Washington, DC: U.S. Department of Health and Human Services (PHS) Alcohol, Drug Abuse, and Mental Health Administration; 1991.
19. Kelly SM, Gryczynski J, Mitchell SG, et al. Validity of brief screening instrument for tobacco, alcohol, and drug use. Pediatrics 2014;133(5):819–26.
20. Benningfield MM, Riggs P, Stephan SH. The role of schools in substance use prevention and intervention. Child Adolesc Psychiatr Clin N Am 2015;24:291–303.
21. Knight JR, Harris SK, Sherritt L, et al. Prevalence of positive substance abuse screen results among adolescent primary care patients. Arch Pediatr Adolesc Med 2007;161(11):1035–41.
22. Agley J, Gassman RA, Jun M, et al. Statewide administration of the CRAFFT screening tool: highlighting the spectrum of substance use. Subst Use Misuse 2015;50(13):1668–77.
23. Carney T, Myers B. Effectiveness of early interventions for substance-using adolescents: findings from a systematic review and meta-analysis. Subst Abuse Treat Prev Policy 2012;7(1):25.
24. Tait RJ, Hulse GK. A systematic review of the effectiveness of brief interventions with substance using adolescents by type of drug. Drug Alcohol Rev 2003;22:337–46.
25. Levy S. Brief interventions for substance use in adolescents: still promising, still unproven. CMAJ 2014;186(8):565–6.
26. Curtis BL, McLellan AT, Gabellini BN. Translating SBIRT to public school settings: an initial test of feasibility. Journal of Substance Abuse Treatment 2014;46:15–21.
27. Mitchell SG, Gryczynski J, Gonzales A, et al. Screening, brief intervention, and referral to treatment (SBIRT) for substance use in a school-based program: services and outcomes. Am J Addict 2012;21:S5–13.
28. Grenard JL, Ames SL, Wiers RW, et al. Brief intervention for substance use among at-risk adolescents: a pilot study. J Adolesc Health 2007;40:188–91.
29. McCambridge J, Strang J. The efficacy of single-session motivational interviewing in reducing drug consumption and perceptions of drug related risk and harm among young people: results from a multi-site cluster randomized trial. Addiction 2004;99:39–52.

30. McCambridge J, Strang J. Deterioration over time in effect of motivational interviewing in reducing drug consumption and related risk among young people. Addiction 2005;100:470–8.
31. McCambridge J, Slym RL, Strang J. Randomized controlled trial of motivational interviewing compared with drug information and advice for early intervention among young cannabis users. Addiction 2008;103:1809–18.
32. Winters KC, Leitten W. Brief intervention for drug-abusing adolescents in a school setting. Psychol Addict Behav 2007;21(2):249–54.
33. Winters KC, Lee S, Botzet A, et al. One-year outcomes and mediators of a brief intervention for drug abusing adolescents. Psychol Addict Behav 2014;28(2): 464–74.
34. Walker DD, Roffman RA, Stephens RS, et al. Motivational enhancement therapy for adolescent marijuana users: a preliminary randomized controlled trial. J Consult Clin Psychol 2006;74:628–32.
35. Walker DD, Stephens R, Roffman R, et al. Randomized controlled trial of motivational enhancement therapy with nontreatment-seeking adolescent cannabis users: a further test of the teen marijuana check-up. Psychol Addict Behav 2011;25:474–84.
36. Carney T, Bj M, Louw J, et al. Brief school-based interventions and behavioural outcomes for substance-using adolescents. Cochrane Database Syst Rev 2014;(2):CD008969.
37. Riggs P. Treating adolescents for substance abuse and comorbid psychiatric disorders. Sci Pract Perspect 2003;2003:18–28.
38. Hall BC, Stewart DG, Arger C, et al. Modeling motivation three ways: effects of MI metrics on treatment outcomes among adolescents. Psychol Addict Behav 2014; 28(1):307–12.
39. Serafini K, Shipley L, Stewart DG. Motivation and substance use outcomes among adolescents in a school-based intervention. Addict Behav 2016;53:74–9.
40. Stewart DG, Felleman BI, Arger CA. Effectiveness of motivational incentives for adolescent marijuana users in a school-based intervention. J Subst Abuse Treat 2015;58:43–50.
41. Riggs P. Encompass: an integrated treatment intervention for adolescents with co-occurring psychiatric and substance use disorders. Abstract, in scientific proceedings of the American Academy of Child and Adolescent Psychiatry 61st Annual Meeting (AACAP). San Antonio, October 24, 2014.
42. Tripodi SJ, Bender K, Litschge C, et al. Interventions for reducing adolescent alcohol abuse: a meta-analytic review. Arch Pediatr Adolesc Med 2010;164: 85–91.

Continuing Care for Adolescents in Treatment for Substance Use Disorders

Lora L. Passetti, MS[a], Mark D. Godley, PhD[a],*,
Yifrah Kaminer, MD, MBA[b]

KEYWORDS

- Adolescents • Aftercare • Continuing care • Assertive continuing care
- Adaptive treatment • Mutual aid groups

KEY POINTS

- Adolescents who enter treatment for substance use often do not complete the recommended program, return to regular use, and do not initiate continuing care services.
- Assertive approaches (counselor-initiated home or school-based continuing care) increase linkage to continuing care, and rapid initiation of continuing care makes a difference in reducing substance use.
- Findings suggest that continuing care is appropriate for those who successfully complete treatment.
- Evidence is accumulating to suggest that matching adolescents to age-appropriate 12-step and other mutual aid groups can support recovery.
- Adaptive treatment designs hold promise for establishing decision rules as to which individuals need low-intensity continuing care services and which need more intensive care.

INTRODUCTION

Several evidence-based treatments for adolescent substance use have emerged since the early 1990s. Treatments such as Multidimensional Family Therapy, Family Behavior Therapy, the Adolescent Community Reinforcement Approach (A-CRA), Motivational Interviewing, cognitive–behavioral therapy, and contingency management have all been adapted for and tested with adolescents. Randomized clinical trials using singular or integrated protocols of these interventions have demonstrated

The authors have no conflicts of interest.
Funding: NIH, R01AA021118.
[a] Chestnut Health Systems, 448 Wylie Drive, Normal, IL 61761, USA; [b] Alcohol Research Center, University of Connecticut School of Medicine, 263 Farmington Avenue, Farmington, CT 06030, USA
* Corresponding author.
E-mail address: mgodley@chestnut.org

improved short-term substance use outcomes in outpatient clinics, hospital emergency rooms, and school settings.[1–12]

Despite these advancements, adolescent relapse rates during the year after treatment often exceed 60%, and many youth cycle between periods of substance use and abstinence.[1,13–17] These statistics are reinforced by analysis of a large national dataset of adolescents entering outpatient and residential treatment programs for substance use disorders.[18] **Fig. 1** shows that more than one-half of adolescents relapse within 90 days of the end of an acute episode of care.

These data support research that indicates that alcohol and substance use disorders, like other chronic relapsing illnesses (eg, asthma, diabetes), require long-term monitoring and support.[19–23] Research also suggests that addressing substance use problems is a process that involves acute treatment, ongoing management, and multiple continuing interventions as needed.[19,24–27]

Although high rates of adolescent relapse may reflect that youth tend to be less motivated to change substance use than adults, have low problem recognition, and enter treatment because of external pressures,[28,29] it is impossible to know which adolescents are beginning a long-term chronic relapsing illness and which will "age out" or enter long-term remission and recovery through treatment. Regardless of which path will be followed, recent investigation into adolescent brain development points to the importance of treating substance use disorders in youth.[30]

Brain imaging research demonstrates that the human brain is still developing until the early 20s, notably in the prefrontal cortex regions that control executive functioning such as reasoning, decision making, impulse control, and judgment. Therefore, it may be assumed that adolescents entering treatment for substance use disorders have poor executive functioning in the prefrontal cortex and are potentially at higher risk to the effects of drugs.[31,32] They may make emotional and impulsive decisions. Evidence is accumulating that adolescent brains may be more sensitive to the effects

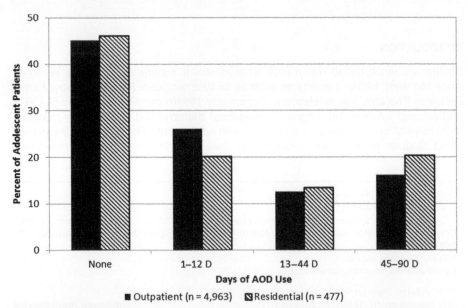

Fig. 1. Adolescent alcohol or drug use in the 90 days after discharge from treatment.

of alcohol in decreasing social discomfort, and they may be less sensitive to its intoxication effects.[33] Furthermore, laboratory research has shown that adolescent rats display significantly more damage from alcohol to their frontal cortex and working memory than adult rats.[33,34] More research is needed, however, to determine the extent to which neurocognitive functions may recover over time with abstinence and to tease out the effects of substances and other independent influences on the brain.[35]

Because substance use disorders can be chronic relapsing conditions that begin in adolescence and adolescent brains may be more vulnerable to the effects of substance use, continuing care services are especially important to help youth maintain treatment gains. Historically, continuing care was referred to as "aftercare" that followed a successful acute treatment episode. "Step-down" care was the first and most common form of aftercare and involved referral to lower intensity treatment (outpatient) upon completion of more intensive services (usually residential or inpatient).

Referral to nonprofessional recovery supports has also become a common continuing care practice. For example, recommendations to attend mutual support groups became increasingly popular following the founding of Alcoholics Anonymous (AA) in 1935, and in the mid-twentieth century, the development of the Minnesota model of treatment relying on 12-step education and meeting attendance.[36-38] Treatment programs have traditionally referred both adults and adolescents to these groups.[39-42]

As aftercare has evolved, there has been a shift from the idea of "aftercare" to the concept of "continuing care." Aftercare is predicated on the assumption that individuals complete a more intensive level of care and step down to a less intensive set of services. In reality, most adolescents do not respond to treatment in this manner. Studies show that a large percentage of adolescents entering treatment will relapse and return to the same or a more intensive level of treatment. It is also common for youth to end treatment prematurely.[13,43-45] Such findings with both adolescents and adults have led the American Society of Addiction Medicine[46] to define continuing care as:

The provision of a treatment plan and organizational structure that will ensure that a patient receives whatever kind of care he or she needs at the time. The treatment program thus is flexible and tailored to the shifting needs of the patient and his or her level of readiness to change. (p. 361)

Research on continuing care with adults has shown promise[21,47-52] and research on adolescent continuing care is still in its early stages and growing. This paper reviews the literature on continuing care and other recovery supports for adolescents and makes recommendations for clinical practice and future research.

RESEARCH ON ADOLESCENT LINKAGE TO CONTINUING CARE SERVICES

Despite evidence of the importance of continuing care and the emphasis placed on continuity of care by the American Society of Addiction Medicine and other organizations, most adolescents do not receive these services. Linkage rates to professional continuing care range from 35% to 45% within 90 days of discharge.[15,43] Less than one-half of youth receive a referral for continuing care because they leave treatment early—usually against staff advice or at staff request.[53] Reports of linkage rates to mutual support groups, typically AA and Narcotics Anonymous (NA), vary widely between studies. They indicate that anywhere from 42% to 75% of adolescents will attend 1 or more 12-step meetings in the first 3 months after discharge from residential treatment.[54–57]

For youth with a planned discharge, those who are referred to continuing care within the same organization are much more likely to connect than those referred to a different organization (89% vs 50%).[15,54] Additional potential influences on linkage rates include distance from a youth's residence to an outpatient clinic or mutual support meeting, transportation problems, treatment fatigue, and caregiver work schedules.[15,53] Lack of follow-through with referrals to and drop-out from mutual support groups can be due to age dissimilarity with other group members or the philosophy of the referring treatment program. It may also be affected by, when compared with adults, the presence of less severe substance use problems, briefer substance use histories, lower motivation for abstinence, and lower problem recognition.[29,41,57,58]

RESEARCH ON CONTINUING CARE FOR ADOLESCENTS AFTER RESIDENTIAL TREATMENT FOR SUBSTANCE USE DISORDERS

Most research on adolescent continuing care has focused on delivery of services after discharge from residential treatment.

Early Studies of Continuing Care

In one of the earliest studies, Ralph and McMenamy[59] examined data from adolescents who had completed an inpatient substance abuse treatment program. These youth were offered an aftercare program that consisted of adolescent and family multigroups for 1 year after discharge. Participation in aftercare was associated with less substance use since discharge and lower amounts of use over 6 months.

In another study, juvenile offenders in detention facilities were committed to a 2-month residential substance abuse treatment program. Those who completed treatment and resided in the county were placed in a 4-month aftercare program. "Prerelease" occurred during residential treatment and included a family assessment, treatment contract, weekly family sessions, and support groups. The "intensive" phase included 2 months of postrelease supervision, daily face-to-face contacts, youth and family support meetings, and youth meetings with an addiction counselor. In the "transitional" phase, youth met with case managers 2 times per week and with an addiction counselor 2 times per month for a total of 2 months. Youth were linked with community services. Family support groups continued, and family therapy was provided as needed.

When compared with a no-aftercare group of youth, participation in aftercare was associated with reduced emotional abuse as well as more drug-related, but not personal-related, delinquency. No evidence of a program effect was found for increasing family supervision, attachment, emotional support, and communication, reducing family violence and drug use, increasing internal locus of control, increasing drug knowledge, decreasing health problems, increasing coping and problem-solving skills, or positive urine tests. Results need to be interpreted with caution, however, owing to significant differences between the comparison groups, low follow-up completion rates, problems with implementation, and low family involvement.[60]

Studies of Standard Continuing Care

In 1 study, a standard recommendation for adolescents who received inpatient care was to attend aftercare sessions with their families at the facility after discharge. Participants could discuss individual concerns and learn about substance use and recovery. Weekly meetings lasted about 1 hour. Although no further detail about these services was provided, findings were that more frequent aftercare meeting attendance was associated with more days of abstinence during the 6-month follow-up period.[61]

Winters and associates[62] found that adolescents who completed an outpatient or residential program based on the Minnesota model were expected to enter a half-year outpatient aftercare program that met 2 to 3 times per week. The purpose of aftercare was to continue the treatment process, provide ongoing assessment, and make referrals for assistance as necessary. Adolescents who attended aftercare at a moderate/regular level were more likely to show improved substance use than those who attended aftercare at a minimum level or did not attend at all.

Assertive Continuing Care

A current approach aimed at increasing continuing care linkage rates is Assertive Continuing Care (ACC). ACC brings continuing care to the adolescent in his/her home community whether or not residential treatment was completed successfully and shifts responsibility of service delivery from the youth to the clinician. ACC services are initiated as soon as possible after discharge from the initial treatment episode, thereby requiring clinicians to coordinate closely with referring treatment programs. At that time, ACC clinicians deliver case management services combined with an evidence-based treatment—A-CRA.

Case management services include: (a) home visits, (b) help linking the adolescent to necessary services, (c) transportation to needed services, a prosocial activity, or potential jobs, (d) advocacy to access services, (e) monitoring lapse cues and attendance at services and activities, and (f) social support for coping with a lapse or other challenging issues.[63]

A-CRA includes sessions with the youth alone, the caregivers alone, and the youth and caregivers together. Using principles of operant learning theory and a positive, nonconfrontational approach, the clinician helps the youth and his or her family to restructure social and recreational activities to compete with time spent using alcohol and drugs. During sessions, the clinician draws from 17 different therapeutic procedures that focus on various skills and life areas. They include relapse prevention, relationship skills, communication skills, problem solving, goal setting and working through barriers to completion, analysis of using behaviors, making non–substance-using friends, engaging in satisfying social and leisure activities that do not involve substance use, sampling new activities, and assignment of homework. On an ongoing basis, the youth fills out a self-assessment to develop and monitor progress toward completion of goals. There are also optional procedures for coping with a lapse, anger management, and job finding.[15,53,64]

ACC has been tested with adolescents in 2 randomized clinical trials after residential treatment. In the first study, 183 youth were aged 12 to 17 years old and met DSM-IV criteria for current alcohol or other drug abuse or dependence. The majority were male (71%), Caucasian (73%), and aged 15 to 18 years (89%). Most were involved with the juvenile justice system (82%) and had 1 or more co-occurring mental health disorders.

After 1 week of residential treatment, participating youth were randomized to attend either ACC or usual continuing care for the first 90 days after discharge. All youth were referred to community outpatient clinics in their home communities. Analyses demonstrated that youth receiving ACC had significantly higher linkage rates to continuing care than those receiving usual continuing care (94% vs 54%). They also received more days of continuing care sessions (18.1 vs 6.3 sessions). A main effect for ACC was demonstrated over the 9-month follow-up period for abstinence from marijuana. The intervention produced medium to large effect sizes. Adolescents in the 2 conditions had the same average duration of residential stay (52 days) and comparable unplanned discharge rates (51% and 53%).[65] There were no differences in 12-step attendance between conditions, with 65% attending 1 or more meetings and an average attendance of approximately 12 meetings during the 90-day period.[53]

The second clinical trial of ACC tested whether or not ACC augmented with motivational incentives would further improve substance use outcomes. Youth (n = 337) were recruited from 2 residential programs and randomized to one of the following conditions for the first 90 days after discharge from residential care: (a) usual continuing care only, (b) motivational incentives only, (c) ACC only, or (d) motivational incentives plus ACC. Motivational incentives in the form of prize drawings were provided weekly contingent upon completion of verifiable prosocial activities and abstinence. The prize bowl contained 510 slips of paper: (a) 150 or 30% of the slips showed a smile face (no prize), (b) 324 or 62.8% of the slips read "small" (prize worth $1), (c) 35 or 7% of the slips read "large" (prize worth $25), and (d) 1 or 0.2% of the slips read "jumbo" (prize worth $100).[66]

Similar to the first trial, youth were aged 12 to 17 years old and met criteria for substance abuse or dependence. The majority were male (63%) and Caucasian (70%). The average age was 15.7 years (SD = 1.2). Most (81%) had 1 or more co-occurring mental health disorders.[66]

Results show that youth receiving any of the 3 experimental conditions were significantly more likely to engage in their continuing care condition (attending ≥4 sessions within 45 days after residential discharge)[67] than youth in usual continuing care only (75%-84% vs 49%). Adolescents in the motivational incentives only and ACC only conditions demonstrated significantly more days of abstinence from substance use over 12 months and were more likely to be in remission at 12 months than those receiving usual continuing care. Furthermore, motivational incentives and ACC resulted in significantly fewer days spent in a controlled environment.[66] Motivational incentives plus ACC did not result in significantly better outcomes.

Research on Continuing Care for Adolescents after Outpatient Treatment for Substance Use Disorders

Although research on continuing care after outpatient treatment is a newer development in the field, there have been a small number of clinical trials.

Active Aftercare

Kaminer and colleagues have been researching the effects of telephone continuing care delivered to adolescents after outpatient treatment. For this trial, 144 youth were randomized to one of 3 conditions for 3 months after completion of group treatment: (a) active aftercare consisting of 5 in-person sessions, (b) active aftercare consisting of 5 brief telephone sessions, or (c) a no aftercare control. Sixty-seven percent were male, 82% were Caucasian, and the average age was 15.9 years (SD = 1.2). Seventy-nine percent were diagnosed with substance abuse or dependence, 58% with an internalizing disorder, and 76% with an externalizing disorder.

Both active aftercare conditions were manual-guided and consisted of 1 session of functional analysis followed by 4 integrated motivational enhancement and cognitive–behavioral therapy sessions.[68] Therapists assessed substance use and motivation to change, identified problem areas, and provided skills guidelines to address problems. In-person sessions were 50 minutes, and telephone sessions were 12 to 15 minutes.[69]

Overall, there was a significant decrease in alcohol abstinence from the end of treatment to the end of aftercare, with those assigned to no active aftercare showing greater decreases than those assigned to active aftercare. In-person and telephone conditions were equal and resulted in higher alcohol abstinence rates (37.5%) than no aftercare (26.8%). Adolescents in active aftercare also had significantly fewer drinking days per month and heavy drinking days per month. There was a significant overall decrease in marijuana abstinence from end of treatment to end of aftercare, but not as a function of condition.[6] Initial results diminished at the 12-month follow-up assessment.[70]

Assertive Continuing Care

In a trial after outpatient treatment, 320 adolescents were randomized to receive ACC or usual continuing care after outpatient discharge. Youth were aged 13 to 18 years old and met criteria for substance abuse or dependence. The majority were male (76%) and Caucasian (73%) with an average age of 15.9 years (SD = 1.2). Most (56%) had 1 or more co-occurring mental health disorders. There were no significant findings for the effectiveness of ACC.[71]

In a different trial, Henderson and colleagues[72] compared 3 months of outpatient A-CRA followed by 3 months of ACC with services as usual provided by a juvenile probation department. One hundred twenty-six youth between 12 and 17 years old were enrolled in the study. Average age was 15.2 years (SD = 1.07), and all screened positive for a moderate to severe alcohol or drug use problem. Most adolescents were male (74%) and Caucasian (79%). Although all participating youth reduced substance use frequency and substance-related problems after outpatient treatment, youth receiving ACC demonstrated a substantially greater decrease in substance-related problems.

ADAPTIVE APPROACHES TO CONTINUING CARE

Because research shows that a large segment of youth who enter treatment do not complete the program and that many do not achieve abstinence or sobriety, it is important to examine continuing care interventions aimed at improving outcomes of poor responders to treatment. Godley and colleagues[65] state that, because several episodes of treatment are the rule rather than the exception, noncompletion of services does not necessarily indicate that youth may fail to benefit from continuing care. Because 94% of adolescents who initiate at least 1 week of abstinence do so by the sixth week of treatment, this suggests that an adaptive approach to continuing care could benefit youth who do not achieve abstinence by this time. That is, it may be more effective to commence continuing care for poor responders at this point rather than follow a fixed, preplanned treatment schedule.[73]

In a recent study, Kaminer and colleagues[74] provided continuing care for adolescents with cannabis use disorders who were poor responders to outpatient treatment. One hundred sixty youth were defined as poor responders because they did not achieve abstinence after 7 weeks of outpatient treatment. These youth were randomized into a 10-week continuing care phase of either an individualized enhanced cognitive-behavioral therapy or A-CRA. Thirty-seven percent of poor responders completed the continuing care phase, and 27% percent achieved abstinence. There was neither a difference in retention rates nor in abstinence rates between the 2 conditions.

Other than the study cited, there is little research guidance on adaptive approaches to continuing care with adolescents; however, McKay[75] presented a series of key questions about individuals who do not respond to treatment: Should they be switched to another treatment? Which one? Or, should another treatment augment what is already being received? One approach that has the potential to increase rates of participation is to admit individuals to the least restrictive appropriate level of care and then "step" them up to more intensive treatment if warranted by poor initial response. Such stepped care may increase cost effectiveness and cost benefit.

Kaminer and Godley[25] described several elements thought to be critical for the design of adaptive treatment protocols. First, tailoring variables need to be identified that assess key markers of progress. For example, a therapist may assess substance use regularly and use that information to make treatment decisions. Second, an adaptive treatment protocol needs to offer a menu of clinical interventions that are meaningfully different on at least 1 dimension, such as frequency or theoretic orientation. For an adaptive strategy to work, treatment options must be different enough that poor response in 1 treatment approach does not strongly predict failure in other options.[75] Finally, decision rules need to be created that link the tailoring variables and the menu of interventions into 1 algorithm, ideally arrived at through expert consensus or experimental study. The adaptive algorithm would then be used to decide what services are provided to which individuals and when.

RESEARCH ON OTHER RECOVERY SUPPORTS FOR ADOLESCENTS

Although most randomized studies of adolescent continuing care have investigated professionally provided programs, there has been research with varying levels of rigor into other recovery support services.

Volunteer Telephone Continuing Care

In 1 quasi-experimental study, 222 adolescents were recruited to participate. These youth were between 13 and 18 years old, met criteria for substance abuse or dependence, had remained in either outpatient treatment for at least 4 sessions within 44 days from the intake session or in residential treatment for at least 2 weeks, and had telephone access.

Over the course of the study, the intervention was delivered by 60 pre-professional volunteers who were recruited primarily from university undergraduate and graduate programs in social work, psychology, and nursing. All volunteers participated in background checks and a training session on selected A-CRA/ACC procedures, recovery support call procedures, ethics, and confidentiality. In addition to documenting call information, volunteers recorded calls for weekly supervision.

Within the first week after discharge from treatment, trained volunteers initiated recovery support calls. During each session, volunteers asked about:

a. Significant events since the last call
b. Substance use, if any, since the last contact
c. Steps recently taken to stay clean and sober
d. Additional ways to stay clean and sober
e. The occurrence of any using thoughts and strategies for dealing with them
f. Prorecovery goals and homework to set for the next week
g. Progress on goals set during the previous call
h. Recovery-related events in communities
i. The use of additional support services

Volunteers made referrals for substance abuse treatment services if relapse occurred and referrals for mental health services if emotional and/or behavioral difficulties were reported.

Telephone calls were typically 15 minutes or less in length. Text messaging was used to remind adolescents of upcoming calls or to complete sessions at the adolescent's request. The goal was to complete sessions with adolescents once per week during the first 90 days after discharge. The frequency of contacts after that time varied depending on adolescents' functioning and preference.

Six-month outcome data from 202 adolescents who had received recovery support calls were compared with 6-month outcome data from a matched comparison sample of adolescents. Results suggested adolescents in the recovery support sample had significantly greater reductions in their recovery environment risk relative to the comparison sample. Analyses also suggested that the reduction in recovery environment risk produced by recovery support calls had indirect impacts on reductions in social risk, substance use, and substance-related problems.[76]

Mutual Support Groups

There is a growing body of research into adolescent participation in mutual support groups. To date, these studies have focused exclusively on the 12-step groups of AA and NA. Correlational studies suggest that youth who attend AA and/or NA after residential treatment for substance use are more likely to remain abstinent and use substances less frequently.[41,56,57,77–80]

Despite this preliminary yet inconclusive evidence of benefit, clinicians have expressed concerns anecdotally when referring youth to these groups. Most group members will be significantly older, with longer substance use histories and different life challenges owing to their age.[42] This age difference has also given rise to concerns about safety. Worries include the belief that older male members with criminal histories may intimidate or engage youth in illegal or predatory activities.[81] Although the majority of youth in 1 study reported feeling very safe at AA or NA meetings, 22% reported at least 1 negative experience, such as feeling intimidated, threatened, or sexually harassed. Reports were more common among those who went to NA. However, youth did not report safety concerns as a reason to stop attending.[82] On the other hand, some clinicians felt that certain youth benefitted from the wisdom and praise of adults at meetings.[81]

Additional research regarding age indicates that youth who attend 12-step meetings with at least a substantial proportion of people their age after inpatient treatment have better substance use outcomes.[58] Unfortunately, youth-oriented meetings are not accessible to a large percentage of adolescents owing to limited availability.

WHICH ADOLESCENTS BENEFIT MOST FROM CONTINUING CARE?

Existing research with adults and adolescents provides preliminary ideas for which youth might benefit most from particular continuing care services. In the adult literature, when Lynch and colleagues[83] compared telephone monitoring plus counseling with treatment as usual with telephone monitoring only, they found that telephone monitoring was more beneficial than treatment as usual for women and participants with lower readiness to change. McKay and colleagues[51] discovered that adults with high scores on a composite risk indicator had better total abstinence outcomes for up to 21 months if they received standard counseling rather than the telephone intervention, whereas those with lower scores had higher abstinence rates in the telephone intervention than in standard counseling. McKay and colleagues[84] found that, for adults with alcohol dependence only, the telephone-based monitoring and brief counseling interventions produced better alcohol use outcomes than standard group counseling on all measures examined and better outcomes than relapse prevention on some of the measures.

In the adolescent literature, Godley and Godley[53] reanalyzed data from the first ACC clinical trial. They compared youth assigned to the ACC group who failed to link with any continuing care services with those in the usual continuing care condition who failed to link with any continuing care despite receiving referrals from their residential treatment counselors. There were no demographic or clinical differences between the 2 groups. Although typical referrals to continuing care failed to work, within the ACC subgroup, all but 6 participants received varying levels of the ACC intervention delivered by a clinician via home or other community visits. Clinical outcome comparisons between these 2 subgroups revealed that the ACC subgroup was significantly more likely to remain abstinent from all drugs during the ACC phase and significantly more likely to remain abstinent from marijuana over the total 9-month follow-up period.

Godley and Godley[15] analyzed data from adolescents who did not complete residential treatment. Of noncompleters assigned to usual continuing care, 33% received continuing care within 14 days of discharge. Of those assigned to an assertive condition (ACC and/or motivational incentives), 64% did. Those who received additional services within 14 days of discharge were more likely to have superior alcohol and marijuana abstinence outcomes, even if they did not complete residential treatment, regardless of condition. Within an assertive condition, residential completers and noncompleters that received services within 14 days of discharge were significantly more likely to be abstinent from alcohol than noncompleters who did not.

Finally, analyses of volunteer telephone continuing care data demonstrated that the effects of recovery support calls did not differ by gender, but were significantly greater for adolescents with lower levels of treatment readiness.[76]

Taken together, these data suggest that future research is needed to better examine whether telephone continuing care could especially benefit individuals with lower readiness to change, only alcohol dependence, and lower risk. They also indicate that continuing care, especially using an assertive approach to reaching and engaging youth, may work well for individuals who do not complete treatment or follow through on typical continuing care referral advice.

SUMMARY

Research shows that many adolescents who enter substance use treatment do not complete the program and, after discharge, do not initiate continuing care services. Furthermore, the majority of adolescents will return to some level of substance use either during or after treatment. As youth return to use and problems occur, many will re-enter treatment, and some will do so several times. This pattern of disjointed treatment episodes remains the norm in contemporary practice rather than the intended plan of a course of treatment followed by continuing care. The studies reviewed in this paper offer prospective continuing care options consistent with expert consensus.[46]

Our review found 10 outcome studies of continuing care treatment for adolescents, 6 of which used randomized designs. Although there are only 6 prospective, well-controlled continuing care studies, 5 resulted in clinical improvement for youth receiving the experimental continuing care approaches. Four of the controlled studies used ACC (2 postresidential and 2 postoutpatient), and 3 of these found a clinical advantage for ACC, suggesting its effectiveness.

Key findings of these trials are that more assertive approaches can increase linkage rates to continuing care.[75] Another key finding of some trials was that rapid initiation of continuing care (ie, linking to ongoing services within 14 days of discharge from treatment) made a difference in reducing substance use. Thus, rapid provision of continuing care is likely to prevent or assist in terminating a relapse. Both ACC and motivational incentive approaches can be used to facilitate rapid linkage.[85] Contrary to aftercare programs that require treatment completion, multiple studies support providing continuing care to those who do not complete.[53,65,66,74] This suggests that continuing care is appropriate for those who successfully complete treatment and can improve outcomes for individuals who do not.

In contrast, the effectiveness of continuing care approaches, especially those that are more labor intensive like ACC, may not be necessary for all adolescents. Research using adaptive treatment designs similar to that used by Kaminer and colleagues[74] holds promise for establishing decision rules as to which individuals need low-intensity continuing care and which need more intensive home-based continuing care such as ACC. Although using decision rules is proving useful to assess who may need continuing care, providers may not have ready access to good follow-up outcome information, especially for individuals discharged early from residential treatment.

Although there are no randomized controlled studies of adolescent participation in mutual aid groups, evidence is accumulating in the published literature suggesting that matching adolescents to age appropriate 12-step and other mutual aid groups can support recovery. Referrals to meetings that are predominantly attended by adults should be assessed carefully to ensure a safe match. The lower cost of continuing care delivered through recovery coaches and other volunteers is promising, but controlled prospective studies are required before these approaches can be recommended.[76,86–88]

Additional continuing care research is needed in several areas. Studies are needed to assess whether patient intake variables (such as substance and/or co-occurring problem severity), treatment process variables (such as treatment completion or attainment of 1 or more treatment goals), and variables measuring parental involvement in treatment serve as valid predictors of who needs low- or high-intensity monitoring, support, counseling, and/or case management. Research accessible to therapists serving a broad range of individuals is needed that establishes decision rules using clinical and treatment variables that prove useful in matching level of continuing care services to individuals. Conducting research to establish more accessible predictor variables may be best accomplished through multisite research collaborations with sufficiently large samples to use adaptive treatment designs. Particularly for adolescents, more data regarding technology-based interventions would be useful because of its inherent appeal to this population. Research on low-cost and sustainable continuing care delivery methods would help to inform treatment programs trying to implement services with shrinking budgets or issues with service reimbursement. Investigation into the use of incentives for continuing care linkage and retention and continuing care research with youth who have co-occurring psychiatric disorders is sorely needed. Finally, with the promise of continuing care research to date and the potential of low-cost approaches, incorporating these interventions into adaptive continuing care studies to establish cost-effective decision rules should be a fruitful area for further examination.

REFERENCES

1. Dennis ML, Godley SH, Diamond GS, et al. The Cannabis Youth Treatment (CYT) study: main findings from two randomized trials. J Subst Abuse Treat 2004;27: 197–213.

2. Diamond GS, Godley SH, Liddle HA, et al. Five outpatient treatment models for adolescent marijuana use: a description of the Cannabis Youth Treatment interventions. Addiction 2002;97:S70–83.

3. Donohue B, Azrin NA. Treating adolescent substance abuse using family behavior therapy: a step-by-step approach. Hoboken (NJ): John Wiley and Sons; 2012.

4. Godley SH, Godley MD. Behavioral treatments for adolescents with substance use disorders. In: Miller PM, editor. Interventions for addiction: comprehensive addictive behaviors and disorders. San Diego (CA): Academic Press; 2013. p. 167–75.

5. Kaminer Y. Contingency management reinforcement procedures for adolescent substance abuse. J Am Acad Child Adolesc Psychiatry 2000;39:1324–6.

6. Kaminer Y, Burleson JA, Burke RH. Efficacy of outpatient aftercare for adolescents with alcohol use disorders: a randomized controlled study. J Am Acad Child Adolesc Psychiatry 2008;7:1405–12.

7. Monti PM, Colby SM, O'Leary TA, editors. Adolescents, alcohol, and substance abuse: reaching teens through brief interventions. New York: Guilford Press; 2001.

8. Petry NM. A comprehensive guide to the application of contingency management procedures in general clinic settings. Drug Alcohol Depend 2000;58:9–25.

9. Stanger C, Budney AJ, Kamon J, et al. A randomized trial of contingency management for adolescent marijuana abuse and dependence. Drug Alcohol Depend 2009;105:240–7.

10. Wagner EF, Macgowan MJ. School-based group treatment for adolescent substance abuse. In: Liddle HA, Rowe CL, editors. Adolescent substance abuse: research and clinical advances. Cambridge (UK): Cambridge University Press; 2006. p. 333–56.

11. Waldron HB, Turner CW. Evidence-based psychological treatments for adolescent substance abuse. J Clin Child Adolesc Psychol 2008;37:238–61.

12. Winters KC, Leitten W. Brief intervention for drug-abusing adolescents in a school setting. Psychol Addict Behav 2007;21:349–54.

13. Brown SA, Vik PW, Creamer VA. Characteristics of relapse following adolescent substance abuse treatment. Addict Behav 1989;14:291–300.

14. Chung T, Maisto SA. Review and reconsideration of relapse as a change point in clinical course in treated adolescents. Clin Psychol Rev 2006;26:149–61.

15. Godley MD, Godley SH. Assertive continuing care for adolescents. In: Kelly JF, White WL, editors. Addiction recovery management: theory, research and practice. New York: Springer Science; 2011. p. 103–26.

16. Kaminer Y, Burleson J, Goldberger R. Psychotherapies for adolescent substance abusers: short-and long-term outcomes. J Nerv Ment Dis 2002;190:737–45.

17. Williams RJ, Chang SY. An assertive and comparative review of adolescent substance abuse treatment outcome. Clin Psychol 2000;7:138–66.

18. GAIN Coordinating Center. Briefing book slides on all grantees in the 2012 SAMHSA/CSAT summary analytic file [electronic version]. Normal (IL): Chestnut Health Systems; 2013. Available at: www.gaincc.org/slides. Accessed April 14, 2016.

19. McLellan AT, Lewis DC, O'Brien CP, et al. Drug dependence, a chronic medical illness: implications for treatment, insurance, and outcomes evaluation. JAMA 2000;284:1689–95.

20. McLellan AT, McKay JR, Forman R, et al. Reconsidering the evaluation of addiction treatment: from retrospective follow-up to concurrent recovery monitoring. Addiction 2005;100:447–58.

21. Scott CK, Foss MA, Dennis ML. Utilizing recovery management checkups to shorten the cycle of relapse, treatment reentry, and recovery. Drug Alcohol Depend 2005;78:325–38.
22. Weisner C, McLellan T, Barthwell A, et al. Report of the Blue Ribbon Task Force on health services research at the National Institute on Drug Abuse. Rockville (MD): National Institute on Drug Abuse; 2004.
23. White WL, Boyle M, Loveland D. Recovery from addiction and recovery from mental illness: shared and contrasting lessons. In: Ralph R, Corrigan P, editors. Recovery and mental illness: consumer visions and research paradigms. Washington, DC: American Psychological Association; 2004. p. 233–58.
24. Dennis ML, Scott CK. Managing addiction as a chronic condition. Addict Sci Clin Pract 2007;4:45–55.
25. Kaminer Y, Godley M. From assessment reactivity to aftercare for adolescent substance abuse: are we there yet? Child Adolesc Psychiatr Clin N Am 2010;19:577–90.
26. Miller WR. What is relapse? Fifty ways to leave the wagon. Addiction 1996;91:S15–27.
27. White WL, Boyle M, Loveland D. Addiction as chronic disease: from rhetoric to clinical application. Alcohol Treat Q 2002;20(3/4):107–30.
28. Battjes RJ, Gordon MS, O'Grady KE, et al. Factors that predict adolescent motivation for substance abuse treatment. J Subst Abuse Treat 2003;24:221–32.
29. Tims FM, Dennis ML, Hamilton N, et al. Characteristics and problems of 600 adolescent cannabis abusers in outpatient treatment. Addiction 2002;97(Suppl 1):S46–57.
30. Winters KC. Adolescent brain development and drug abuse. Loughborough (UK): The Mentor Foundation; 2008.
31. Giedd JN. Structural magnetic resonance imaging of the adolescent brain. Ann N Y Acad Sci 2004;1021:77–85.
32. Rutherford HJV, Mayes LC, Potenza MN. Neurobiology of adolescent substance use disorders: implications for prevention and treatment. Child Adolesc Psychiatr Clin N Am 2010;19(3):479–92.
33. Spear LP. Alcohol's effects on adolescents. Alcohol Health Res World 2002;26(4):287–91.
34. Brown SA, Tapert SF, Granholm E, et al. Neurocognitive functioning of adolescents: effects of protracted alcohol use. Alcohol Clin Exp Res 2000;242:164–71.
35. Gonzalez R, Swanson JM. Long-term effects of adolescent-onset and persistent use of cannabis. Proc Natl Acad Sci U S A 2012;109(40):15970–1.
36. Godley MD, White WL. The history and future of "aftercare". Counselor 2003;4(1):19–21.
37. Jainchill N. Therapeutic communities for adolescents: the same and not the same. In: De Leon G, editor. Community as method: therapeutic communities for special population and special settings. Westport (CT): Praeger Publishers/Greenwood Publishing Group; 1997. p. 161–77.
38. White WL, Dennis ML, Tims FM. Adolescent treatment: its history and current renaissance. Counselor 2002;3:20–4.
39. Drug Strategies. Treating teens: a guide to adolescent drug programs. Washington, DC: Author; 2003.
40. Humphreys K, Wing S, McCarty D, et al. Self-help organizations for alcohol and drug problems: toward evidence-based practice and policy. J Subst Abuse Treat 2004;26:151–8.

41. Kelly JF, Myers MG. Adolescents' participation in Alcoholics Anonymous and Narcotics Anonymous: review, implications and future directions. J Psychoactive Drugs 2007;39:259–69.

42. Passetti LL, White WL. Recovery support meetings for youths: considerations when referring young people to 12-step and alternative groups. J Groups Addict Recover 2008;2(2–4):97–121.

43. Godley SH, Godley MD, Dennis ML. The assertive aftercare protocol for adolescent substance abusers. In: Wagner E, Waldron H, editors. Innovations in adolescent substance abuse interventions. New York: Elsevier Science; 2001. p. 311–29.

44. Godley SH, Passetti LL, Funk RR, et al. One-year treatment patterns and change trajectories for adolescents participating in outpatient treatment for the first time. J Psychoactive Drugs 2008;40:17–27.

45. Office of Applied Studies. Treatment episode data set (TEDS): 2002. Discharges from substance abuse treatment services, DASIS Series S-25, DHHS Publication No. (SMA) 04–3967. Rockville (MD): SAMHSA; 2005. Available at: www.dasis.samhsa.gov/teds02/2002_teds_rpt_d.pdf. Accessed April 7, 2016.

46. American Society of Addiction Medicine (ASAM). Patient placement criteria for the treatment of substance-related disorders. 2nd edition. Chevy Chase (MD): ASAM; 2001.

47. Dennis ML, Scott CK, Funk RR. An experimental evaluation of recovery management check-ups (RMC) for people with chronic substance use disorders. Eval Program Plann 2003;26:339–52.

48. Godley MD, Coleman-Cowger VH, Titus JC, et al. A randomized controlled trial of telephone continuing care. J Subst Abuse Treat 2010;38:74–82.

49. Gustafson DH, McTavish FM, Chih MY, et al. A smartphone application to support recovery from alcoholism: a randomized clinical trial. JAMA Psychiatry 2014; 71(5):566–72.

50. Hubbard RL, Leimberger JD, Haynes L, et al. Telephone enhancement of long-term engagement (TELE) in continuing care for substance abuse treatment: a NIDA clinical trials network (CTN) study. Am J Addict 2007;16:495–502.

51. McKay JR, Lynch KG, Shepard DS, et al. The effectiveness of telephone-based continuing care for alcohol and cocaine dependence: 24 month outcomes. Arch Gen Psychiatry 2005;62:199–207.

52. McKay JR, Van Horn D, Oslin D, et al. Extended telephone-based continuing care for alcohol dependence: 24 month outcomes and subgroup analyses. Addiction 2011;106:1760–9.

53. Godley MD, Godley SH. Continuing care following residential treatment: history, current practice, and emerging approaches. In: Jainchill N, editor. Understanding and treating adolescent substance use disorders. Kingston (NJ): Civic Research Institute; 2012. p. 14-22–14-24.

54. Chun JS, Godley MD, Funk RR, et al. Residential treatment and continuing care for adolescent substance abusers: an analysis of CSAT's ART initiative. Paper presented at: 2006 Joint Meeting on Adolescent Treatment Effectiveness (JMATE). Baltimore (MD), March 26–29, 2006.

55. Godley MD, Godley SH, Dennis ML, et al. A review of usual, innovative, and assertive continuing care approaches. Paper presented at: 2005 Joint Meeting on Adolescent Treatment Effectiveness (JMATE). Washington, DC, March 21–23, 2005.

56. Kelly JF, Myers MG, Brown SA. A multivariate process model of adolescent 12-step attendance and substance use outcome following inpatient treatment. Psychol Addict Behav 2000;14(4):376–89.

57. Kelly JF, Myers MG, Brown SA. Do adolescents affiliate with 12-step groups? A multivariate process model of effects. J Stud Alcohol 2002;63:293–304.

58. Kelly JF, Myers MG, Brown SA. The effects of age composition of 12-step groups on adolescent 12-step participation and substance use outcome. J Child Adolesc Subst Abuse 2005;15:63–72.

59. Ralph N, McMenamy C. Treatment outcomes in an adolescent chemical dependency program. Adolescence 1996;31:91–107.

60. Sealock MD, Gottfredson DC, Gallagher CA. Drug treatment for juvenile offenders: some good and bad news. J Res Crime Delinq 1997;34:210–36.

61. Whitney SD, Kelly JF, Myers MG, et al. Parental substance use, family support and outcome following treatment for adolescent psychoactive substance use disorders. J Child Adolesc Subst Abuse 2002;11:67–81.

62. Winters KC, Stinchfield RD, Latimer WW, et al. Long-term outcome of substance dependent youth following 12-step treatment. J Subst Abuse Treat 2007;33:61–9.

63. Godley SH, Godley MD, Karvinen T, et al. The Assertive Continuing Care protocol: a clinician's manual for working with adolescents after residential treatment of alcohol and other substance use disorders. 2nd edition. Bloomington (IL): Lighthouse Institute; 2006.

64. Godley SH, Meyers RJ, Smith JE, et al. DHHS Publication No. (SMA) 01-3489, Cannabis youth treatment (CYT) manual series. The adolescent community reinforcement approach (ACRA) for adolescent cannabis users, vol. 4. Rockville (MD): Center for Substance Abuse Treatment; Substance Abuse and Mental Health Services Administration; 2001.

65. Godley MD, Godley SH, Dennis ML, et al. The effect of assertive continuing care (ACC) on continuing care linkage, adherence and abstinence following residential treatment for adolescents. Addiction 2006;102:81–93.

66. Godley MD, Godley SH, Dennis ML, et al. A randomized trial of assertive continuing care and contingency management for adolescents with substance use disorders. J Consult Clin Psychol 2014;82:40–51.

67. Garnick DW, Lee MT, Chalk M, et al. Establishing the feasibility of performance measures for alcohol and other drugs. J Subst Abuse Treat 2002;23:375–85.

68. Kaminer Y, Napolitano C. Dial for therapy: aftercare for adolescent substance use disorders. J Am Acad Child Adolesc Psychiatry 2004;43:171–4.

69. Kaminer Y, Napolitano C. Brief telephone continuing care therapy for adolescents. Center City (MN): Hazelden; 2010.

70. Burleson JA, Kaminer Y, Burke RH. Twelve-month follow-up of aftercare for adolescents with alcohol use disorders. J Subst Abuse Treat 2012;42(1):78–86.

71. Godley SH, Garner BR, Passetti LL, et al. Adolescent outpatient treatment and continuing care: main findings from a randomized clinical trial. Drug Alcohol Depend 2010;110(1–2):44–54.

72. Henderson CE, Wevodau AL, Henderson SE, et al. An independent replication of the Adolescent community reinforcement approach with justice-involved youth. Am J Addict 2016;25(3):233–40.

73. Brown PC, Budney AJ, Thostenson JD, et al. Initiation of abstinence in adolescents treated for marijuana use disorders. J Subst Abuse Treat 2013;44:384–90.

74. Kaminer Y, Ohannessian CM, Burke RH. Adolescents with cannabis use disorders: Adaptive treatment for poor responder outcomes. Paper presented at:

2016 College on Problems of Drug Dependence (CPDD) annual meeting. Palm Springs (CA), June 11–16, 2016.

75. McKay JR. Treating substance use disorders with adaptive continuing care. Washington, DC: American Psychological Association; 2009.

76. Garner BR, Godley MD, Passetti LL, et al. Recovery support for adolescents with substance use disorders: the impact of recovery support telephone calls provided by pre-professional volunteers. J Subst Abus Alcohol 2014;2(2):1010.

77. Chi FW, Kaskutas LA, Sterling S, et al. Twelve-step affiliation and three-year substance use outcomes among adolescents: social support and religious service attendance as potential mediators. Addiction 2009;104:927–39.

78. Kelly JF, Myers MG, Rodolico J. What do adolescents exposed to Alcoholics Anonymous think about 12-step groups? Subst Abuse 2008;29:53–62.

79. Kelly JF, Dow SJ, Yeterian JD, et al. Can 12-step group participation strengthen and extend the benefits of adolescent addiction treatment? A prospective analysis. Drug Alcohol Depend 2010;110:117–25.

80. Kelly JF, Urbanoski K. Youth recovery contexts: the incremental effects of 12-step attendance and involvement on adolescent outpatient outcomes. Alcohol Clin Exp Res 2012;36(7):1219–29.

81. Passetti LL, Godley SH. Adolescent substance abuse treatment clinicians' self-help meeting referral practices and adolescent attendance rates. J Psychoactive Drugs 2008;40:29–40.

82. Kelly JF, Dow SJ, Yeterian JD, et al. How safe are adolescents at Alcoholics Anonymous and Narcotics Anonymous meetings? A prospective investigation with outpatient youth. J Subst Abuse Treat 2011;40:419–25.

83. Lynch KG, Van Horn D, Drapkin M, et al. Moderators of response to extended telephone continuing care for alcoholism. Am J Health Behav 2010;34(6): 788–800.

84. McKay JR, Lynch KG, Shepard DS, et al. The effectiveness of telephone-based continuing care in the clinical management of alcohol and cocaine use disorders: 12-month outcomes. J Consult Clin Psychol 2004;72:967–79.

85. Stanger C, Budney AJ. Contingency management approaches for adolescent SUD. Child Adolesc Psychiatr Clin N Am 2010;19:547–62.

86. Douglas-Siegel JA, Ryan JP. The effect of recovery coaches for substance-involved mothers in child welfare: impact on juvenile delinquency. J Subst Abuse Treat 2013;45:381–7.

87. Ryan JP, Choi S, Hong J, et al. Recovery coaches and substance exposure at birth. Child Abuse Negl 2008;32(11):1072–9.

88. White WL. Sponsor, recovery coach, addiction counselor: the importance of role clarity and role integrity. Philadelphia: Philadelphia Department of Behavioral Health and Mental Retardation Services; 2006.

The Role of Pharmacotherapy in the Treatment of Adolescent Substance Use Disorders

 CrossMark

Christopher J. Hammond, MD

KEYWORDS

- Adolescence • Development • Substance use disorder • Addiction
- Pharmacotherapy • Medication

KEY POINTS

- Pharmacotherapy, when used in conjunction with psychosocial substance use disorder (SUD) treatment interventions, may improve outcomes compared with psychosocial treatment alone.
- Compared with ample research in adults, relatively few randomized controlled medication trials have been conducted in adolescents with SUD.
- Results suggest that a number of medications may improve adolescent SUD treatment outcomes, including nicotine replacement therapy and bupropion (tobacco use disorders), N-acetylcysteine (cannabis use disorders), and buprenorphine-naloxone (opioid use disorders).

INTRODUCTION

Despite national efforts, substance use disorders (SUDs) and the excessive use of alcohol and other drugs remains a significant public health issue that has been estimated to cost the United States over $400 billion annually.[1] More than 90% of US adults who develop SUDs started using alcohol and other drugs during adolescence.[2,3] Growing evidence suggests that SUDs can be viewed as developmental disorders with genetic, temperamental, and environmental antecedents that emerge

Conflict of Interest and Financial Disclosures: Dr C.J. Hammond currently receives research support from the American Academy of Child and Adolescent Psychiatry (AACAP) and the National Institute on Drug Abuse (NIDA) in the form of a career development award (K12DA000357).
Behavioral Pharmacology Research Unit, Johns Hopkins Bayview Medical Campus, 50 Nathan Shock Drive, Baltimore, MD 21224, USA
E-mail address: chammo20@jhmi.edu

Child Adolesc Psychiatric Clin N Am 25 (2016) 685–711
http://dx.doi.org/10.1016/j.chc.2016.05.004
1056-4993/16/$ – see front matter © 2016 Elsevier Inc. All rights reserved.

childpsych.theclinics.com

Abbreviations	
AUD	Alcohol use disorder
AWS	Alcohol withdrawal syndrome
CM	Contingency management
CO	Carbon monoxide
CUD	Cannabis use disorder
DSM	*Diagnostic and Statistical Manual of Mental Disorders*
FDA	US Food and Drug Administration
GABA	Gamma-aminobutyric acid
MI	Motivational interviewing
MMT	Methadone maintenance therapy
NAC	*N*-acetylcysteine
NRT	Nicotine replacement therapy
OUD	Opioid use disorder
OWS	Opioid withdrawal syndrome
RCT	Randomized, controlled trial
SR	Sustained release
SUD	Substance use disorder
XL	Extended release

during early childhood.[4] Substance use initiation, progression to regular use, and the development of SUDs peaks during adolescence and young adulthood, and decreases throughout the rest of the lifespan.[5,6] SUDs represent a major source of morbidity and mortality in the teenage years.[7–11]

Many youth meet criteria for SUDs and a major treatment gap exists, with fewer than 1 in 10 adolescents who are in need of treatment receiving it.[12] Data on national admissions to substance use treatment between 2002 and 2012 found that 75% of all adolescent SUD treatment admissions were related to cannabis, 13% to alcohol, 3% to opioids, 3% to methamphetamines or amphetamines, and 1% to cocaine.[13]

A number of psychosocial interventions have demonstrated short-term efficacy in clinical trials, but effect sizes for these interventions remain small to moderate, and few youth achieve sustained abstinence.[14–20] In light of the limited treatment response and increased morbidity and mortality associated with adolescent SUDs, the field of addiction science is focused on expanding treatment approaches that may enhance treatment response and improve outcomes.[15] A potential approach to improve treatment response is to use adjunctive pharmacotherapy.

Growing evidence indicates that pharmacotherapy when added to psychosocial interventions improves treatment outcomes in adult SUDs.[21,22] As such, a primary question for the field is can pharmacotherapies, when added to psychosocial interventions, improve outcomes for adolescent SUDs? To address this question, this article presents a comprehensive clinical review of the state of the evidence of pharmacotherapy for adolescent SUDs. It focuses on recent randomized, controlled trials (RCTs) using medications in combination with psychosocial interventions to treat SUDs in individuals aged 13 to 25 years (**Table 1**).

The Role of Pharmacotherapy in the Treatment of Substance Use Disorders

Medication assisted treatments are defined as the use of a US Food and Drug Administration (FDA)-approved medication in combination with evidence-based psychosocial intervention to provide a 'whole patient' approach to the treatment of SUDs.[21] Numerous controlled trials in adults have shown that medications targeting alcohol use disorders (AUD),[23] tobacco use disorders,[24] and opioid use disorders (OUD)[25,26] have been associated with improved treatment outcomes,[23–25] reductions

Table 1
Pharmacotherapy for adolescent substance use disorders

Drug	Sample(s)	Study Design(s)	Intervention Dosing and Duration	Outcome Measures	Level of Evidence[a]
AWS					
Benzodiazepines		Consensus guidelines; there are no controlled treatment studies examining pharmacotherapy for adolescent AW or AWS			Grade C (level 3 evidence) for AWS
AUD					
Naltrexone (oral)	Outpatient, treatment-seeking, adolescents (mean age = 13.2 y); non–treatment-seeking heavy drinkers (ages 15–19); 2 studies, n = 27 total subjects	6-wk, open-label, clinical study; 4-wk double-blind, placebo controlled cross-over study using EMA	Naltrexone, oral, flexible dose, 25–50 mg/d; naltrexone, oral, fixed dose, 50 mg/d	Self-report alcohol use (time-line follow-back methods and EMA); A-OCDS; alcohol craving; subjective-response to alcohol	Grade C (level 3 evidence) for AUD
Disulfiram	Postdetoxification, outpatient, treatment-seeking adolescents (ages 16–19); 1 study, n = 26 subjects	90-d, randomized double-blind, placebo controlled study	Disulfiram, oral, fixed dose, 200 mg/d	Self-report alcohol use	Grade C (level 3 evidence) for AUD
Ondansetron	Outpatient, treatment-seeking, adolescents (ages 14–20); 1 study, n = 12 subjects	8-wk, open-label, clinical study	Ondansetron, oral, fixed dose, 4 µg/kg 2 times per day	Self-report alcohol use; adverse events	Grade C (level 3 evidence) for AUD

(continued on next page)

Table 1
(continued)

Drug	Sample(s)	Study Design(s)	Intervention Dosing and Duration	Outcome Measures	Level of Evidence[a]
Topiramate	Non–treatment-seeking, heavy drinkers (mean age = 19 y); 1 study, n = 13 subjects	5-wk, randomized, placebo controlled, pilot study using EMA	Topiramate, oral, escalating dose, up to 200 mg per day	Self-report alcohol use (EMA); alcohol craving; subjective-response to alcohol	Grade C (level 3 evidence) for AUD
TUD					
Nicotine replacement therapy (patch, gum, nasal spray)	Outpatient, treatment-seeking adolescents (ages 12–19), smoking ≥5 CPD[b]; 5 studies, n = 728 total subjects	Metaanalysis, 12-wk randomized double-blind, double-placebo controlled study comparing nicotine patch with nicotine gum; 10-wk randomized double-blind placebo-controlled study of nicotine patch; 6- to 9-week randomized, double-blind placebo controlled study of nicotine patch; 8-wk open-label clinical study of nicotine nasal spray	Nicotine patch, fixed dose 21 mg (participants smoking ≥20 CPD) or 14 mg (<20 CPD) Nicotine patch, fixed taper dosing, starting dose 21 mg (participants smoking >15 CPD) or 14 mg (10–14 CPD) tapered over 10 wk Nicotine gum, 4 mg (participants smoking ≥24 CPD) or 2 mg (<24 CPD) Nicotine nasal spray, 1 mg dosing as needed	CO-confirmed PPA at EOT; cotinine-confirmed PPA at EOT; nicotine craving; nicotine withdrawal	*Nicotine patch:* grade B (level 2 evidence) for TUD *Nicotine gum and nasal spray:* grade C (level 3 evidence) for TUD
Varenicline	Outpatient, treatment-seeking adolescents (ages 14–20), smoking ≥5 CPD; 1 study, n = 29 subjects	8-wk, randomized double-blind controlled study comparing Varenicline to bupropion XL	Varenicline, oral, 1 mg 2 times per day or bupropion XL, oral, 300 mg/d	Self-report smoking reduction; cotinine confirmed PPA at EOT	Grade B (level 2 evidence) for TUD

Buproprion	Outpatient, treatment-seeking adolescents (ages 12–21), smoking ≥5 CPD[b], 4 studies, n = 688 total subjects	Metaanalysis, 8-wk, randomized, double-blind, placebo controlled add-on to nicotine patch; 6-wk, randomized, double-blind, placebo controlled dose comparison study (150 mg vs 300 mg) study; 6-wk, randomized double-blind, placebo controlled study with added ± CM; 8-wk, randomized double-blind comparison with varenicline	Buproprion SR, oral, fixed dose, 150 mg/d or 300 mg/d	Cotinine-confirmed PPA at EOT; CO-confirmed PPA at EOT; self-report smoking reduction	Grade B (level 2 evidence) for TUD
CUD					
NAC	Outpatient, treatment-seeking, adolescents (ages 15–21); 2 studies, n = 134 total subjects	8-wk, randomized, double-blind, placebo controlled study added to brief cessation counseling and CM; 4-wk open-label pilot study	NAC, oral, fixed dose, 1200 mg 2 times per day (2400 mg/d)	Negative urine cannabinoid test, self-report cannabis use, cravings for cannabis	Grade B (level 2 evidence) for CUD
Topiramate	Outpatient, treatment-seeking, youth (ages 15–24); 1 study, n = 66	6-wk, randomized, double-blind, placebo controlled pilot study medication added to 3 sessions of motivational enhancement therapy	Topiramate, oral, fixed dose, titrated to 200 mg/d over 4 wk and maintained at 200 mg/d over 2 wk	Positive urine cannabinoid test, self-report cannabis use (% days of cannabis use, grams of cannabis use per day), treatment retention, adverse events, neurocognitive functioning	Grade C (level 3 evidence) for CUD

(continued on next page)

Table 1
(continued)

Drug	Sample(s)	Study Design(s)	Intervention Dosing and Duration	Outcome Measures	Level of Evidence[a]
OWS					
Buprenorphine and buprenorphine–naloxone	Outpatient detoxification, treatment-seeking, adolescents (ages 13–18); 2 studies, n = 188 total subjects	Systematic review; 28-d randomized, double-blind, double-placebo, controlled study comparing clonidine and buprenorphine detoxification regimens; 12-wk randomized multisite clinical trial comparing 2-wk detoxification with 12-wk maintenance	Buprenorphine, sublingual, fixed taper dosing, starting dose 8 or 6 mg (age based); buprenorphine–naloxone (2 mg/ 0.05 mg ratio), oral, fixed taper dosing, up to 24 mg/d	Opiate negative urine tests, treatment retention, self-report HIV-risk behavior, opiate withdrawal symptoms	Grade B (level 2 evidence) for OWS
Clonidine (patch)	Outpatient detoxification, treatment-seeking, adolescents (ages 13–18); 1 study, n = 36 subjects	28-d randomized, double-blind, double-placebo, controlled study comparing clonidine and buprenorphine detoxification regimens	Buprenorphine, sublingual, fixed taper dosing, starting dose 8 or 6 mg (age based); clonidine, transdermal patch, fixed taper dosing, starting dose 0.1–0.3 mg/d	Opiate-negative urine tests, treatment retention, self-report HIV-risk behavior, opiate withdrawal symptoms	Grade B (level 2 evidence) for OWS

OUD					
Methadone	Inpatient detoxification and specialized opioid treatment programs, treatment-seeking, adolescents (ages ≤20); 9 studies, n = 6263 total subjects	Systematic review; naturalistic study comparing methadone maintenance, detoxification, therapeutic community, and abstinence-based treatments; naturalistic studies of methadone maintenance or methadone detoxification treatment without comparator groups; methadone-based short-term detoxification (30-d) vs long-term detoxification (up to 6-mo)	Methadone, oral, flexible dosing, for 30-d detoxification or up to 6-mo maintenance treatment	Treatment retention, self-report opioid use	Grade C (level 3 evidence) for OUD
Buprenorphine–naloxone	Outpatient, treatment-seeking, adolescents (ages 15–21); 1 study, n = 152 subjects	Systematic review; 12-wk, randomized, multisite, controlled study comparing 2-wk buprenorphine–naloxone detoxification to 12-wk buprenorphine–naloxone maintenance/extended treatment	Buprenorphine–naloxone (2 mg/ 0.05 mg ratio), oral, fixed taper dosing, up to 24 mg/d	Opiate-positive urine tests	Grade B (level 2 evidence) for OUD

(continued on next page)

Table 1
(continued)

Drug	Sample(s)	Study Design(s)	Intervention Dosing and Duration	Outcome Measures	Level of Evidence[a]
Extended-release injectable naltrexone (intramuscular)	Residential treatment transitioning to outpatient treatment, treatment-seeking, adolescents (ages 16–20); 1 study, n = 16 subjects	Retrospective, open-label, case series	XR-naltrexone, intramuscular injection, 380 mg once every 4 wk	Treatment retention, abstinence, opioid use of (chart abstraction of self-report and urine drug screen data)	Grade C (level 3 evidence) for OUD
Opioid overdose					
Naloxone (intranasal)		Consensus guidelines; there have been no studies examining pharmacotherapy for opioid overdose in adolescents	Naloxone, intranasal, 2 mg/2 mL prefilled Luer-lock needleleless syringe		Grade C (level 3 evidence) for opioid overdose

Abbreviations: A-OCDS, alcohol obsessive compulsive drinking scale; AUD, alcohol use disorder; AW, alcohol withdrawal; AWS, alcohol withdrawal syndrome; bupropion SR, sustained release bupropion; bupropion XL, extended release bupropion; CM, contingency management; CO, carbon monoxide; cotinine, urine cotinine level (ng/dL); CPD, cigarettes per day; CUD, cannabis use disorder; EMA, ecological momentary assessment; EOT, end of treatment; HIV, human immunodeficiency virus; NAC, N-acetylcysteine; NRT, nicotine replacement therapy; OUD, opioid use disorder; OWS, opioid withdrawal syndrome; PPA, point prevalence abstinence; TUD, tobacco use disorder; XR-naltrexone, Extended-release injectable Naltrexone.

[a] Levels of evidence presented are based on the US Preventative Services Task Force Strength of Recommendation Taxonomy approach to grading evidence in medical literature.[103] Levels of evidence include: Level 1: good-quality, patient-oriented evidence including systematic reviews, metaanalyses, and well-designed randomized controlled trials with consistent findings; Level 2: limited-quality, patient-oriented evidence including lower-quality/less consistent systematic reviews, metaanalyses, or clinical trials as well as cohort and case-control series; Level 3: other evidence in the form of consensus guidelines, disease-oriented evidence, and case series. These levels of evidence are used to determine a strength of recommendation grade, which include A (good-quality, patient-oriented evidence); B (limited-quality, patient-oriented evidence); C (other evidence); and no recommendation.

[b] For the adolescent TUD pharmacotherapy studies, and specifically the 5 NRT and 4 bupropion studies, all studies had CPD-based inclusionary criteria, which ranged from ≥5 to ≥10 CPD.

in total treatment costs,[27–29] and reduction in SUD-related morbidity and mortality.[23–26] As such, treatments that combine pharmacotherapies with psychosocial interventions (ie, medication-assisted treatments) are now thought of as a central component of SUD management for adults with those disorders. Because the term "medication-assisted therapy" has been used primarily in relation to the treatment of OUDs with medications and psychosocial treatments, in this article we use the term "pharmacotherapy."

Pharmacotherapy research has focused on developing medications to (1) reduce craving and the urge to drink or use drugs, (2) decrease acute and postacute/protracted withdrawal symptoms, and (3) decrease impulsive or situational alcohol or drug use.[23,24] Studies in adults suggest that integrating FDA-approved SUD pharmacotherapy with psychosocial treatments can have a synergistic effect on improving treatment outcomes.[23–26] Despite positive findings in the adult SUD pharmacotherapy literature, it is unclear if adjunctive pharmacotherapy improves outcomes in a similar way in adolescents with SUDs.

Treatment of Adolescents Versus Adults: Developing Brains and Different Pharmacokinetics and Pharmacodynamics

A major problem with extrapolating adolescent treatment guidelines from adult SUD pharmacotherapy trials is that adolescents are not just "little adults." Adolescents with SUDs differ from their adult counterparts in important ways. Developmental differences may impact the biological or physiologic effects of the substance of abuse and the psychotropic medication. Developmental differences may also influence psychological aspects of drug and medication taking and subjective drug and medication experience, such as expectancies and medication adherence.[30] These differences likely impact adolescent response to both the substances of abuse as well as the psychotropic medication prescribed to treat the SUD.

Adolescence is a period of marked changes in bodily systems.[31] Developmental differences exist in neurobiology, pharmacodynamics, and pharmacokinetics when comparing children and adolescents to adults.[31,32] Age-related changes in the body fat, extracellular water, and hepatic and renal function alter the bioavailability, metabolism, and clearance of drugs, leading to different pharmacokinetic profiles by age.[33,34] Neurotransmitter systems, including dopaminergic, serotonergic, noradrenergic, gamma-aminobutyric acid (GABA)ergic, and glutamatergic systems, mature across adolescence.[35,36] These developmental changes affect biochemical and physiologic effects of medications, which may explain age-related differences in therapeutic response and medication side effect profiles.[33,37,38]

PHARMACOTHERAPY FOR ALCOHOL USE DISORDERS

Alcohol is the most common drug of abuse used by adolescents,[3] and the second most common drug for which adolescents present for SUD treatment.[13] The pathophysiology of AUDs involves allostatic brain changes in glutamatergic and GABAergic neurotransmission, altering excitatory-to-inhibitory balance with repeated heavy drinking episodes.[39] Pharmacotherapy for alcohol withdrawal syndrome (AWS) targets the neuronal hyperexcitability and GABA–glutamate imbalance that produce the core withdrawal symptoms. Maintenance pharmacotherapies for AUD act to decrease alcohol cravings, postacute/protracted withdrawal symptoms, and the rewarding effects of alcohol, thereby decreasing alcohol use and reducing the likelihood of relapse. To date, the FDA has approved 4 medications for the treatment of AUD in adults:

1. Naltrexone (oral),
2. Extended-release injectable naltrexone (XR-naltrexone) (intramuscular),
3. Disulfiram, and
4. Acamprosate.

Additionally, nonbenzodiazepine anticonvulsants, including gabapentin and topiramate, have emerged as potential pharmacotherapy options in adults.[40] There are limited safety and efficacy data available on these medications in adolescent samples.

Pharmacotherapy for Alcohol Withdrawal Syndrome

Alcohol withdrawal and AWS is rare in adolescents, and clinical guidelines and treatment principles are extrapolated from the adult literature.[41] To date, no controlled studies have examined pharmacotherapy interventions for AWS in adolescents. Among adolescents with AUDs, 5% to 10% report experiencing withdrawal symptoms.[42] A minority of these cases will present with severe AWS, which represents a life-threaten emergency owing to the risk for AWS-related seizures or delirium tremens. As such, all youth who present for AUD treatment should be evaluated for symptoms of alcohol withdrawal and risk stratified. Treatment principles from adult AWS treatment should guide management.[43]

Benzodiazepines

Although a number of nonbenzodiazepine anticonvulsants are being studied for the treatment of AWS and AUD in adults,[40] benzodiazepines currently remain the first line of pharmacotherapy for treatment of AWS.[43] Consensus guidelines suggest that adolescents with severe AUD who present with moderate to severe AWS should be treated with benzodiazepines in inpatient treatment settings.[41,44]

Pharmacotherapy for Maintenance Treatment of Alcohol Use Disorders

To date, RCTs examining the short-term efficacy of maintenance pharmacotherapy for adolescent AUDs have been completed for naltrexone (oral) and disulfiram. Small open-label and randomized pilot studies exist for ondansetron and topiramate. Collectively, these studies include 5 small trials, and a total of 78 subjects.

Naltrexone

Naltrexone is a long-acting opiate receptor antagonist. When combined with psychosocial interventions, naltrexone has been shown to reduce relapse rates during active treatment and follow-up, and is associated with reductions in drinking days, drinks per drinking day, and alcohol consumption during treatment of adults with AUDs.[45,46] Alcohol's reinforcing effects are, in part, mediated by endogenous opioid activity in the midbrain dopaminergic system.[23] Naltrexone acts by attenuating the rewarding effects of alcohol and reducing alcohol cravings in alcoholics, enhancing abstinence and reducing heavy drinking.[47]

Two small pilot studies provide preliminary evidence for naltrexone's tolerability, safety, and efficacy in adolescents AUDs. First, Deas and colleagues[48] (2005) completed an outpatient-based 6-week open-label pilot study of naltrexone (flexible dosing 25–50 mg/d) for the treatment of adolescents meeting *Diagnostic and Statistical Manual of Mental Disorders* (DSM)-IV criteria for alcohol dependence. Average drinks per day and alcohol-related obsessions and compulsions decreased significantly and naltrexone was well-tolerated in all subjects. Deas and colleagues have followed-up that open-label pilot study with a 12-week randomized double-blind placebo-controlled study of naltrexone for adolescent AUD, but the results are pending at this time. Second, Miranda and colleagues[49] (2013) completed a small randomized double-blind placebo-controlled cross-over study using self-reported alcohol use collected in real-time using ecological momentary assessment approaches and laboratory-based subjective-response and cue-reactivity to alcohol as outcome measures. Twenty-eight non–treatment-seeking heavy drinking youth (ages 15–19 years) were randomized to receive naltrexone (oral, 50 mg/d) or placebo for 8 to 10 days followed by a washout period and then switch to the opposite medication for 8 to 10 days. Naltrexone as compared with placebo decreased the likelihood of heavy drinking (odds ratio [OR], 0.5), drinking on a study day (OR, 0.7), and attenuated alcohol cravings and subjective response to alcohol in the laboratory protocol.

Disulfiram

Disulfiram is FDA approved for the treatment of AUDs in adults, and known as an alcohol-sensitizing/aversive agent. It irreversibly binds to aldehyde dehydrogenase, leading to a rapid increase in acetaldehyde when alcohol is consumed, resulting in aversive symptoms.[23] Emerging data suggests that disulfiram also acts in the central nervous system by altering dopaminergic function, via inhibition of dopamine beta-hydroxylase, which may contribute to its efficacy.[50]

Niederhofer and Staffen[51] (2003) completed a randomized double-blind placebo-controlled study in treatment-seeking adolescents (ages 16–19 years) with a DSM-IV diagnosis of alcohol dependence who were admitted to inpatient detoxification. Participants underwent detoxification for AWS and were randomized to either disulfiram (200 mg/d) or placebo after 5 days of alcohol abstinence and then followed weekly for 90 days. The disulfiram group compared with placebo had significant greater mean cumulative days of abstinence (69 vs 30) and significantly more participants who remained abstinent at 90 days (7 vs 2). Participants tolerated disulfiram and reported few side effects.

Ondansetron

Ondansetron is a selective serotonin 5-HT$_3$ receptor antagonist that is FDA-approved for treatment of nausea and vomiting. An early RCT examining ondansetron for adults with AUDs discovered that individuals with early-onset adult AUD had a better treatment response, and subsequently a number of pharmacogenetics and translational studies have examined ondansetron in relation to serotonin gene function and age of AUD onset.[52–55]

No RCTs of ondansetron have been conducted in adolescents with AUD. However, a small (n = 12) 8-week open-label pilot study of ondansetron in alcohol-dependent adolescents receiving weekly individual motivational interviewing (MI) with cognitive–behavioral therapy reported that ondansetron to be relatively well-tolerated, with mild transient side effects of fatigue, nausea, and reduced appetite reported. Given the open-label design and lack of a comparison group, it is unclear to whether ondansetron contributed to the reported reduction in drinks per day (−1.7) beyond the effects MI with cognitive–behavioral therapy/psychosocial treatment alone.

Topiramate

Topiramate is an nonbenzodiazepine anticonvulsant that is FDA approved for the treatment of seizure disorders and migraines in both children and adults. Its mechanisms of action includes blocking voltage-dependent sodium channels and L-type calcium channels, inhibiting carbonic anhydrase, and increasing GABAergic transmission via direct action on α-amino-3-hydroxy-5-methyl-4-isoxazoleproprionic acid/kainite receptors and GABA$_A$ receptors.[56,57] Topiramate has been shown to be efficacious for reducing heavy drinking and relapse to alcohol for AUD in adults in a number of

RCTs and prospective longitudinal studies as described in a recent systematic review.[40]

Monti and colleagues[58] (2010) recently presented preliminary findings from a small, 5-week, randomized double-blind placebo-controlled pilot study comparing topiramate (escalating dose up to 200 mg/d) versus placebo for non–treatment-seeking adolescent and young adult heavy drinkers (ages 14–24). Topiramate was well-tolerated with no serious adverse events and few side effects. Over 5 weeks, the topiramate group reported an average reduction of –1.8 drinks per week (range, 3.8–2.0) compared with the placebo group, whose drinking did not decrease from baseline levels.

Summary of evidence for alcohol use disorders

Taken together, these preliminary studies suggest that naltrexone, disulfiram, ondansetron, and topiramate may be relatively safe and well-tolerated medications that show some promise as adjunctive treatment for adolescents with AUDs. Larger RCTs are warranted.

PHARMACOTHERAPY FOR TOBACCO USE DISORDERS

Tobacco use continues to be the number one preventable cause of death in the United States and internationally, and more than 90% of adults with TUDs report first smoking before 18 years of age.[59] In adults with TUDs, metaanalyses show that the combination of psychopharmacology and evidence-based psychosocial interventions is more effective for smoking cessation than either medication or psychosocial intervention alone.[24] Consensus guidelines recommend that practitioners encourage all adult patients attempting to quit to use effective medications except when contraindicated.[24] Seven medications are FDA approved for the treatment of TUDs in adults:

1. Nicotine replacement therapy (NRT) in 5 different formulations
   a. Nicotine patch,
   b. Nicotine nasal spray,
   c. Nicotine inhaler,
   d. Nicotine lozenge, and
   e. Nicotine gum;
2. Bupropion sustained-release (SR); and
3. Varenicline.

Compared with adult tobacco use disorders pharmacotherapy trials, adolescent studies have reported more mixed findings to date.

Kim and colleagues[60] (2011) published a metaanalysis examining the safety and efficacy of pharmacotherapies for adolescent smokers (ages 12–20). Six RCTs conducted between 1991 and 2009 including 816 participants were included in the review. Pharmacotherapies were not associated with lower rates of smoking cessation compared with controls (relative risk, 1.38; 95% CI, 0.92–2.07; 6 RCTs). The authors concluded that the quality of the evidence was low, owing to the small sample size of most studies. A number of pharmacotherapy RCTs for adolescent smoking cessation have been published since 2009. To date, 8 RCTs have examined pharmacotherapies for adolescent TUDs and smoking cessation.

Nicotine Replacement Therapy

NRT is an agonist-based pharmacotherapy approach that is available over the counter, and is FDA approved for individuals ages 18 and older for smoking cessation. The use of NRT (monotherapy or combined) is associated with increased likelihood of successful tobacco cessation (ORs of 1.5–3.5) and abstinence rates (19%–37%) compared with placebo in adult smokers.[24] To date, 5 studies including a total of 728 subjects have examined NRT for the treatment of tobacco cessation in adolescents. Hanson and colleagues[61] conducted the first study of NRT in adolescent smokers (ages 13–19 years), a 10-week, randomized double-blind placebo-controlled study comparing nicotine patch and placebo, with both treatment groups receiving weekly CBT and contingency management (CM). They found no significant differences between the nicotine patch group and placebo group in end-of-treatment abstinence confirmed by carbon monoxide (CO) breathalyzer (28% vs 24%). This was followed by a 12-week randomized double-blind, double-dummy placebo-controlled study comparing nicotine patch, nicotine gum, and placebo conditions (placebo patch and placebo gum), added to group CBT, in 120 adolescents with TUDs.[62] Both NRT formulations (patch and gum) were well-tolerated, but nicotine gum compliance was poor. CO breathalyzer-confirmed abstinence for end of treatment and follow-up arms of the study were achieved by 21% of the nicotine patch group compared with 9% of the nicotine gum and 5% of placebo groups. The differences in abstinence observed between nicotine patch and placebo were statistically significant.

A recent study by Scherphof and colleagues[63,64] (2014), used a randomized double-blind, placebo-controlled design and followed adolescents for 6 to 9 weeks, to examine the efficacy of nicotine patch versus placebo in adolescent smokers. Although the nicotine patch was associated with increased abstinence compared with placebo at week 2 (32% vs 21%),[63] there were no differences in end of treatment abstinence (15% vs 13%) or in abstinence at the 6-month (8% vs 6%) or 12-month (4% vs 7%) posttreatment follow-up visits.[64] A secondary analysis examining a subgroup of highly compliant patch users showed increased end of treatment abstinence rates for nicotine patch versus placebo patch (22% vs 15%).[65]

The efficacy of nicotine nasal spray for adolescent tobacco use disorders was examined in a small, 10-week, open-label pilot study that included a nicotine nasal spray group (1 mg intranasal as needed) and a no nasal spray control group, with both groups receiving weekly counseling.[66] Nasal spray compliance was poor, and no significant group differences were observed between the nicotine nasal spray and no nasal spray groups in end of treatment CO breathalyzer-confirmed abstinence (0% vs 12%).

These findings collectively suggest that nicotine patch, but not nicotine gum or nasal spray, has short-term efficacy for tobacco cessation in adolescents, but that relapse after discontinuation of NRT remains elevated.

Bupropion

Bupropion SR is FDA approved in adults for the treatment of TUDs. Preclinical studies suggest that bupropion acts as an inhibitor of dopamine and norepinephrine reuptake and as a nicotinic acetylcholinergic receptor antagonist.[67] These mechanisms are thought to attenuate withdrawal symptoms (dopaminergic and noradrenergic neurotransmission) and the reinforcing effects of nicotine (nicotinic antagonism), thereby reducing the likelihood of relapse.

Four RCTs, including a total of 688 subjects, have examined bupropion for the treatment of adolescent smoking cessation published to date. Killen and colleagues[68] completed the first study, an 8-week double-blind placebo-controlled RCT comparing bupropion SR and placebo, added on to nicotine patch treatment in 211 adolescent daily smokers (ages 15–18 years). All youth also received weekly group skills training. No differences in abstinence were found between treatment groups at end of treatment or 6-month posttreatment follow-up visit. CO breathalyzer-confirmed end of treatment abstinence was 23% in the bupropion SR + nicotine patch group, and 28% in the placebo + nicotine patch group. At the 6-month posttreatment follow-up, 8% versus 7% were abstinent. Although bupropion did not improve abstinence rates, potential efficacy may have been masked by the NRT that both treatment groups received. A second randomized double-blind placebo-controlled study compared 2 doses of bupropion SR (300 and 150 mg) versus placebo, added to weekly individual counseling, for 312 adolescents with TUDs (ages 14–17 years), over a 6-week treatment interval.[69] They found urine cotinine-confirmed end of treatment abstinence was 14% for the bupropion 300 mg/d treatment group, 11% for the bupropion 150 mg/d treatment group, and 6% for the placebo group. At the 6-month posttreatment follow-up, CO breathalyzer-confirmed abstinence rates were 14% versus 3% versus 10%, respectively, for the bupropion 300 mg/d, bupropion 150 mg/d, and placebo groups. Bupropion 300 mg/d was statistically superior to placebo at end of treatment (OR, 2.6; P = .02) and statistically superior to bupropion 150 mg/d at 6-month follow-up (OR, 1.5; P = .05). Secondary analyses of predictors of outcome demonstrated that medication compliance, noted to be highest in the bupropion 300 mg/d group, was associated with elevated CO breathalyzer-confirmed abstinence rates (21% vs 0% abstinence in high vs low compliance group).[70] Gray and colleagues[71] (2011) recently completed a 6-week double-blind placebo-controlled RCT examining if abstinence-incentivized CM would increase the efficacy of bupropion SR 300 mg. One hundred thirty-six adolescents (ages 12–21 years) were randomized into 4 different treatment arms: bupropion 300 mg + CM, placebo + CM, bupropion 300 mg + no CM, and placebo + no CM for 6 weeks of treatment. All groups received weekly brief individual counseling and medication management. Urine cotinine-confirmed end of treatment abstinence was superior in the combined bupropion + CM group (27%) compared with bupropion + no CM (8%), placebo + CM (10%), and placebo + no CM (9%) groups. Abstinence rates were 11%, 6%, 0%, and 6% respectively, at the 6-week posttreatment follow-up, with no statistically significant between-group differences observed.

In sum, bupropion SR at the 300 mg/d dosing may improve tobacco abstinence in adolescents with TUDs, especially when combined with psychosocial interventions and CM.

Varenicline

Varenicline is an α4β2 nicotinic receptor partial agonist that is FDA approved for tobacco cessation in adults. It is thought to aid in cessation by modulating dopaminergic neurotransmission to counteract nicotine withdrawal symptoms (nicotinic agonism) while at the same time reducing smoking satisfaction (nicotinic antagonism).[72]

To date, 2 published studies have examined varenicline for the treatment of adolescent TUDs. An open-label pharmacokinetic dose-finding pilot study demonstrated tolerability and safety at standard adult dosing (2 mg/d).[73] This was followed by a recent 8-week RCT comparing varenicline with bupropion for adolescent smoking cessation.[74] Gray and colleagues randomized 29 adolescent smokers to receive varenicline (2 mg/d) or extended-release bupropion (bupropion XL, 300 mg/d), added to brief weekly individual counseling and medication management. CO breathalyzer-confirmed end of treatment abstinence was 27% for the varenicline group and 14% for the bupropion XL group, with reductions in cigarettes per day in both treatment groups. Although there were no statistically significant between-group differences on any of the outcome measures, given the sample size the study was underpowered.

Currently, 2 large-scale randomized double-blinded placebo-controlled studies of varenicline for adolescent smoking cession are underway.

Postmarketing surveillance reports of suicidality and psychiatric adverse events led the FDA to add warning labels to both varenicline and bupropion SR. Large-scale controlled trials and naturalistic studies have not confirmed the association between varenicline and bupropion SR with serious psychiatric adverse events.[75] In light of the FDA warning labels, practitioners should be cautious, ask about cooccurring psychiatric disorders, and monitor for changes in psychiatric symptoms and suicidality, especially when prescribing for adolescents.

Summary of Evidence for Tobacco Use Disorders

Growing evidence exists for improved adolescent tobacco cessation rates during active treatment when psychosocial interventions are combined with nicotine patch and bupropion SR. Still, the impact of these pharmacotherapy approaches on long-term abstinence remains unclear, and real-world effectiveness studies are needed. Although initial data are promising for varenicline, results need to be replicated. Practitioners may consider trials of nicotine patch or bupropion SR in adolescent smokers who fail to response to psychosocial treatments.

PHARMACOTHERAPY FOR CANNABIS USE DISORDERS

Cannabis remains the most commonly used illicit drug in the United States,[3] and is the most common drug for which adolescents present for SUD treatment.[13] No FDA-approved medications exist for cannabis use disorders (CUDs). Cannabis use modulates glutamatergic[76] and GABAergic[77,78] activity, and drugs that target these systems represent promising CUD pharmacotherapies. Although a number of potential pharmacotherapies for CUDs have been examined, N-acetylcysteine (NAC; a glutamatergic modulator)[79,80] and gabapentin (a GABAergic modulator)[81] are the only medications with positive findings. Three studies examining adolescent CUD pharmacotherapies have been published to date, including one open-label pilot study and 2 controlled pharmacotherapy trials, which enrolled a combined total of 200 subjects.

N-Acetylcysteine

NAC is a cysteine prodrug that modulates intracellular and extracellular glutamate by way of the cysteine-glutamate exchanger.[82] Preclinical studies suggest that it may normalized frontostriatal function and prevent relapse to chronic drug use.[83] It is safe and well-tolerated in humans, and has been studied in a number of neuropsychiatric disorders.[84]

Gray and colleagues[79] initially completed a 4-week open-label pilot study of NAC (1200 mg twice daily) in 24 cannabis-dependent young adults (ages 18–21 years) finding that it was safe and well-tolerated, and associated with a significant reduction in self-reported cannabis use and cannabis-related cravings. This pilot study was then followed by a large (n = 116) 8-week randomized double-blind placebo-controlled trial.[80] Adolescents (ages 15–21 years) meeting DSM-IV-TR criteria for cannabis dependence were randomized to receive NAC (1200 mg twice daily) or placebo, added to brief weekly counseling. All participants also received a CM intervention. NAC, compared with placebo, was associated with superior treatment outcomes and significant reductions in cannabis. Odds of a negative urine cannabinoid test during study visits was 41% for participants in the NAC + CM group and 27% for participants in the placebo + CM group (OR, 2.4; $P = .03$). Urine cannabinoid-confirmed end of treatment abstinence from cannabis was 36% in the NAC group and 21% in the placebo group (OR, 2.3; P = .05).

The National Institute on Drug Abuse Clinical Trials Network is currently completing a 12-week, multisite, randomized double-blind placebo-controlled trial for CUD in adults.[85] If the findings for this adult CUD study are positive, this will provide further support for NAC pharmacotherapy for CUDs. The preliminary adolescent findings suggest that NAC may enhance cannabis cessation outcomes when combined with psychosocial interventions and CM.

Topiramate

A recent randomized double-blind placebo-controlled pilot study examined the potential efficacy of topiramate plus MI for treatment of adolescent heavy cannabis users (ages 15–24 years).[86] Sixty-six participants were randomized to receive either topiramate (titrated over 4 weeks to 200 mg/d and stabilized at 200 mg/d for 2 weeks) or placebo, added to 3 MI sessions, over a 6-week treatment interval. Topiramate was poorly tolerated in the study. Only 48% (19 participants) randomized to topiramate completed the 6-week study, compared with 77% (20 participants) randomized to placebo. Adverse medication side effects were the most commonly reported reason for treatment dropout. The topiramate + MI group, compared with the placebo + MI group, was significantly more likely to report depression, anxiety, difficulty with coordination or balance, weight loss, and paresthesia. Latent growth models showed that topiramate + MI compared with placebo + MI, was associated with a reduction in the number of grams of cannabis smoked per day, but was not associated with abstinence, days of cannabis use, or urine cannabis testing. In light of the poor tolerability and inconsistent effect on cannabis use outcome measures, topiramate likely does not have a role in the treatment of adolescent CUDs.

Summary of Evidence for Cannabis Use Disorders

Early stage evidence for CUD pharmacotherapy is promising. Preliminary data from an open-label pilot study and a large RCT suggest that NAC may reduce cannabis use in adolescents with CUDs. Results of the National Institute on Drug Abuse Clinical Trials Network study should guide future clinical practice guidelines for this medication.

PHARMACOTHERAPY FOR OPIOID USE DISORDERS

Over the past decade, opioid use has increased significantly among adolescents and young adults owing to a large increase in prescription opioid misuse.[3,87] Because OUDs among adolescents are associated with increased morbidity and mortality in comparison with other adolescent SUDs,[88] identifying and treating these youth is of vast importance.

Pharmacotherapy in OUDs is used for acute detoxification of the opioid withdrawal syndrome (OWS) and for maintenance OUD treatment. Consensus guidelines for treatment of adult OUDs recommend detoxification for OWS, followed by OUD maintenance pharmacotherapy plus psychosocial interventions.[89,90] Buprenorphine, methadone, and alpha-2-agonists, such as clonidine, are commonly used to treat OWS in adults.[91] OUD maintenance pharmacotherapy can be categorized as agonist-based versus antagonist-based treatments. OUD maintenance therapy in adults is associated with reductions in opiate use, human immunodeficiency virus risk behaviors, opioid withdrawal syndrome, opioid overdoses, and associated morbidity and mortality.[25,26,89–91] The FDA has approved 5 medications for the maintenance treatment of OUDs in adults:

1. Methadone,
2. Buprenorphine,
3. Buprenorphine–naloxone,
4. Naltrexone (oral), and
5. XR-naltrexone.

Although there have been a number of open-label and observational treatment studies in adolescents with OUDs, few controlled studies exist. Only 2 RCTs have been published to date.

Pharmacotherapy for Opioid Withdrawal Syndrome

Clonidine and buprenorphine

A small (n = 36) randomized double-blind double-dummy parallel-group study compared buprenorphine versus clonidine for treatment of OWS in adolescents with DSM-IV opioid dependence during a 28-day outpatient detoxification.[92] All participants received behavioral counseling 3 times weekly and opioid negative urine incentivized CM. Outcomes included treatment retention, opiate abstinence, human immunodeficiency virus risk behaviors, and opioid withdrawal. Buprenorphine was superior to clonidine across a number of treatment outcomes. Seventy-two percent of participants in the buprenorphine group were retained in treatment compared with 39% of participants in the clonidine group. The buprenorphine participants, compared with the clonidine participants, had a significantly higher percentage of opiate-negative urine screens (64% vs 32%) and significant reductions in human immunodeficiency virus risk behaviors. There were no differences in opioid withdrawal between the groups. At the end of detoxification, 61% of the buprenorphine group compared with 5% of the clonidine group initiated naltrexone maintenance therapy. Buprenorphine's efficacy for treatment of OWS in adolescents with opiate dependence was confirmed as a secondary outcome by another RCT comparing extended- and short-term treatment.[93]

Minozzi and colleagues[94] (2014) recently published a Cochrane Systematic Review of detoxification treatments for adolescent OUDs, but was unable to draw conclusions across studies, because only 1 controlled study for adolescent OWS has been published. Current evidence suggests that buprenorphine, rather than clonidine, should be used for OWS treatment in adolescents with OUDs.

Pharmacotherapy for Maintenance Treatment of Opioid Use Disorders

A recent Cochrane Systematic Review of maintenance treatments for opiate-dependent adolescents was completed in 2014 analyzing data from 2 RCTs, including 189 participants.[95] Like the opioid detoxification review,[94] the authors could not draw conclusions, because differences in study design and outcome precluded the ability to metaanalyze the data. Evidence from observational studies and a single RCT suggests that agonist therapies, including methadone and buprenorphine, may be effective during active treatment. Still, agonist-based therapy is controversial in adolescents owing to concerns over the impact of chronic opioid agonism on brain and endocrine system development, and the effects of inducing a prolonged state of physical dependence in youth.[96]

Methadone

To date, no controlled studies have examined methadone maintenance therapy (MMT) for the treatment of adolescent OUD. Hopfer and colleagues[97] completed a systematic review of the treatment and descriptive literature for adolescent heroin use, and found 9 treatment studies including a total of 6263 adolescents and young adults with heroin use. Most of the studies were completed in the 1970s and used naturalistic or observational designs. Few compared across different treatments. A large observational study by Sells and Simpson[98] (1979) compared MMT, detoxification, therapeutic community, and abstinence-based treatments for 5407 adolescents (age ≤19) across multiple US drug abuse treatment programs. They found that daily opiate using adolescents were more likely to require MMT, and that MMT was associated with higher treatment retention rates.

Methadone for OUD maintenance therapy can only be prescribed in licensed and regulated specialty clinics. Adolescents, even those under the age of 16 years, can be treated with MMT, but the Department of Health and Human Services regulations require documentation of 2 treatment failures of drug-free detoxification followed by psychosocial interventions before they may be referred.

Buprenorphine

Buprenorphine is a μ-opioid receptor partial agonist that is FDA approved for the treatment of individuals, ages 16 years and older, with an OUD. As an FDA schedule III medication, it can be prescribed by trained licensed physicians in outpatient clinical settings.

The National Institute on Drug Abuse Clinical Trials Network recently completed a large (n = 152) multisite RCT in adolescents meeting DSM-IV criteria for opioid dependence comparing 2-week short-term buprenorphine–naloxone detoxification versus 12-week extended pharmacotherapy with buprenorphine–naloxone.[93] All participants received behavioral counseling, and the outcome measures were percentage of opioid-positive urine tests at weeks 4, 8, and 12. Although adolescents randomized to extended-treatment buprenorphine–naloxone had significantly fewer opioid positive urine tests at weeks 4 (26% vs 61%) and 8 (23% vs 54%), by week 12, after the buprenorphine–naloxone had been tapered and discontinued, there were no between-group differences in opioid-negative urine tests (43% vs 51%). Rates of opioid relapse were high in both groups. By 12 months posttreatment, 53% of participants randomized to buprenorphine–naloxone extended treatment and 72% participants randomized to detoxification had relapsed. An analysis of predictors of treatment response observed lower end of treatment opioid use for adolescents with higher opioid use severity, psychiatric comorbidity, and those with opioid withdrawal syndrome.[99] Results suggest that combined maintenance pharmacotherapy with buprenorphine–naloxone and counseling is more effective than detoxification followed by behavioral counseling, but that after the buprenorphine–naloxone is discontinued, opioid-dependent youth quickly relapse and there are no differences in 12-month outcomes. Thus, maintenance or long-term treatment with buprenorphine–naloxone may be necessary to sustain treatment gains. This result would be consistent with findings from adult studies, where maintenance as compared with short-term treatment is associated with improved outcomes.[90,91] Because higher risk youth had better treatment outcomes, pharmacotherapy with buprenorphine–naloxone may be appropriate for this subgroup of adolescents with OUDs. Future controlled studies should examine pharmacotherapy with buprenorphine–naloxone in this subgroup.

Naltrexone

Naltrexone is an effective FDA-approved OUD maintenance pharmacotherapy for adults. To date, a single open-label prospective case series has examined XR-naltrexone for the treatment of adolescent and young adult OUD.[100] Sixteen youth meeting DSM-IV criteria for OUD were admitted to inpatient detoxification at a community substance use treatment center and started on XR-naltrexone (380 mg intramuscular injection once per month). Clinical data from chart review on opioid use, side effects, and tolerability were examined. XR-naltrexone was well-tolerated and associated with clinical improvements. There are currently 2 controlled studies examining XR-naltrexone for the treatment of adolescents (ages 15–21 years) with OUDs that are underway.

Pharmacotherapy for Opiate Overdose

Rates of opioid overdose deaths have increased dramatically in the past decade.[101] Although the majority of opioid overdose deaths occur in individuals aged 25 to 54, many opioid users started using before 18 years of age and adolescents with OUDs are at increased risk for overdose-related deaths.[88]

Intranasal naloxone

Naloxone is an opioid antagonist rescue agent used to treat opioid overdose. The World Health Organization strongly recommends that people likely to witness an opioid overdose (ie, family and friends) should have access to naloxone and be trained to administer it for emergency management of suspected opioid overdose, as manifested by respiratory or central nervous system depression.[102] In November 2015, the FDA approved intranasal naloxone for opioid overdose.[103] Practitioners who treat adolescents with OUDs should strongly consider prescribing intranasal naloxone, and provide education and training about the signs and symptoms of opioid intoxication and what to do in the event of a suspected overdose.[104]

Summary of evidence for Opioid Use Disorders

The current standard of treatment for adolescent OUD remains medically assisted detoxification followed by behavioral counseling. Results from the current literature suggest that buprenorphine is more effective than clonidine for treatment of OWS and may be associated with improvements in treatment retention. With regard to OUD maintenance treatment, there may be a role for outpatient-based pharmacotherapy approaches including buprenorphine–naloxone combined with counseling for adolescents, ages 16 years and older, with more severe opioid addiction, intravenous drug use, comorbid psychiatric disorders, and those who fail detoxification plus behavioral counseling. MMT is also an option for youth if they have more than 2 documented treatment failures after detoxification and behavioral counseling. Additional studies are need to clarify the efficacy naltrexone in adolescent samples.

SUMMARY

Adolescent SUDs remain a major public health burden, and clinical strategies that enhance treatment response are necessary to improve long-term outcomes. Combining pharmacotherapies with evidence-based psychosocial interventions may be an effective enhancement strategy. Over the past decade, an increasing number of studies have begun to examine pharmacotherapies for adolescent SUDs. To date, the results of these studies have been promising, but the quality of the evidence is poor. Most studies are not adequately powered, did not include posttreatment follow-up, and some lacked biochemically verified outcomes. Medication compliance varied across studies but was, in general, associated with better outcomes.[65,70] Use of adequately powered, controlled study designs with randomization, allocation concealment, proper blinding, intention-to-treat analyses, biochemically verified endpoints, and adequate follow-up are necessary to improve the quality of the evidence base for adolescent SUD pharmacotherapy. Additional research is needed to clarify appropriate treatment settings, target symptoms, and patient-level predictors of outcomes for pharmacotherapies with preliminary positive findings.

Early evidence for the short-term efficacy of adding pharmacotherapies to psychosocial interventions is encouraging. Psychotropic medications across a broad range of classes, mechanisms of action, and side effect profiles seem to be safe and well-tolerated among adolescents with SUDs. These studies indicate that, like in adults, combining pharmacotherapy and behavioral interventions may synergistically reduce substance use.[71] Consistent with adult SUD studies, preliminary evidence indicates that medications may improve substance-specific outcomes when used adjunctively with psychosocial interventions in adolescents with TUDs (nicotine patch; bupropion SR), OUDs (buprenorphine–naloxone), and to a lesser extent, CUDs (NAC).

Practitioners providing SUD treatment to adolescents who do not respond adequately to psychosocial interventions may consider a medication trial using the described pharmacotherapies to enhance treatment response and reduce risk of relapse (**Box 1**). To date buprenorphine is the only pharmacotherapy to date with an FDA-approved indication for the treatment of adolescent SUDs. As such, the use of other medications described in this article, although evidence based, would be

---

Box 1
Rationale for adolescent SUD pharmacotherapy and clinical considerations

When to consider pharmacotherapy for SUDs in adolescents

- Moderate to severe SUD
- Comorbid/cooccurring psychiatric disorders[a]
- Youth has failed psychosocial interventions (eg, ≥2 prior detoxification attempts for adolescent OUDs to consider methadone)
- Youth is engaged in psychosocial interventions but is not improving (no change in drug use, no functional improvement)
- High risk for morbidity and mortality (intravenous drug use, drunk or drugged driving, unprotected sexual intercourse, accidents)
- Family or parents/guardians are engaged in treatment planning and willing to monitor medication

What factors should be considered in choosing a medication

- Patient's past experience with SUD maintenance medications
- Patient and family's opinions and beliefs
- Family and parent/guardian involvement in treatment plan (for monitoring)
- Level of motivation for abstinence
- Health status (medical and psychiatric history, and allergies)
- Contraindications for medications
- Safety profile of medication and drug-to-drug interactions between medication and drugs of abuse
- History of medication compliance

Abbreviations: OUD, opiate use disorder; SUD, substance use disorder.
[a] For patients with comorbid substance use and psychiatric disorders, pharmacotherapy should be initially directed at treating the co-occurring psychiatric symptoms and disorders (See Robinson Z, Riggs PD: Co-occurring Psychiatric and Substance Use Disorders, in this issue).

considered "off-label" use. Concerns about potential short- and long-term medication side effects should be weighed against the risk of continued drug use and related morbidity and mortality. Medications should only be prescribed in the context of appropriate psychosocial interventions and regularly monitored for safety and emergent adverse side effects. Developing a monitoring plan with families, and providing incentives for medication compliance (ie, CM), is recommended, because compliance may improve outcomes.[71,105,106]

REFERENCES

1. Uhl GR, Grow RW. The burden of complex genetic brain disorders. Arch Gen Psychiatry 2004;61:223–9.
2. Healthday. Addiction starts early in American Society. US News World Rep 2011. Available at: http://consumer.healthday.com/mental-health-information-25/addiction-news-6/addiction-starts-early-in-american-society-report-finds-654 435.html. Accessed March 1, 2016.
3. Eaton LK, Kann I, Kinchen S. Youth risk behavior surveillance—United States: 2007, surveillance summaries. MMWR Surveill Summ 2008;57(SS04):1–131.
4. Tarter RE, Vanyukov M. Alcoholism: a developmental disorder. J Consult Clin Psychol 1994;62(6):1096–107.
5. Lopez-Quintero C, Perez de los Cobos J, Hasin DS, et al. Probability and predictors of transition from first use to dependence on nicotine, alcohol, cannabis, and cocaine: results of the National Epidemiologic Survey on Alcohol and Related Conditions (NESARC). Drug Alcohol Depend 2011;115(1–2):120–30.
6. Wagner FA, Anthony JC. From first drug use to drug dependence - developmental periods of risk for dependence upon marijuana, cocaine, and alcohol. Neuropharmacology 2002;26(4):479–88.
7. Centers for Disease Control and Prevention (CDC). Mental health surveillance among children - United States, 2005-2011. MMWR 2013;62(Suppl 2):1–17.
8. Arendt M, Munk-Jorgensen P, Sher L, et al. Mortality among individuals with cannabis, cocaine, amphetamine, MDMA, and opioid use disorders: a nationwide follow-up study of Danish substance users in treatment. Drug Alcohol Depend 2011;114(2–3):134–9.
9. Hall W, Solowij N. Adverse effects of cannabis. Lancet 1998;352(9140):1611–6.
10. Volkow ND, Baler RD, Compton WM, et al. Adverse health effects of marijuana use. N Engl J Med 2014;370(23):2219–27.
11. Lisdahl KM, Gilbart ER, Wright NE, et al. Dare to delay? The impacts of adolescent alcohol and marijuana use onset on cognition, brain structure, and function. Front Psychiatry 2013;4:53.
12. Substance Abuse and Mental Health Services Administration (SAMHSA). Results from the 2013 National survey on drug use and health: summary of national findings. Rockville (MD): Substance Abuse and Mental Health Services Administration (SAMHSA); 2014.
13. Substance Abuse and Mental Health Services Administration (SAMHSA). Treatment episode data set (TEDS): 2002-2012. National admissions to substance abuse treatment services. Rockville (MD): Substance Abuse and Mental Health Services Administration (SAMHSA); 2014.
14. Waldron HB, Turner CW. Evidence-based psychosocial treatments for adolescent substance abuse. J Clin Child Adolesc Psychol 2008;37(1):238–61.
15. Winters KC, Tanner-Smith EE, Bresani E, et al. Current advances in the treatment of adolescent drug use. Adolesc Health Med Ther 2014;5:199–210.

16. Stanger C, Budney AJ. Contingency management approaches for adolescent substance use disorders. Child Adolesc Psychiatr Clin N Am 2010;19(3): 547–62.
17. Stanger C, Ryan SR, Scherer EA, et al. Clinic- and home-based contingency management plus parent training for adolescent cannabis use disorders. J Am Acad Child Adolesc Psychiatry 2015;54(6):445–53.e2.
18. Dennis M, Godley SH, Diamond G, et al. The Cannabis Youth Treatment (CYT) Study: main findings from two randomized trials. J Subst Abuse Treat 2004; 27(3):197–213.
19. Cornelius JR, Maisto SA, Pollock NK, et al. Rapid relapse generally follows treatment for substance use disorders among adolescents. Addict Behav 2003;28: 381–6.
20. Brown PC, Budney AJ, Thostenson JD, et al. Initiation of abstinence in adolescents treated for marijuana use disorders. J Subst Abuse Treat 2013;44(4): 384–90.
21. Mann C, Frieden T, Hyde PS, et al. Medication assisted treatment for substance use disorders. Center for Medicaid and CHIP services information bulletin. 2014. Available at: www.medicaid.gov/federal-policy-guidance/downloads/cib-07-11-2014.pdf. Accessed January 15, 2016.
22. Volkow ND, Frieden T, Hyde PS, et al. Medication-assisted therapies - tackling the opioid-overdose epidemic. N Engl J Med 2014;370(22):2063–6.
23. Center for Substance Abuse Treatment. Incorporating alcohol pharmacotherapies into medical practice. Vol HHS Publ No. (SMA) 09–4380. Rockville (MD): Substance Abuse and Mental Health Services Administration; 2009.
24. Fiore MC, Jaen CR. Tobacco Use and Dependence Guideline Panel. Treating tobacco use and dependence: 2008 update. Rockville, MD: US Department of Health and Human Services; 2008. p. 106–30.
25. Thomas CP, Fullerton CA, Kim M, et al. Medication-assisted treatment with buprenorphine: assessing the evidence. Psychiatr Serv 2014;65(2):158–70.
26. Fullerton CA, Kim M, Thomas CP, et al. Medication-assisted treatment with methadone: assessing the evidence. Psychiatr Serv 2014;65(2):146–57.
27. Holder HD. Costs benefits of substance abuse treatment: an overview of results from alcohol and drug abuse. J Ment Health Policy Econ 1998;1(1):23–9.
28. Jones HE, Kaltenbach K, Heil SH. Neonatal abstinence syndrome after methadone or buprenorpine exposure. N Engl J Med 2010;363:2320–31.
29. Baser O, Chalk M, Rawson R, et al. Alcohol dependence treatments: comprehensive healthcare costs, utilization outcomes, and pharmacotherapy persistence. Am J Manag Care 2011;17:222–34.
30. Deas D, Riggs PR, Langenbucher J, et al. Adolescents are not adults: developmental considerations in alcohol users. Alcohol Clin Exp Res 2000;24(2):232–7.
31. Hammond CJ, Mayes LC, Potenza MN. Neurobiology of adolescent substance use and addictive behaviors: prevention and treatment implications. Adolesc Med State Art Rev 2014;25(1):15–32.
32. Fernandez E, Perez R, Hernandez A, et al. Factors and mechanisms for pharmacokinetic differences between pediatric population and adults. Pharmaceutics 2011;3(1):53–72.
33. Vitiello B. Developmental aspects of pediatric psychopharmacology. In: Findling RL, editor. Clinical manual of child & adolescent psychopharmacology. Arlington (VA): American Psychiatric Association; 2008. p. 1–31.
34. van den Anker JN, Schwab M, Kearns GL. Developmental pharmacokinetics. Handb Exp Pharmacol 2011;205:51–75.

35. Paus T, Keshavan M, Giedd JN. Why do so many psychiatric disorders emerge during adolescence? Nat Neurosci 2008;9:947–57.
36. Shaw P, Kabani NJ, Lerch JP, et al. Neurodevelopmental trajectories of the human cerebral cortex. J Neurosci 2008;28(14):3586–94.
37. Vitiello B. Pediatric psychopharmacology and the interaction between drugs and the developing brain. Can J Psychiatry 1998;43(6):582–4.
38. Spear LP. Adolescent alcohol exposure: are there separable vulnerable periods within adolescence? Physiol Behav 2015;148:122–30.
39. Cui C, Noronha A, Morikawa H, et al. New insights on neurobiological mechanisms underlying alcohol addiction. Neuropharmacology 2013;67:223–32.
40. Hammond CJ, Niciu MJ, Drew S, et al. Anticonvulsants for the treatment of alcohol withdrawal syndrome and alcohol use disorders. CNS Drugs 2015; 29(4):293–311.
41. Clark DB. Pharmacotherapy for adolescent alcohol use disorders. CNS Drugs 2012;26(7):559–69.
42. Martin CS, Kaczynski NA, Maisto SA, et al. Patterns of DSM-IV alcohol abuse and dependence symptoms in adolescent drinkers. J Stud Alcohol 1998;56: 672–80.
43. Mayo-Smith MF. Pharmacological management of alcohol withdrawal: a meta-analysis and evidence based practice guideline. American Society of Addiction Medicine Working Group on Pharmacological Management of Alcohol Withdrawal. JAMA 1997;287(2):144–51.
44. The National Clinical Guideline Centre for acute and Chronic Conditions. Alcohol use disorders: diagnosis and clinical management of alcohol-related physical complications. Clinical guideline 100. London (United Kingdom): National Clinical Guidelines Centre at the Royal College of Physicians; 2010.
45. Bouza C, Angeles M, Munoz A, et al. Efficacy and safety of naltrexone and acamprosate in the treatment of alcohol dependence: a systematic review. Addiction 2004;99(7):811–28.
46. Roozen HG, de Waart R, van der Windt DA, et al. A systematic review of the effectiveness of naltrexone in the maintenance treatment of opioid and alcohol dependence. Eur Neuropsychopharmacol 2006;16(5):311–23.
47. Monti PM, Rohsenow DJ, Hutchinson KE, et al. Naltrexone's effect on cue-elicited craving among alcoholics in treatment. Alcohol Clin Exp Res 1999; 23(8):1386–94.
48. Deas D, May K, Randall CL, et al. Naltrexone treatment of adolescent alcoholics: an open-label pilot study. J Child Adolesc Psychopharmacol 2005;15(5):723–8.
49. Miranda R, Ray L, Blanchard A, et al. Effects of naltrexone on adolescent alcohol cue reactivity and sensitivity: an initial randomized trial. Addict Biol 2014;19(5):941–54.
50. Schroeder JP, Cooper DA, Schank JR, et al. Disulfiram attenuates drug-primed reinstatement of cocaine seeking via inhibition of dopamine beta-hydroxylase. Neuropsychopharmacology 2010;35(12):2440–9.
51. Niederhofer H, Staffen W. Comparison of disulfiram and placebo in treatment of alcohol dependence of adolescents. Drug Alcohol Rev 2003;22(3):295–7.
52. Kranzler HR, Pierucci-Lagha A, Feinn R, et al. Effects of ondansetron in early- versus late-onset alcoholics: a prospective, open-label study. Alcohol Clin Exp Res 2003;27(7):1150–5.
53. Johnson BA, Roache JD, Javors MA. Ondansetron for reduction of drinking among biologically predisposed alcohol patients: a randomized controlled trial. JAMA 2000;284(8):963–71.

54. Johnson BA, Roache JD, Ait-Daoud N, et al. Ondansetron reduces the craving of biologically predisposed alcoholics. Psychopharmacology (Berl) 2002; 160(4):408–13.

55. Johnson BA, Ait-Daoud N, Seneviratne C, et al. Pharmacogenetic approach at the serotonin transporter gene as a method of reducing the severity of alcohol drinking. Am J Psychiatry 2011;168(3):265–75.

56. White HS. Mechanism of action of newer anticonvulsants. J Clin Psychiatry 2004;64(Suppl 8):5–8.

57. Perucca E. Clinical pharmacology and therapeutic use of the new antiepileptic drugs. Fundam Clin Pharmacol 2001;15:405–17.

58. Monti PM, Miranda R, Justus A, et al. Biobehavioral mechanisms of topiramate and drinking in adolescents: preliminary findings. Neuropharmacology 2010;35: S164.

59. Backinger CL, Fagan P, Matthews E, et al. Adolescent and young adult tobacco prevention and cessation: current status and future directions. Tob Control 2003; 12(Suppl IV):iv46–53.

60. Kim Y, Myung SK, Jeon YJ, et al. Effectiveness of pharmacologic therapy for smoking cessation in adolescent smokers: meta-analysis of randomized controlled trials. Am J Health Syst Pharm 2011;68(3):219–26.

61. Hanson K, Allen S, Jensen S, et al. Treatment of adolescent smokers with the nicotine patch. Nicotine Tob Res 2003;5(4):514–26.

62. Moolchan ET, Robinson ML, Ernst M, et al. Safety and efficacy of the nicotine patch and gum for the treatment of adolescent tobacco addiction. Pediatrics 2005;115(4):e407–414.

63. Scherphof CS, van den Eijnden RJ, Engels RC, et al. Short-term efficacy of nicotine replacement therapy for smoking cessation in adolescents: a randomized controlled trial. J Subst Abuse Treat 2014;46(2):120–7.

64. Scherphof CS, van den Eijnden RJ, Engels RC, et al. Long-term efficacy of nicotine replacement therapy for smoking cessation in adolescents: a randomized controlled trial. Drug Alcohol Depend 2014;140:217–20.

65. Scherphof CS, van den Eijnden RJ, Lugtig P, et al. Adolescents' use of nicotine replacement therapy for smoking cessation: predictors of compliance trajectories. Psychopharmacology (Berl) 2014;231(8):1743–52.

66. Rubinstein ML, Benowitz NL, Auerback GM, et al. A randomized trial of nicotine nasal spray in adolescent smokers. Pediatrics 2008;122(3):e595–600.

67. Warner C, Shoaib M. How does bupropion work as a smoking cessation aid? Addict Biol 2005;10(3):219–31.

68. Killen JD, Robinson TN, Ammerman S, et al. Randomized clinical trial of the efficacy of bupropion combined with nicotine patch in the treatment of adolescent smokers. J Consult Clin Psychol 2004;72(4):729–35.

69. Muramoto ML, Leischow SJ, Sherill D, et al. Randomized double-blind, placebo controlled trial of 2 dosages of sustained-release bupropion for adolescent smoking cessation. Arch Pediatr Adolesc Med 2007;161:1068–74.

70. Leischow SJ, Muramoto ML, Matthews E, et al. Adolescent smoking cessation with bupropion: the role of adherence. Nicotine Tob Res 2016;18(5):1202–5.

71. Gray KM, Carpenter MJ, Baker NL, et al. Bupropion SR and contingency management for adolescent smoking cessation. J Subst Abuse Treat 2011;40(1): 77–86.

72. Cahill K, Stead LF, Lancaster T. Nicotine receptor partial agonists for smoking cessation. Cochrane Database Syst Rev 2012;(4):CD006103. 1–121.

73. Faessel HM, Obach RS, Rollema H, et al. A review of the clinical pharmacokinetics and pharmacodynamics of varenicline for smoking cessation. Clin Pharmacokinet 2010;49(12):799–816.

74. Gray KM, Carpenter MJ, Lewis AL, et al. Varenicline versus bupropion XL for smoking cessation in older adolescents: a randomized, double-blind pilot trial. Nicotine Tob Res 2012;14(2):234–9.

75. Thomas KH, Martin RM, Davies NM, et al. Smoking cessation treatment and risk of depression, suicide, and self harm in the Clinical Practice Research Datalink: prospective cohort study. BMJ 2013;347:f5704.

76. Suarez I, Bodega G, Fernandez-Ruiz J, et al. Down-regulation of the AMPA glutamate receptor subunits GLUR1 and GLUR2/3 in the rat cerebellum following pre- and perinatal delta-9-tetrahydrocanninol exposure. Cerebellum 2003;2:66–74.

77. Behan AT, Hryniewiecka M, O'Tuathaigh CM, et al. Chronic adolescent exposure to delta-9-tetrahydrocannabinol in COMT mutant mice: impact on indices of dopaminergic, endocannabinoid and GABAergic pathways. Neuropsychopharmacology 2012;37(7):1773–83.

78. Moreira FA, Jupp B, Belin D, et al. Endocannabinoids and striatal function: implications for addiction-related behaviours. Behav Pharmacol 2015;26(1–2): 59–72.

79. Gray KM, Watson NL, Carpenter MJ, et al. N-acetylcysteine (NAC) in young marijuana users: an open-label pilot study. Am J Addict 2010;19(2):187–9.

80. Gray KM, Carpenter MJ, Baker NL, et al. A double-blind randomized controlled trial of N-acetylcysteine in cannabis-dependent adolescents. Am J Psychiatry 2012;169(8):805–12.

81. Mason BJ, Crean R, Goodell V, et al. A proof-of-concept randomized controlled study of gabapentin: effects on cannabis use, withdrawal and executive function deficits in cannabis-dependent adults. Neuropsychopharmacology 2012; 37(7):1689–98.

82. Lewerenz J, Hewett SJ, Huang Y, et al. The cysteine/glutamate antiporter system x(c)(-) in health and disease: from molecular mechanisms to novel therapeutic opportunities. Antioxid Redox Signal 2013;18(5):522–55.

83. Baker DA, McFarland K, Lake RW, et al. Neuroadaptations in cystine-glutamate exchange underlie cocaine relapse. Nat Neurosci 2003;6(7):743–9.

84. Deepmala, Slattery J, Kumar N, et al. Clinical trials of N-acetylcysteine in psychiatry and neurology: a systematic review. Neurosci Biobehav Rev 2015;55: 294–321.

85. McClure EA, Sonne SC, Winhusen T, et al. Achieving cannabis cessation – evaluating N-acetylcysteine treatment (ACCENT): design and implementation of a multi-site, randomized controlled study in the National Institute on Drug Abuse Clinical Trials Network. Contemp Clin Trials 2014;39(2):211–23.

86. Miranda R Jr, Treloar H, Blanchard A, et al. Topiramate and motivational enhancement therapy for cannabis use among youth: a randomized placebo-controlled pilot study. Addiction Biology 2016. [Epub ahead of print].

87. Fiellin DA. Treatment of adolescent opioid dependence: no quick fix. JAMA 2008;300(17):2057–9.

88. Subramaniam GA, Stitzer ML, Woody G, et al. Clinical characteristics of treatment-seeking adolescents with opioid versus cannabis/alcohol use disorders. Drug Alcohol Depend 2009;99(1–3):141–9.

89. Mattick RP, Breen C, Kimber J, et al. Buprenorphine maintenance versus placebo or methadone maintenance for opioid dependence. Cochrane Database Syst Rev 2014;2:CD002207.

90. Mattick RP, Breen C, Kimber J, et al. Methadone maintenance therapy versus no opioid replacement therapy for opioid dependence. Cochrane Database Syst Rev 2009;(3):CD002209. 1–34.

91. Stotts AL, Dodrill CL, Kosten TR. Opioid dependence treatment: options in pharmacotherapy. Expert Opin Pharmacother 2009;10(11):1727–40.

92. Marsch L, Bickel WK, Badger GL, et al. Comparison of pharmacological treatments for opioid-dependent adolescents. Arch Gen Psychiatry 2005;62: 1157–64.

93. Woody G, Poole SA, Subramaniam G, et al. Extended vs short-term buprenorphine-naloxone for treatment of opioid-addicted youth. JAMA 2008;300(17): 2003–11.

94. Minozzi S, Amato L, Bellisario C, et al. Detoxification treatments for opiate dependent adolescents. Cochrane Database Syst Rev 2014;(4):CD006749. 1–36.

95. Minozzi S, Amato L, Bellisario C, et al. Maintenance treatments for opiate-dependent adolescents. Cochrane Database Syst Rev 2014;(6):CD007210. 1–34.

96. Lowinson JH, Marion IL, Joseph H, et al. Methadone maintenance. In: Lowinson JH, Ruiz P, Millman RB, editors. Substance abuse: a comprehensive textbook. 2nd edition. Baltimore (MD): Williams and Wilkins; 1992. p. 405–14.

97. Hopfer CJ, Khuri E, Crowley TJ. Treating adolescent heroin use. J Am Acad Child Adolesc Psychiatry 2003;42(5):609–11.

98. Sells SB, Simpson DD. Evaluation of treatment outcome for youths in the drug abuse reporting program (DARP): a followup study. In: Beschner GM, Friedman AS, editors. Youth drug abuse: problems, issues, and treatment. Lexington (MA): Lexington Books; 1979. p. 571–628.

99. Subramaniam G, Warden D, Minhajuddin A, et al. Predictors of abstinence: National Institute on Drug Abuse multisite buprenorphine/naloxone treatment trial in opioid-dependent youth. J Am Acad Child Adolesc Psychiatry 2011;50(11): 1120–8.

100. Fishman MJ, Winstanley EL, Curran E, et al. Treatment of opioid dependence in adolescents and young adults with extended release naltrexone: preliminary case-series and feasibility. Addiction 2010;105(9):1669–76.

101. Centers for Disease Control and Prevention. National vital statistics system mortality data. 2015. Available at: www.cdc.gov/nchs/deaths.htm.

102. World Health Organization (WHO). Community management of opioid overdose. Geneva (Switzerland): WHO Press; 2014.

103. US Food and Drug Administration (FDA). FDA moves quickly to approve easy-to-use nasal spray to treat opioid overdose 2015; FDA Informational Bulletin. Available at: www.fda.gov/NewsEvents/Newsroom/PressAnnouncements/ucm 473505.htm. Accessed January 15, 2016.

104. Substance Abuse and Mental Health Services Administration (SAMHSA). SAMHSA Opioid overdose prevention toolkit. Rockville (MD): Substance Abuse and Mental Health Services Administration (SAMHSA); 2014. Vol HHS Publ No. (SMA) 14-4742.

105. O'Farrell TJ, Bayog RD. Antabuse contracts for married alcoholics and their spouses: a method to maintain antabuse ingestion and decrease conflict about drinking. J Subst Abuse Treat 1986;3:1–8.

106. Ebell MH, Siwek J, Weiss BD, et al. Simplifying the language of evidence to improve patient care: strength of Recommendation taxonomy (SORT): a patient-centered approach to grading evidence in the medical literature. J Fam Pract 2010;53(2):111–20.

Cooccurring Psychiatric and Substance Use Disorders

Zachary D. Robinson, MD[a],*, Paula D. Riggs, MD[b]

KEYWORDS

- Adolescents • Treatment • Cooccurring disorders • Comorbidity
- Substance use disorders

KEY POINTS

- Psychiatric disorders commonly cooccur in adolescents with substance use disorders and are associated with poorer substance treatment outcomes.
- There is considerable consensus among clinicians and researchers that treatment of adolescents with cooccurring substance and nonsubstance psychiatric disorders should be integrated, but few receive it.
- National health care reforms are reducing longstanding systemic and economic barriers to progress toward more widespread integrated behavioral health services.
- A growing body of research is providing an empirical foundation from which evidence-based principles of integrated treatment can be derived.
- This research has informed the development of at least 1 evidence-based integrated treatment model.

INTRODUCTION

Research has shown that adolescence is a particularly vulnerable developmental period for the onset of mental illness and substance use disorders (SUDs).[1] Approximately one-half of all psychiatric disorders begin before age 15, and three-quarters by age 24. Most adults who suffer from chronic addiction report initiating substance use as adolescents.[2] This increased vulnerability is thought to be due, in part, to rapid brain development that occurs throughout adolescence into young adulthood.[1,3] A

Disclosure Statement/Conflicts of Interest: The authors have no conflicts to disclose.
[a] Child and Adolescent Psychiatry, Children's Hospital Colorado, University of Colorado Hospital, University of Colorado School of Medicine, 13001 East 17th Place, Campus Box F546, Building 500, Room E2322, Aurora, CO 80045, USA; [b] Division of Substance Dependence, Department of Psychiatry, University of Colorado School of Medicine, Building 400, Mail Stop F478, Aurora, CO 80045, USA
* Corresponding author.
E-mail address: zachary.robinson@ucdenver.edu

Child Adolesc Psychiatric Clin N Am 25 (2016) 713–722
http://dx.doi.org/10.1016/j.chc.2016.05.005
1056-4993/16/$ – see front matter © 2016 Elsevier Inc. All rights reserved.
childpsych.theclinics.com

Abbreviations	
ADHD	Attention deficit hyperactivity disorder
CBT	Cognitive–behavioral therapy
CDRS-R	Childhood Depression Rating Scale-Revised
CM	Contingency management
MDD	Major depressive disorder
MET	Motivational enhancement therapy
OROS- MPH	Safety Assessment of Potential Interactions Between IV Methamphetamine and Osmotic-Release Methylphenidate
SUD	Substance use disorder

number of childhood-onset psychiatric disorders have been shown to increase the risk of adolescent-onset SUD, including depression, anxiety, and disruptive behavior disorders.[4–9] Substance abuse during adolescence may also exacerbate preexisting mental health problems and increase the risk of developing new psychiatric disorders.[10] Longitudinal studies have shown that regular cannabis use during adolescence is associated with significant reductions in adult IQ and persistent neurocognitive deficits that may not be fully reversible, even with abstinence.[11–15] Other prospective studies have shown that regular cannabis use during adolescence approximately quadruples the risk of developing psychosis and doubles the risk of depression or anxiety disorders in early adulthood.[16–19]

The high prevalence of comorbidity between SUDs and other psychiatric disorders does not mean that one "causes" the other. Some studies suggest that shared or common genetic and/or environmental risk factors (eg, chronic maltreatment) may increase risk for both mental illness and SUD.[20–22] Genetic factors contribute to about half of the risk for addiction.[22,23] Several studies have also shown that similar brain regions and neural circuits are involved in SUD and other psychiatric disorders.[24] Repeated drug use may also alter gene expression and transcription in ways that can produce long-term changes in brain structure that may increase the risk of developing depression and/or anxiety disorders.[25–27] Taken together, this body of research suggests that risk and vulnerability to addiction and mental illness is due to complex interactions among multiple genes and environmental factors.[22,23] Although the mechanisms are still not well-understood, the high prevalence of cooccurring mental illness and SUD is well-established, and adolescence is a time of heightened vulnerability to the onset of both.

In nationally representative samples, nearly one-third of adolescents (32%) with a SUD also meet criteria for a nonsubstance psychiatric disorder.[28–30] Psychiatric comorbidity is even more common among adolescents who are referred to substance treatment including conduct disorder (60%–80%); attention deficit hyperactivity disorder (ADHD; 30%–50%); and major depressive disorder (MDD; 24%–50%).[31–33] Comorbidity has important clinical implications. Numerous studies have shown that adolescents with SUD and other cooccurring psychiatric disorders have poorer treatment outcomes compared with noncomorbid youth.[34–36] Based on this research, the National Institute on Drug Abuse has emphasized the importance of providing integrated or concurrent treatment for SUD and psychiatric comorbidity as a key principle of drug addiction treatment.[37] The Substance Abuse and Mental Health Services Association also strongly endorses the importance of integrated substance and mental health treatment for cooccurring disorders. In 2010, the Substance Abuse and Mental Health Services Association's Integrated Treatment for Co-Occurring Disorders KIT identifies core components of integrated treatment, which include cross-trained practitioners, stage-wise treatment, motivational interventions, a cognitive–behavioral approach, multiple formats, and integrated medication services.[38] Despite the considerable clinical consensus and empirical support for integrated treatment, such treatment remains critically lacking in most treatment settings. Barriers to progress toward integrated treatment include longstanding systemic and economic barriers and limited research to inform development of integrated treatment approaches. This article reviews the growing body of research from which empirically based principles of integrated mental health and substance treatment can be derived and that have informed the development of at least 1 evidence-based integrated treatment model.

Evidence-Based Adolescent Substance Treatment Interventions

In the past 2 decades, there has been considerable progress toward the development of evidence-based substance treatment interventions for adolescents. These include motivational enhancement therapy (MET), both group and individual format with cognitive–behavioral therapy (CBT), contingency management (CM), combined MET/CBT + CM, and family-based interventions such as multisystemic therapy, multidimensional family therapy, brief strategic family therapy, and adolescent community reinforcement approach.[33,39,40] Metaanalyses and comparative effectiveness studies indicate that these evidence-based interventions produce superior outcomes compared with less structured "treatment as usual" comparison conditions.[39–42]

Overall, these interventions have comparable effect sizes and each has been shown to be efficacious based on the results of at least 2 randomized controlled trials. Although efficacious, taken together, these interventions produce only modest reductions in substance use and relatively low rates of abstinence. Based on the results of adolescent and adult studies, individual MET/CBT is most consistently associated with sustained or even emerging posttreatment effect size. However, acute treatment effects attenuate over time and few remain abstinent 1 year after treatment.[39,40] Ample research in adults and an increasing number of studies in adolescents have reported higher rates of abstinence when CM/abstinence-based incentives are added to MET/CBT or other psychosocial treatment interventions.[43–46]

Although there has been progress in evidence-based substance treatment interventions, such treatment remains in critical shortage. Another important limitation of existing evidence-based substance treatment interventions is the lack of concurrent assessment and treatment of other cooccurring (nonsubstance) psychiatric disorders. National service use surveys continue to report that fewer than 10% of adolescents who could benefit from substance treatment receive it, and even fewer receive integrated treatment for cooccurring substance and psychiatric disorders.[47]

PROGRESS TOWARD INTEGRATION OF MENTAL HEALTH AND SUBSTANCE TREATMENT

The Mental Health and Addiction Parity Act in 2008 and the Affordable Care Act in 2010 initiated a significant national health care reform movement and has begun to dismantle the longstanding systemic and economic barriers to integrated mental health and addiction treatment services and the integration of behavioral health into mainstream medicine. A growing body of adolescent substance abuse research in the past decade now provides an empirical foundation for deriving evidence-based principles for integrating mental health and substance treatment. Perhaps most informative in this regard are a handful of controlled trials of combined pharmacotherapy and behavioral interventions conducted in adolescents with SUD and other psychiatric comorbidities. Results of these studies and the research-based integrated treatment principles derived from them are discussed below.

TREATMENT OF DEPRESSION IN ADOLESCENTS WITH SUBSTANCE USE DISORDERS

Riggs and colleagues[48] conducted a randomized controlled trial of fluoxetine with CBT in adolescents with SUD and MDD. In this study, 126 adolescents (ages 13–17) meeting DSM-IV diagnostic criteria for MDD, lifetime conduct disorder, and at least 1 nontobacco SUD were randomized to a 20 mg/d dose of fluoxetine or matching placebo. Participants in both groups received weekly, individual MET/CBT as outpatient substance treatment throughout the 16-week medication trial. Fluoxetine showed greater efficacy than placebo on reductions in Childhood Depression Rating Scale-Revised (CDRS-R) scores (primary outcome measure). Substance use decreased significantly in both groups but there was not a statistically significant difference between groups.[48]

Rates of depression remission (defined as final CDRS-R raw score ≤28) were unexpectedly high in both the fluoxetine (70%) and placebo (52%) treatment groups. This led investigators to speculate that CBT (targeting substance abuse), received by participants in both groups, may have contributed to depression treatment response despite primary focus on substance abuse. Similar findings in adult studies have been reported.[49,50] A metaanalysis of controlled antidepressant medication trials (mostly serotonin reuptake inhibitors/selective serotonin reuptake inhibitors) in adults with cooccurring depression and SUD, concluded that mixed findings were due in part to an unusually high "placebo response" in studies in which participants received concurrent individual CBT as outpatient substance treatment.[49]

TREATMENT OF ATTENTION DEFICIT HYPERACTIVITY DISORDER IN ADOLESCENTS WITH SUBSTANCE USE DISORDERS

An estimated 30% to 50% of adolescents referred to substance treatment meet criteria for ADHD.[33,51] Left untreated, ADHD symptoms such as poor concentration, frustration tolerance, and impulsivity may contribute to poorer substance treatment outcomes. Yet, clinicians may be reluctant to treat ADHD with first-line psychostimulants owing to concerns about the potential for scheduled medication abuse or diversion and the lack of research addressing medication safety and efficacy in substance abusing adolescents.

To address these clinically important questions, a multisite randomized controlled trial of osmotic-release methylphenidate (Safety Assessment of Potential Interactions Between IV Methamphetamine and Osmotic-Release Methylphenidate [OROS-MPH]) was conducted in the National Institute on Drug Abuse Clinical Trials Network. In this landmark study, 303 adolescents (ages 13–17) meeting DSM-IV diagnostic criteria for ADHD and SUD were randomized to OROS-MPH or matching placebo across 11 participating sites. Participants in both groups received individual, manual-standardized MET/CBT as outpatient substance treatment throughout the 16-week medication trial. Results showed significant decreases in ADHD symptom severity and substance use in both groups but no difference between groups on either primary ADHD or substance outcome measures. However, some secondary outcomes indicated that treatment of ADHD with OROS-MPH "added benefit" compared with placebo. Participants treated with OROS-MPH had significantly more negative urine drug screens and reported significant improvement in coping and problem-solving skills related to their substance use compared with participants treated with placebo who reported no improvement.[52]

A second similarly designed 12-week placebo-controlled trial of atomoxetine versus placebo in 70 adolescents (ages 13–18) meeting diagnostic criteria for ADHD and SUD reported similar findings. Participants in both groups participated in weekly individual

MET/CBT outpatient substance treatment throughout the trial. Both groups showed clinically and statistically significant decreases in ADHD symptom severity (ADHD rating scale scores) and substance use (days of past 28-day substance use), but no difference between groups on these primary outcome measures.[53]

The higher than expected placebo response rates in these adolescent studies, coupled with similar findings in 3 controlled psychostimulant medication trials in adults with ADHD participating in weekly, individual MET/CBT (outpatient substance treatment),[54–56] begs the question of whether MET/CBT (targeting substance abuse) contributes to reductions in ADHD symptom severity. This is in contrast with the results of 2 randomized controlled medication trials in adolescents (pemoline) and adults (atomoxetine) with ADHD and SUD reporting significantly greater reductions in ADHD symptom severity in participants who received pemoline or atomoxetine, respectively, compared with placebo in participants who did not receive concurrent MET/CBT or other psychosocial substance treatment during the trials.[57,58]

Several studies have demonstrated the efficacy of CBT for ADHD in adults who do not have cooccurring SUD.[59,60] Ample research has also demonstrated the efficacy of CBT for depression and anxiety disorders in both adolescents and adults without cooccurring SUD.[61] However, to our knowledge no controlled trials have yet examined the potential impact of substance treatment with CBT (targeting SUD) on reductions in symptoms of cooccurring ADHD, depression, and/or anxiety disorders in adults or adolescents with SUD. Clearly, studies that are designed specifically to examine the separate and combined effects of MET/CBT (targeting SUD) with and without pharmacotherapy on reductions in cooccurring psychiatric symptom severity are warranted.

IMPLICATIONS FOR CLINICAL PRACTICE, INTEGRATED TREATMENT, AND FUTURE RESEARCH

Taken together these studies have important implications for clinical practice. The similar design, methodology, measures, and results of these studies can also inform integrated approaches for treating cooccurring substance and other psychiatric disorders:

1. Each of these studies included a semistructured diagnostic evaluation to establish valid substance and psychiatric diagnoses at baseline. Diagnostic validity is important in such studies to ensure that study participants meet criteria for diagnoses required for study inclusion (eg, MDD, ADHD). In clinical practice, it is equally important to establish valid diagnoses to guide treatment.
2. Each of the studies also used psychometrically valid repeated measures to establish baseline psychiatric symptom severity (eg, MDD/CDRS-R; ADHD/ADHD-RS) and track changes in symptom severity at regular intervals (at least monthly) during treatment to assess treatment response. Changes in substance use were similarly tracked using standardized timeline followback procedures (calendar method) to determine the number of days of nontobacco substance use in the past 28 days at baseline. CBT therapists also used calendar-based timeline followback procedures to document and track self-reported substance use at each weekly visit accounting for all days during treatment. Urine drug screens were also ascertained weekly as a biological measure of substance use. Similar measures can and should be used by clinicians as a sound approach for systematically assessing response to treatment.
3. Manual standardized MET/CBT was used to standardize the "background" substance treatment for participants in both medication and placebo arms in each of the 3 trials. Because all participants received MET/CBT it is not possible to

determine its potential contribution to reductions in depression or ADHD symptoms. However, similar findings (ie, high placebo response rates with MET/CBT) reported in several adult studies suggests that individual MET/CBT may tentatively be considered as a first-line psychosocial substance treatment modality for individual with cooccurring substance and psychiatric comorbidity at this time. More confident and definitive recommendations in this regard are not possible in the absence of controlled studies specifically designed to determine the separate and combined effects of MET/CBT on cooccurring psychiatric symptom severity. However, such studies are clearly warranted.

4. In each of the 3 studies, participants received $25 per week as compensation as research participants and completion of research assessments. These payments may have contributed to high rates of treatment completion and compliance in these studies. In an integrated treatment model, known as *Encompass* (www.ucdenver.edu/academics/colleges/medicalschool/departments/psychiatry/Research/Subdep/ENCOMPASS/Pages/default.aspx) that was developed based on the integrated approach used in these studies, CM was added to MET/CBT as a "research-to-practice" adaptation or replacement for weekly research payments. Adolescents earn opportunities to draw for prizes for treatment compliance (CBT session attendance), negative urine drug screens (abstinence-based incentives, escalating scale), and for completing prosocial nondrug activities (2 such activities are negotiated weekly; 1 prize draw is earned with documentation of each completed activity). CM procedures as used in the *Encompass* intervention are based on well-established principles of behavioral reinforcement and controlled trials in adults and adolescents showing that the addition of CM/incentives to MET/CBT or other psychosocial substance treatment interventions can increase significantly the rates of abstinence achieved during treatment compared with MET/CBT or psychosocial treatment alone (without CM).[45,46]

SUMMARY

This article has reviewed the foundational research supporting an informed and integrated approach for treating cooccurring SUD and other psychiatric disorders. Unfortunately, establishing an evidence-based treatment framework is only the first step to improving treatment outcomes. State, county, and city mental health authorities often encounter policies related to organizational structure, financing, regulations, and licensing that work against the functional integration of mental health and substance abuse services.[62] Although an integrated clinical philosophy and a practical approach to the treatment of cooccurring disorders have been delineated clearly for more than a decade, educational institutions rarely teach this approach. Consequently, mental health clinicians typically lack training in treatment of cooccurring disorders and have to rely on informal, self-initiated opportunities for learning current interventions.[63,64] Because of a lack of training, administrators of clinics, centers, and programs often lack the experience necessary to develop and implement integrated treatment models, quality assurance procedures, and outcome measures needed to implement cooccurring treatment programs. Efforts to increase access significantly and the availability of substance or integrated behavioral health treatment will require significant expansion of the workforce.

Clinical training programs will need to be enhanced significantly and transformed to address the critical shortage of clinicians with dual training in mental health and addiction prevention and treatment, as identified by the Institute of Medicine. Mental health clinician training should include training in systematic assessment of biological and developmental processes, environmental risk, and protective factors associated with adolescent-onset substance abuse; training in evidence-based prevention and treatment interventions that have been shown to reduce risk and enhance resilience or protective factors; training in evidence-based approaches to integrated or coordinated treatment; and training in continuing care and coordinated care models for youth with cooccurring substance abuse and mental health problems.

REFERENCES

1. Giedd JN. Structural magnetic resonance imaging of the adolescent brain. In: Dahl RE, Spear LP, editors. Adolescent brain development: vulnerabilities and opportunities. vol. 1021. New York: Annals of the New York Academy of Sciences; 2004. p. 77–85.
2. Chen CM, Yi H , Falk DE, et al. Alcohol and Alcohol use disorders in the United States: Main findings from the 2001-2002 National Epidemiologic survey on Alcohol and Related Conditions (NESARC). U.S. Alcohol Epidemiologic Data Reference Manual. 2006.
3. Casey BJ, Jones RM, Hare TA. The adolescent brain. Ann N Y Acad Sci 2008; 1124:111–26.
4. Krueger RF, Hicks BM, Patrick CJ. Etiologic connections among substance dependence, antisocial behavior, and personality: modeling the externalizing spectrum. J Abnorm Psychol 2002;111(3):411–24.
5. Bukstein OG. Disruptive behavior disorders and substance use disorders in adolescents. J Psychoactive Drugs 2000;32:67–79.
6. Clark DB, Winters KC. Measuring risks and outcomes in substance use disorders prevention research. J Consult Clin Psychol 2002;70:1207–23.
7. White HR, Xie M, Thompson W. Psychopathology as a predictor of adolescent drug use trajectories. Psychol Addict Behav 2001;15:210–8.
8. Burke JD, Burke KC, Rae DS. Increased rates of drug abuse and dependence after onset of mood or anxiety disorders in adolescence. Hosp Community Psychiatry 1994;45(5):451–5.
9. Deas–Nesmith D, Campbell S, Brady K. Substance use disorders in an adolescent inpatient psychiatric population. J Natl Med Assoc 1998;90:233–8.
10. Deas D. Adolescent substance abuse and psychiatric comorbidities. J Clin Psychiatry 2006;67(Suppl 7):18–23.
11. Meier MH, Caspi A, Ambler A, et al. Persistent cannabis users show neuropsychological decline from childhood to midlife. Proc Natl Acad Sci U S A 2012;2: 109–40.
12. Pope HG Jr, Yurgelun-Todd D. The residual cognitive effects of heavy marijuana use in college students. JAMA 1996;275:521–7.
13. Pope HG Jr. Early-onset cannabis use and cognitive deficits: what is the nature of the association? Drug Alcohol Depend 2003;69:303–10.
14. Pope HG Jr, Gruber AJ, Hudson JI, et al. Neuropsychological performance in long-term cannabis users. Arch Gen Psychiatry 2001;58:909–15.
15. Jager G, Ramsey NF. Long-term consequences of adolescent cannabis exposure on the development of cognition, brain structure and function: an overview of animal and human research. Curr Drug Abuse Rev 2008;1:114–23.
16. Bagot KS, Milin R, Kaminer Y. Adolescent initiation of cannabis use and early-onset psychosis. Subst Abus 2015;36(4):524–33.

17. Doody GA, Murray RM, Jones PB, et al. Cannabis use, gender and age of onset of schizophrenia: data from the ÆSOP study. Psychiatry Res 2014;215(3): 528–32.
18. Arseneault L, Cannon M, Poulton R, et al. Cannabis use in adolescence and risk for adult psychosis: longitudinal prospective study. BMJ 2002;325(7374):1212–3.
19. Patton GC, Coffey C, Carlin JB, et al. Cannabis use and mental health in young people: cohort study. BMJ 2002;325(7374):1195–8.
20. Felitti V, Anda R. The relationship of adverse childhood experiences to adult medical disease, psychiatric disorders, and sexual behavior: implications for health care. In: Lanius R, Vermetten E, Pain C, editors. The impact of early life trauma on health and disease. Cambridge (United Kingdom): Cambridge University Press; 2010. p. 77–87.
21. Fergusson DM, Lynskey MT. Physical punishment/maltreatment during childhood and adjustment in young adulthood. Child Abuse Negl 1997;21(7):617–30.
22. Young SE, Rhee SH, Stallings MC, et al. Genetic and environmental vulnerabilities underlying adolescent substance use and problem use: general or specific? Behav Genet 2006;36(4):603–15.
23. Rhee SH, Hewitt JK, Young SE, et al. Genetic and environmental influences on substance initiation, use, and problem use in adolescents. Arch Gen Psychiatry 2003;60(12):1256–64.
24. Brady KT, Sinha R. Co-occurring mental and substance use disorders: the neurobiological effects of chronic stress. Am J Psychiatry 2005;162(8):1483–93.
25. Nestler EJ. Molecular basis of neural plasticity underlying addiction. Nat Rev Neurosci 2001;2(2):119–28.
26. Nestler EJ. The neurobiology of cocaine addiction. Sci Pract Perspect 2005;3(1): 4–10.
27. Renthal W, Kumar A, Xiao G, et al. Genome-wide analysis of chromatin regulation by cocaine reveals a role for sirtuins. Neuron 2009;62(3):335–48.
28. Merikangas KR, He JP. Lifetime prevalence of mental disorders in U.S. Adolescents: results from the national comorbidity survey replication-adolescent supplement (NCS-A). J Am Acad Child Adolesc Psychiatry 2010;49(10):980–9.
29. Merikangas KR, He JP. Service utilization for lifetime mental disorders in U.S. adolescents: results of the National Comorbidity Survey- Adolescent Supplement (NCS-A). J Am Acad Child Adolesc Psychiatry 2011;50(1):32–45.
30. Swendsen J, Burstein M. Use and abuse of alcohol and illicit drugs in US adolescents: results of the National Comorbidity Survey-Adolescent Supplement. Arch Gen Psychiatry 2012;69(4):390–8.
31. Bukstein OG, Glancy LJ, Kaminer Y. Patterns of affective comorbidity in a clinical population of dually diagnosed adolescent substance abusers. J Am Acad Child Adolesc Psychiatry 1992;31(6):1041–5.
32. Kaminer Y, Burleson JA, Goldberger R. Cognitive-behavioral coping skills and psychoeducation therapies for adolescent substance abuse. J Nerv Ment Dis 2002;190(11):737–45.
33. Riggs P, Levin F, Green AI, et al. Comorbid psychiatric and substance abuse disorders: recent treatment research. Subst Abus 2008;29(3):51–63.
34. Humfleet GL, Prochaska JJ, Mengis M. Preliminary evidence of the association between the history of childhood attention-deficit/hyperactivity disorder and smoking treatment failure. Nicotine Tob Res 2005;7(3):453–60.
35. Ercan ES, Coskunol H, Varan A, et al. Childhood attention deficit/hyperactivity disorder and alcohol dependence: a 1-year follow-up. Alcohol Alcohol 2003; 38(4):352–6.

36. White AM, Jordan JD, Schroeder KM. Predictors of relapse during treatment and treatment completion among marijuana-dependent adolescents. Subst Abus 2004;25(1):53–9.
37. National Institute on Drug Abuse. Homepage on the Internet. Available at: http://www.drugabuse.gov.
38. Substance Abuse and Mental Health Services Administration (SAMHSA). Co-occurring disorders. Available at: http://media.samhsa.gov/co-occurring.
39. Tanner-Smith EE, Wilson SJ, Lipsey MW. The comparative effectiveness of outpatient treatment for adolescent substance abuse: a meta-analysis. J Subst Abuse Treat 2013;44(2):145–58.
40. Belendiuk KA, Riggs P. Treatment of adolescent substance use disorders. Curr Treat Options Psychiatry 2014;1(2):175–88.
41. Tripodi SJ, Bender K, Litschge C, et al. Interventions for reducing adolescent alcohol abuse: a meta-analytic review. Arch Pediatr Adolesc Med 2010;164(1):85–91.
42. Waldron H, Turner C. Evidence-based psychosocial treatments for adolescent substance abuse. J Clin Child Adolesc Psychol 2008;37:238–61.
43. Prendergast M, Podus D, Finney J, et al. Contingency management for treatment of substance use disorders: a meta-analysis. Addiction 2006;101(11):1546–60.
44. Silverman K, Roll JM, Higgins ST. Introduction to the special issue on the behavior analysis and treatment of drug addiction. J Appl Behav Anal 2008;41(4):471–80.
45. Stanger C, Budney AJ, Kamon JL, et al. A randomized trial of contingency management for adolescent marijuana abuse and dependence. Drug Alcohol Depend 2009;105(3):240–7.
46. Stanger C, Ryan SR, Scherer EA, et al. Clinic- and home-based contingency management plus parent training for adolescent cannabis use disorders. J Am Acad Child Adolesc Psychiatry 2015;54(6):445–53.
47. Dicola LA, Gaydos LM, Druss BG, et al. Health insurance and treatment of adolescents with co-occurring major depression and substance use disorders. J Am Acad Child Adolesc Psychiatry 2013;52(9):953–60.
48. Riggs PD, Mikulich SK, Davies RD, et al. A randomized controlled trial of fluoxetine and cognitive behavioral therapy in adolescents with major depression, behavior problems, and substance use disorders. Arch Pediatr Adolesc Med 2007;161(11):1026–34.
49. Nunes EV, Levin FR. Treatment of depression in patients with alcohol or other drug dependence: a meta-analysis. JAMA 2004;291(15):1887–96.
50. Carroll KM, Fenton LR, Ball SA. Efficacy of disulfiram and cognitive behavior therapy in cocaine-dependent outpatients: a randomized placebo-controlled trial. Arch Gen Psychiatry 2004;61(3):264–72.
51. Zulauf CA, Sprich SE, Safren SA, et al. The complicated relationship between attention deficit/hyperactivity disorder and substance use disorders. Curr Psychiatry Rep 2014;16(3):436.
52. Riggs PD, Winhusen T, Davies RD. Randomized controlled trial of osmotic-release methylphenidate with cognitive-behavioral therapy in adolescents with attention-deficit/hyperactivity disorder and substance use disorders. J Am Acad Child Adolesc Psychiatry 2011;50(9):903–14.
53. Thurstone C, Riggs PD, Salomonsen-Sautel S, et al. Randomized, controlled trial of atomoxetine for attention deficit/hyperactivity disorder in adolescents with substance use disorder. J Am Acad Child Adolesc Psychiatry 2010;49:573–82.

54. Levin FR, Evans SM, Brooks DJ, et al. Treatment of methadone-maintained patients with adult ADHD: double-blind comparison of methylphenidate, bupropion, and placebo. Drug Alcohol Depend 2006;81:137–48.
55. Levin FR, Evans SM, Brooks DJ, et al. Treatment of cocaine dependent treatment seekers with adult ADHD: double-blind comparison of methylphenidate and placebo. Drug Alcohol Depend 2007;87:20–9.
56. Schubiner H, Saules KK, Arfken CL, et al. Double-blind placebo controlled trial of methylphenidate in the treatment of adult ADHD patients with comorbid cocaine dependence. Exp Clin Psychopharmacol 2002;10:286–94.
57. Riggs PD, Hall SK, Mikulich-Gilbertson SK, et al. A randomized controlled trial of pemoline for attention-deficit/hyperactivity disorder in substance-abusing adolescents. J Am Acad Child Adolesc Psychiatry 2004;43(4):420–9.
58. Wilens TE, Gignac M, Swezey A, et al. Characteristics of adolescents and young adults with ADHD who divert or misuse their prescribed medications. J Am Acad Child Adolesc Psychiatry 2006;45:408–14.
59. Solanto MV, Marks DJ, Wasserstein J, et al. Efficacy of meta-cognitive therapy (MCT) for adult ADHD. Am J Psychiatry 2010;167(8):958–68.
60. Safren SA, Sprich S, Mimiaga MJ, et al. Cognitive behavioral therapy vs relaxation with educational support for medication-treated adults with ADHD and persistent symptoms: a randomized controlled trial. JAMA 2010;304(8):875–80.
61. Butler AC, Chapman JE, Forman EM, et al. The empirical status of cognitive-behavioral therapy: a review of meta-analyses. Clin Psychol Rev 2006;26(1):17–31.
62. Ridgely M, Goldman H, Willenbring M. Barriers to the care of persons with dual diagnoses: organizational and financing is-sues. Schizophr Bull 1990;16:123–32.
63. Minkoff K. An integrated treatment model for dual diagnosis of psychosis and addiction. Hosp Community Psychiatry 1989;40:1031–6.
64. Carey KB, Purnine DM, Maisto SM. Treating substance abuse in the context of severe and persistent mental illness: clinicians' perspectives. J Subst Abuse Treat 2000;19:189–98.

Substance Abuse and Trauma

Shannon Simmons, MD, MPH[a],*, Liza Suárez, PhD[b]

KEYWORDS

- Trauma - PTSD - Substance abuse - Chemical dependency - Integrated treatment

KEY POINTS

- Traumatic experiences and substance abuse are both common among teenagers. When they occur together, complex and challenging clinical presentations can result.
- The relationship between posttraumatic stress disorder (PTSD) and substance use disorders can be bidirectional, and the 2 issues can reinforce each other.
- An integrated, multisystem treatment approach for teens with cooccurring PTSD and substance use disorders is recommended.

INTRODUCTION

Substance use disorders (SUDs) are highly comorbid with posttraumatic stress disorder (PTSD). The relationship between substance abuse and trauma is complex and bidirectional, with shared social risk factors and biological pathways. Youth with cooccurring PTSD and SUD often have more severe challenges than teens with either disorder alone, with treatment needs that may involve multiple community systems. Integrated treatment principles and recommendations are discussed. Two clinical cases are reviewed to illustrate these treatment principles.

EPIDEMIOLOGY

At least 1 in 4 children experiences a significant traumatic event during childhood; some estimates are significantly higher.[1] The lifetime prevalence of drug abuse or dependence in teens has been found to range from 3.3% to 9.8%.[2] Substance use rates among teens remain high, although rates of teen alcohol use have decreased

The authors have nothing to disclose.

[a] Department of Psychiatry and Behavioral Sciences, University of Washington, Seattle Children's Hospital, 4800 Sand Point Way Northeast, Seattle, WA 98105, USA; [b] Department of Psychiatry, Institute for Juvenile Research, University of Illinois at Chicago, 1747 West Roosevelt Road #192, Chicago, IL 60612, USA
* Corresponding author.
E-mail address: Shannon.simmons@seattlechildrens.org

Child Adolesc Psychiatric Clin N Am 25 (2016) 723–734
http://dx.doi.org/10.1016/j.chc.2016.05.006
1056-4993/16/$ – see front matter © 2016 Elsevier Inc. All rights reserved.

childpsych.theclinics.com

Abbreviations	
CRF	Corticotrophin-releasing factor
DSM-V	Diagnostic and Statistical Manual of Mental Disorders, fifth edition
PTSD	Posttraumatic stress disorder
SUD	Substance use disorder

somewhat in recent years. **Table 1** shows the 2011 and 2014 lifetime and past-month rates of alcohol and cannabis use in 12-grade students.[3]

A multitude of studies have observed a link between traumatic experiences and substance abuse. In the National Survey of Adolescents, 24% of girls and almost 30% of boys with PTSD had comorbid substance abuse or dependence. Out of boys and girls with substance abuse or dependence, 13% and 25%, respectively, also had PTSD.[4] In a retrospective study of more than 8000 adults, respondents with more than 5 adverse childhood experiences were 7 to 10 times more likely to report illicit drug use problems. An increasing adverse childhood experience score was associated with earlier initiation of illicit drug use as well as drug addiction.[5]

CLINICAL PRESENTATION
Posttraumatic Stress Disorder

According to the *Diagnostic and Statistical Manual of Mental Disorders, fifth edition* (DSM-V), a diagnosis of PTSD requires symptoms in 4 different clusters: intrusion symptoms, avoidance, negative alterations in cognitions and mood, and marked alterations in arousal and reactivity.[6] However, youth who have experienced trauma may have a wide range of clinical symptoms, and are at an increased risk for a broad array of clinical sequelae and functional impairment, beyond or in addition to PTSD (**Box 1**).[1]

Many youth demonstrate symptoms of PTSD in the first month after a trauma, but fewer than one-third continue to have symptoms thereafter.[1] Interpersonal traumas, such as sexual assault or violence, are more likely to result in PTSD than noninterpersonal traumas. Family adversity, prior traumas, and pretrauma anxiety may predict the onset of PTSD.[7] Complex trauma is defined as multiple simultaneous or sequential traumas within the caretaking environment, beginning in childhood, as well as the multidomain impairment and symptomatology that often result. The domains of impairment include attachment, biology, affect regulation, dissociation, behavioral control, cognition, and self-concept.[8] Beyond problems with PTSD, depression, and substance abuse, youth who have experienced polyvictimization are at greater risk for behavioral and legal problems.[9]

Substance Use Disorder

Many teens experiment with drugs and alcohol. To meet criteria for a SUD, according to the DSM-5, teens must display at least 2 of 11 possible symptoms over a 12-month

Table 1
Rates of alcohol and cannabis use in 12th graders

	Past-Month Alcohol (%)	Lifetime Alcohol (%)	Past-Month Marijuana (%)	Lifetime Marijuana (%)
2011	40	70	22.6	45.5
2014	37.4	66	21.2	44.4

Data from National Institute on Drug Abuse. High School and Youth Trends. Available at: www.drugabuse.gov/publications/drugfacts/high-school-youth-trends. Accessed September 30, 2015.

Box 1
Possible clinical sequelae for youth with posttraumatic stress disorder

- Depression
- Anxiety
- Self-injury
- Suicide attempts
- Psychosis
- Eating disorders
- Affect regulation problems
- Antisocial behavior
- Health problems

---

period. These symptoms are consuming more substance than planned, failed efforts to control use, spending a large amount of time using substances, resultant failure to fulfill obligations, cravings, continued use despite health or relationship problems, repeated use in dangerous situations, reducing life activities because of the substance use, development of tolerance, and withdrawal symptoms.[6]

Adolescents with SUDs also may have a range of dysfunction in the categories shown in **Box 2**. In addition to PTSD, various other psychopathology such as disruptive behavior, mood disorders, and anxiety may predispose youth to SUDs; in contrast, SUDs may result in negative alterations in behavior or in mood or anxiety levels.[2]

POSTTRAUMATIC STRESS DISORDER AND SUBSTANCE USE DISORDER: A BIDIRECTIONAL RELATIONSHIP

The sequence of onset of PTSD and SUD varies. In 1 study of nearly 400 teens, approximately one-half had an SUD before they experienced a significant trauma.[10] This can be explained by the reciprocally reinforcing and bidirectional relationship between substance abuse and posttraumatic symptomatology.

Teens who have experienced trauma may misuse drugs or alcohol in attempts to manage symptoms such as hyperarousal or distressing memories or flashbacks. Withdrawal symptoms may mimic hyperarousal symptoms of PTSD, causing a teen to use increasing amounts of drugs or alcohol in attempts to mask these symptoms. Substance abuse may also promote and reinforce maladaptive avoidant coping strategies; avoidant tendencies may be a preexisting trait that contributes to the development of PTSD and SUD, or may be a feature of PTSD.[11]

Box 2
Possible areas of dysfunction for adolescents with substance use disorders

- Family conflict
- Interpersonal problems
- Academic struggles
- Risky behavior

In contrast, substance abusing teens may find themselves in situations in which they are endangered or easily victimized. They may engage in risky behavior owing to increased impulsivity while intoxicated.[12] Data from the National Survey of Adolescents suggested that earlier initiation of substance abuse predicted exposure to additional traumas.[13] Additionally, substance misuse may contribute to negative cognitions, such as feelings of inadequacy or isolation. Using substances may interfere with one's ability to cope with the trauma effectively, leading more prolonged symptoms of PTSD.[14] This can lead to a cycle of self-medication and retraumatization.

SUDs and PTSD share some social and environmental risk factors, such as inadequate family support and social problems.[1,15] Data from the Adverse Childhood Experiences study indicated that having parental alcohol abuse is associated with a higher rate of adverse childhood experiences, as well as an increased risk of alcoholism and depression in adulthood (although the latter risk is owing to adverse childhood experiences generally, not specific to having a parent with alcoholism).[16]

Youth with comorbid SUD and PTSD have more severe interpersonal difficulties and internalizing symptoms than teens with only SUD.[7] They are more likely to use services in multiple systems, such as juvenile justice, special education, and child protection.[17] For individuals with comorbid SUD and trauma, exposure to reminders of the traumatic event can lead to an increase in substance (particularly alcohol) cravings, with PTSD severity predicting the intensity of the drug cravings.[18–20] Thus, teens with both SUDs and PTSD may have more significant challenges than teens with either issue separately.

NEUROBIOLOGY

The relationship between substance abuse and psychiatric disorders such as PTSD is likely complex, and research points to common neurobiological pathways. Adding to the complexity is that different substances have different effects on neurobiological systems. The hypothalamic–pituitary–adrenal axis is strongly involved in both substance abuse and posttraumatic stress. Traumatic stress results in increased circulating catecholamines, which in turn stimulate the hypothalamus to produce corticotrophin-releasing factor (CRF). CRF increases anxiety and arousal, and stimulates the pituitary gland to produce adrenocorticotropic hormone, which then causes the adrenal glands to produce epinephrine and cortisol.[21] Increased CRF has also been found in association with cocaine or alcohol withdrawal. These findings suggest that an increased CRF level is involved in PTSD symptoms as well as the reinforcing qualities of some substances owing to withdrawal symptomatology.[22]

Additionally, increased noradrenergic activity has been found in PTSD, alcohol withdrawal, and opiate withdrawal. Brain CRF and adrenergic systems interact to modulate each other through various mechanisms. Stress, then, may stimulate a cascade of events resulting in the release of norepinephrine and CRF in several areas of the brain, including the hypothalamus and amygdala, which can lead to increased noradrenergic reactions with subsequent stressors, including substance withdrawal. This may help us to understand the cycle between substance withdrawal symptoms, worsening of PTSD symptoms associated with withdrawal, and attempts to self-medicate those withdrawal and PTSD symptoms through drugs or alcohol.[17]

DIAGNOSTIC CONSIDERATIONS

Before a comprehensive treatment plan is made, a thorough diagnostic assessment should be completed, and the presence of comorbid conditions should be explored. One diagnostic challenge that arises in youth is that a key symptom of PTSD is avoidance. More specifically, one of the diagnostic criteria is efforts to avoid conversations about, or other reminders of, the trauma.[6] Teens may minimize or not disclose traumatic experience because it is too distressing to do so, because of fears of what consequence may follow, or for a variety of other reasons. Substance abuse also is often minimized or hidden. Using a calm, nonjudgmental stance when inquiring about drug use can be helpful. The use of screening instruments or questionnaires can help to hone the diagnosis, and sometimes elicit information that teens are not comfortable sharing verbally. **Table 2** lists some standardized measures for PTSD, and **Table 3** for substance abuse. These are just a few of the many standardized questionnaires available.

TREATMENT OVERVIEW

There is relatively sparse data on treatment outcomes for adolescents with comorbid SUD and PTSD. A study of more than 1100 teens in an outpatient substance abuse treatment program showed that teens with high levels of traumatic stress responded in a similar pattern compared with their nontraumatized peers on overall rates of abstinence from drugs, either at 3 months after program intake or 1 year after intake. This finding was despite the fact that traumatized youth reported relatively higher substance use frequency at intake. The group with high traumatic stress, however, reported overall higher rates of substance problems over time.[31] Another study of 212 adolescents in residential treatment showed that trauma-exposed teens who did not meet criteria for PTSD left treatment sooner than non–trauma-exposed teens or teens with trauma exposure and PTSD, with unclear implications.[32]

Treatment of Posttraumatic Stress Disorder

Several randomized controlled trials have shown trauma-focused cognitive–behavioral therapy to be superior to waitlist controls, standard community care, or supportive therapy in a range of ages and ethnicities. Trauma-focused cognitive–behavioral therapy includes components of stress management training, psychoeducation about posttraumatic symptomatology and experiences, parenting skills, enhancing safety, graduated exposure exercises including constructing a trauma narrative, and cognitive processing. The American Academy of Child and Adolescent Psychiatry practice parameters recommend that trauma-focused therapies be the first-line treatment for youth with PTSD.[1]

Table 2 Standardized measures for PTSD		
Name	**Ages**	**Source**
Trauma Symptom Checklist for Children (TSC-C)[23]	8–16 y, 3rd-grade reading level	www.parinc.com
UCLA PTSD Reaction Index[24]	6–18 y, 7th-grade reading level	http://oip.ucla.edu/ptsd-reaction-index-instrument-licenses
Juvenile Victimization Questionnaire[25]	8–17 y	www.unh.edu/ccrc/jvq/available_versions.html
Child PTSD Symptom Scale (CPSS)[26]	8–18 y	www.aacap.org/App_Themes/AACAP/docs/resource_centers/resources/misc/child_ptsd_symptom_scale.pdf

Abbreviation: PTSD, posttraumatic stress disorder.

Table 3
Standardized measures for substance abuse

Name	Ages	Source
CRAFFT[27]	14–18 y	www.ceasar-boston.org/clinicians/crafft.php
Drug Use Screening Inventory Revised (DUSI-R)[28]	12–18 y, 5th-grade reading level	http://pubs.niaaa.nih.gov/publications/AssessingAlcohol/InstrumentPDFs/32_DUSI-R.pdf
Personal Experience Survey Questionnaire (PESQ)[29]	12–18 y, 4th-grade reading level	http://lib.adai.washington.edu/instruments
Problem Oriented Screening Instrument for Teenagers (POSIT)[30]	Adolescents, 5th-grade reading level	www.emcdda.europa.eu/html.cfm/index4439EN.html

There are limited data to support specific psychopharmacologic interventions for PTSD, although other psychiatric comorbidities may be the target of psychotropic medications. The American Academy of Child and Adolescent Psychiatry Practice Parameters for PTSD discusses the use of medications for PTSD in more detail.

Treatment of Substance Use Disorder

Evidence most strongly supports family therapy approaches for adolescent SUDs. Individual approaches, including CBT, also are supported by empirical data.[2] Components of these therapies include improved communication between parents and children, anger management, understanding of and planning for triggers, problem-solving skills, and contingency management of problematic behaviors. Motivational Interviewing aims to help teens explore and resolve ambivalence, using client-centered approaches and facilitating intrinsic motivation to change. Support groups are considered adjunctive treatments, as are reinforcements such as vouchers and contingency contracting. Twelve-step programs lack empirical evidence to support their efficacy compared with other treatments, and they may not be developmentally appropriate for adolescents.[11] Although abstinence should remain the goal, harm reduction principals are also considered realistic and important. Treatment in the least restrictive safe and effective setting is recommended; ongoing toxicology tests should be an ongoing part of treatment.[2]

Although data in adults support the use of medications in managing cravings, reducing relapse, and increasing abstinence, empirical studies in adolescents are limited. A full discussion of options is beyond the scope of this article. The National Institute on Drug Abuse's Principals of Adolescent Substance Use Disorder Treatment provides an overview.[33]

INTEGRATED TREATMENT

Given the high rates of comorbid SUD and PTSD, surprisingly few integrated treatment models exist. Although a few studies of trauma-focused cognitive–behavioral therapy for comorbid SUD and PTSD have been tested in adults, these do not include contextual factors that are important when planning an integrated treatment approach for teens. This includes but is not limited to the need for family involvement. For teens with both traumatic stress and SUD, treatment that is only focused on one aspect of their impairment (either mental health or substance abuse) will not adequately address their needs.

Barriers to Implementation

There is considerable overlap in the recommend treatment approaches for adolescent PTSD and SUD; however, there are barriers to providing integrating treatment. Therapists who tend to specialize in either SUD or PTSD may not feel equipped to deal with the other issue, or may not be trained to recognize the signs.[11] Funding for addictions treatment can be separate from that for mental health treatment, creating separate, parallel systems. Close coordination between providers is often hindered by logistical, time management, and other systemic challenges. Additionally, by the time youth with cooccurring trauma and substance abuse problems are connected to services, they may need higher levels of care, and integrated programs are often not available to meet this need.

Treatment Components

Youth with PTSD and SUD experience a wide range of problems, and providers will benefit from guidelines to organizing care.[34] Initial phases of treatment should emphasize engagement, reducing barriers to participation in treatment, and stabilization interventions aimed at maximizing safety and increasing available supports. This should be followed by skill building components where the youth gains mastery in managing negative emotions and substance use cravings. Once the youth experiences success managing emotions and cravings, the final stages of treatment should emphasize processing the trauma narrative, learning to gradually face memories and reminders of traumatic experiences, and gaining a new perspective about themselves and others during the process.

Judith Cohen and her colleagues, in a 2003 review article, recommended components of integrated PTSD and SUD treatment strategy. These included:

1. Establishing a trusting therapeutic relationship with the adolescent and family,
2. Stress management skills,
3. Affect modulation skills,
4. Cognitive restructuring,
5. Problem-solving, drug refusal, and safety skills,
6. Social skills,
7. Gradual exposure to create a trauma narrative,
8. Parenting skills,
9. Psychoeducation,
10. Random drug screens with planned consequences for positive screens,
11. Adjunctive psychopharmacology, and
12. Considering referral to an adolescent 12-step program.[11]

Integration of Systems

This high-needs population is often underidentified and underserved. Suarez and colleagues[17] described the following recommendations for integrated treatment from a systems-of-care perspective.

1. *Systematic screening and assessment for trauma exposure, traumatic stress, and substance abuse across service systems.* Given the wide range of potential problems within this population, comprehensive assessments should tailor treatment to the specific needs of youth and families. These should be responsive to the level of clinical severity, safety and stability in the home and community environment, cultural factors, and supports available within the community.

2. *A wide range of community-based services that can accommodate needs for higher levels of care.* Youth with trauma and substance abuse problems are likely to need more intensive services, including home-based and crisis support services in the community; support and services for parents who may be experiencing their own physical, emotional or social problems; and connection to needed community assistance, including school advocacy, recreational and life skill development opportunities, and access to quality mentorship to improve school and social functioning.
3. *Structural resources to facilitate coordination between providers.* Mental health and substance abuse service systems must be adjusted to allow for the provision of an integrated and coordinated continuum of care where teams can be composed of providers across agencies, disciplines, and service systems. Examples include developing formal and informal partnerships across agencies and providers, using multidisciplinary and multiagency team meetings focused on the individual needs of youth and families, and the provision of case management services to assist youth and families in navigating many service systems.
4. *Cross-training to increase understanding of both trauma and substance abuse.* To minimize challenges of youth being required to overcome one of their problems before receiving services for another, providers across service systems and treatment settings should be prepared through additional training to understand and treat both traumatic stress and substance abuse. Even if fully integrated services are not available, cross training can lead to trauma-informed substance use services, and substance use–informed trauma and mental health services.

Cultural Competence

The National Child Traumatic Stress Network recommends careful consideration of culture and context when working with adolescents. They provide several recommendations for culturally competent care, including using linguistically appropriate educational materials, having bilingual providers or interpreter services readily available, working within a defined family structure, understanding different social customs, and respecting diverse views. Additionally, using a "strength-based" approach can capitalize on each teen's individual family, community, religious, and social resources.[35]

CASE DISCUSSIONS
Sebastian

Case summary
Sebastian is a 16-year-old Latino male who witnessed domestic violence between the ages of 4 and 8. Both parents have a history of alcohol and drug use. Sebastian's parents separated when he was 8 years old and his father passed away when he was 12 owing to a drug overdose. Sebastian's mother has been alcohol and drug free for 7 years, and she works long hours to support the family. As long as Sebastian can remember, he has experienced anxiety and emotional distress, and adults have noticed he has low self-esteem with poor school performance despite having a lot of academic potential. He began using alcohol and marijuana when he was 14 and recently got in trouble for showing up to school under the influence. He was referred to a diversion program that included mentoring, sports activities, and academic support, but he has been refusing to attend. When his mother tried to encourage him to attend, he mentioned to her that the mentor he had been assigned to reminds him

too much of his own father. He was caught by the diversion program staff getting high right outside the facilities.

Treatment recommendations

Sebastian's apprehension to participate in his mentoring program is an indication that there is strong link between trauma-related cues (reminders of loss of his father) and his substance use cravings and use. In his case, the school was able to recognize that he was a youth with a lot of potential and that he needed additional resources and support, but his ongoing and seemingly unaddressed trauma-related distress is getting in the way of participation in opportunities that would be greatly beneficial to him. Also, his diversion program screened him as having untreated mental health issues that needed treatment. He should be referred to therapeutic interventions that provided simultaneous attention to distress associated with past trauma and current trauma reminders, ongoing anxiety, and urges to self-medicate with substances. Psychoeducation will be important for Sebastian and his mother to understand the links between his symptoms of substance use, avoidance, and emotional distress. Building a trusting therapeutic relationship is an important first step for Sebastian's treatment providers; working to understand his motivations and goals may facilitate his engagement in his own treatment. Ongoing communication between his school, diversion program, and mental health program may help him to feel supported and make progress in treatment.

Grace

Case summary

Grace is a 15-year-old Caucasian female who was referred to treatment because she was having extreme academic difficulties, suicidal ideation, self-harm, and trouble sleeping at night. She started using marijuana 2 years ago, but her adoptive parents did not learn about this until recently when she got arrested along with other teenagers who were hanging out in an abandoned house. As a result of the arrest, she was placed on probation. Grace was removed from her birth parents' home when she was 3 years old owing to extreme neglect and parental substance use. She was exposed prenatally to substances in utero and shows signs of verbal expression and comprehension problems that get in the way of her performance at school. She was placed in the care of her extended family members and eventually adopted by her aunt and uncle. She experienced sexual abuse by an older cousin between the ages of 3 and 10, and did not disclose this until she was 13, when her cousin was arrested for unrelated problems. Although it is clear that Grace and her adoptive parents care for each other, they have frequent arguments. Parents complain about Grace's school performance and lack of regard for rules and safety. Grace resents the way they put her down when they criticize her academic challenges and her peer group. Arguments are often followed by episodes of self-mutilation. Grace has begun to spend more time with friends after school to avoid being around her parents, and her marijuana use has increased. Ongoing suicidal thoughts are associated with fears that her cousin would hurt her when he is released from jail, as he had threatened to hurt her if she disclosed the abuse to anyone else.

Treatment recommendations

Grace seems to be experiencing high levels of distress associated with many years of unaddressed trauma and exacerbated by ongoing academic difficulties and family conflict. Given that she is exhibiting self-injurious behaviors, the treatment team must consider what the appropriate level of care she needs, with an emphasis of maximizing safety. Given her fears about retaliation from her cousin, it will be important to provide advocacy and connect her with victim support services. Additionally, her ongoing academic difficulties seem to be related to prenatal drug exposure, along with other environmental and biological influences. Advocacy to ensure she undergoes proper testing and academic accommodations will be important, and should help to minimize some of the conflict at home regarding her schoolwork. During treatment, Grace will need coping tools to address ongoing stressors (emotional regulation, interpersonal and communication skills), and parents will need assistance with achieving a balance between limit setting and being supportive. The treatment team should work with the caregivers to provide guidance on helpful responses to conflict, with particular attention to eliminating risk for self-harm. Finally, the treatment team should coordinate with the probation officer once assigned to increase access to more prosocial after school alternatives.

SUMMARY

Adolescents with cooccurring PTSD and SUDs experience greater problem severity and functional impairment compared with youth diagnosed with only one of these conditions. Although there has been considerable progress in the development of effective interventions to address these problems separately, mental health and substance abuse service systems still operate independently, and coordination and integration of care is uncommon. More research is needed to evaluate the impact of interventions targeting youth with multiple problems. Finally, service programs and youth in the community will benefit from nonfragmented and multidimensional approaches that provide flexibility and a range of resources and expertise to meet these needs.

REFERENCES

1. Cohen J, Bukstein O, Walter H, et al. Practice parameters for the assessment and treatment of children and adolescents with posttraumatic stress disorder. J Am Acad Child Adolesc Psychiatry 2010;49:414–30.

2. Bukstein O, Bernet W, Arnold V, et al. Practice parameter for the assessment and treatment of children and adolescents with substance use disorders. J Am Acad Child Adolesc Psychiatry 2005;44(6):609–21.

3. National Institute on Drug Abuse. High school and youth trends. Available at: www.drugabuse.gov/publications/drugfacts/high-school-youth-trends. Accessed September 30, 2015.

4. Kilpatrick D, Ruggiero K, Acierno R, et al. Violence and risk of PTSD, major depression, substance abuse/dependence, and comorbidity: results from the National Survey of Adolescents. J Consult Clin Psychol 2003;71(4):692–700.

5. Dube S, Felitti V, Dong M, et al. Childhood abuse, neglect, and household dysfunction and the risk of illicit drug use: the Adverse Childhood Experiences study. Pediatrics 2003;111(3):564–72.

6. American Psychiatric Association. Diagnostic and statistical manual of mental disorders, 5th edition. Washington, DC: American Psychiatric Press; 2013.

7. Copeland W, Keeler G, Angold A, et al. Traumatic events and posttraumatic stress in childhood. Arch Gen Psychiatry 2007;64(5):577–84.

8. Cook A, Blaustein M, Spinazzola J, et al. Complex trauma in children and adolescents: a white paper. National Child Traumatic Stress Network; Complex Trauma Task Force; 2002. Available at: www.nctsnet.org/nctsn_assets/pdfs/edu_materials/ComplexTrauma_All.pdf. Accessed October 20, 2015.

9. Ford JD, Elhai J, Connor D, et al. Poly-victimization and risk of post traumatic, depressive and substance use disorders and involvement in delinquency in a national sample of adolescents. J Adolesc Health 2010;45(6):545–52.

10. Giaconia R, Reinherz H, Carmola Hauf A, et al. Comorbidity of substance use and post-traumatic stress disorders in a community sample of adolescents. Am J Orthopsychiatry 2000;70(2):253–62.

11. Cohen J, Mannarino A, Zhitova A, et al. Treating child abuse-related posttraumatic stress and comorbid substance abuse in adolescents. Child Abuse Negl 2003;27:1345–65.

12. National Child Traumatic Stress Network. Making the connection: trauma and substance abuse 2008. Available at: www.nctsn.org/sites/default/files/assets/pdfs/SAToolkit_1.pdf. Accessed September 30, 2015.

13. Kingston S, Chitra R. Relationship of sexual abuse, early initiation of substance use, and adolescent trauma to PTSD. J Trauma Stress 2009;22(1):65–8.

14. Brown P, Wolf J. Substance abuse and post-traumatic stress disorder comorbidity. Drug Alcohol Depend 1994;35:51–9.

15. Weinberg N. Risk factors for adolescent substance abuse. J Learn Disabil 2001; 34(4):343–51.

16. Anda R, Whitfield C, Felitti V, et al. Adverse childhood experiences, alcoholic parents, and later risk of alcoholism and depression. Psychiatr Serv 2002;53(8): 1001–9.

17. Suarez L, Belcher H, Briggs E, et al. Supporting the need for an integrated system of care for youth with co-occurring traumatic stress and substance abuse problems. Am J Community Psychol 2012;49:430–40.

18. Saladin M, Drobes D, Coffe S, et al. PTSD symptom severity as a predictor of cue-elicited drug cravings in victims of violent crimes. Addict Behav 2003;28: 1611–29.

19. Coffey S, Schumacher J, Stasiewicz P, et al. Craving and physiological reactivity to trauma and alcohol cues in posttraumatic stress disorder and alcohol dependence. Exp Clin Psychopharmacol 2010;18(4):340–9.

20. Coffey S, Saladin M, Drobes D, et al. Trauma and substance cue reactivity in individuals with comorbid posttraumatic stress disorder and cocaine or alcohol dependence. Drug Alcohol Depend 2002;65:115–27.

21. Wilson K. The traumatic stress response in child maltreatment and resultant neuropsychological effects. Aggress Violent Beh 2011;16(2):87–97.

22. Brady K, Sinha R. Co-Occurring mental and substance use disorders: the neurobiological effects of chronic stress. Am J Psychiatry 2005;162(8):1483–93.

23. Sadowski C, Friedrich W. Psychometric properties of the trauma symptom checklist for children with psychiatrically hospitalized adolescents. Child Maltreat 2000; 5(4):364–72.

24. Steinberg A, Brymer M, Kim S, et al. Psychometric properties of the UCLA PTSD reaction index, part I. J Trauma Stress 2013;26(1):1–9.

25. Hamby S, Finkelhor D, Ormrod R, et al. The Juvenile Victimization Questionnaire (JVQ): administration and scoring manual. Durham (NH): Crimes Against Children Research Center; 2005.

26. Review of Child and Adolescent Trauma Screening Tools. Available at: www.childsworld.ca.gov/res/pdf/KatieA/ChildAdolescentTraumaScreenTools.pdf. Accessed September 30, 2015.

27. Knight JR, Sherritt L, Shrier L, et al. Validity of the CRAFFT substance abuse screening test among adolescent clinic patients. Arch Pediatr Adolesc Med 2002;156(6):607–14.

28. Kirisci L, Mezzich A, Tarter R. Norms and sensitivity of the adolescent version of the drug use screening inventory. Addict Behav 1995;20(2):149–57.
29. Winters K, Kaminer Y. Screening and assessing adolescent substance use disorders in clinical populations. J Am Acad Child Adolesc Psychiatry 2008;47(7): 740–4.
30. Santisteban DA, Tejeda M, Dominicis C, et al. An efficient tool for screening for maladaptive family functioning in adolescent drug abusers: the problem oriented screening instrument for teenagers. Am J Drug Alcohol Abuse 1999;25(2): 197–206.
31. Williams J, Smith D, An H, et al. Clinical outcomes of traumatized youth in adolescent substance abuse treatment: a longitudinal multisite study. J Psychoactive Drugs 2008;40(1):77–84.
32. Jaycox L, Ebener P, Damesek L, et al. Trauma exposure and retention in adolescent substance abuse treatment. J Trauma Stress 2004;17(2):113–21.
33. National Institute on Drug Abuse. Principles of adolescent substance use disorder treatment: a research based guide. Addictions medications 2014. Available at: www.drugabuse.gov/publications/principles-adolescent-substance-use-disor der-treatment-research-based-guide/evidence-based-approaches-to-treating-ad olescent-substance-use-disorders/addiction-medications. Accessed September 30, 2015.
34. Suárez L, Ellis B, Saxe G. Integrated treatment of traumatic stress and substance abuse problems among adolescents. In: Ehrenreich-May J, Chu B, editors. Transdiagnostic treatments for children and adolescents. New York: Guilford Press; 2013. p. 339–62.
35. National Child Traumatic Stress Network. Treatment for youth with traumatic stress and substance abuse problems. 2008. Available at: www.nctsnet.org/ nctsn_assets/pdfs/SAToolkit_4.pdf. Accessed September 30, 2015.

Substance Use Among College Students

Chloe R. Skidmore, MS, Erin A. Kaufman, MS, Sheila E. Crowell, PhD*

KEYWORDS

- Substance use • College students • Risk factors • Transition to college • Review

KEY POINTS

- Substance use is a significant problem among college students and is associated with a host of consequences, including increased risk of mortality.
- Important differences exist between college students and their non–college-attending peers with regard to rates and types of substance use.
- Athletes, students associated with Greek organizations, sexual minorities, those who suffer from depression and/or anxiety, and white men seem to be at particular risk for substance use during college.

INTRODUCTION

Substance use is among the most critical problems facing college students in the United States.[1,2] Recent epidemiologic research indicates approximately 26% of male and 19.2% of female full-time college students report current illicit drug use.[3] Alcohol use on college campuses has also been a significant concern for decades[1] and current estimates indicate that most college students engage in this behavior (79%).[4] Although certain substances have recently decreased in popularity (eg, cigarette smoking), the rates of many other substances have remained stable or increased over time. For example, daily marijuana use in 2014 was at its highest rate since 1980[4] and nonmedical use of prescription drugs has increased substantially in recent years.[5,6] Though substance use is widely considered to be a normative part of the college experience and most students will outgrow drug use and heavy drinking without treatment,[7] such behavior is far from benign. Although college students are less likely to develop substance use disorders than their non–college-attending peers, the consequences of substance use are significant. Substance use in college students is

The contents of this article have not been published elsewhere, nor are they being submitted simultaneously for publication via another outlet. The authors have obtained approval from all coauthors for submitting the article and there are no conflicts of interest to report.
Department of Psychology, University of Utah, 380 South 1530 East, Room 502, Salt Lake City, UT 84112, USA
* Corresponding author.
E-mail address: sheila.crowell@psych.utah.edu

Child Adolesc Psychiatric Clin N Am 25 (2016) 735–753
http://dx.doi.org/10.1016/j.chc.2016.06.004
1056-4993/16/© 2016 Elsevier Inc. All rights reserved.
childpsych.theclinics.com

associated with poor academic performance (eg, lower class attendance and grades), unintentional injuries, health problems, heightened rates of engagement in other risky behaviors (eg, unprotected sex), legal problems, increased risk of substance use and abuse in adulthood, and mortality.[1,8]

This article reviews current evidence surrounding substance use among college students, presents statistics regarding the use of specific substances, and discusses differences between college-attending emerging adults and their non–college-attending peers. Risk and protective factors, substance use in special populations of college students, and the current status of prevention and intervention programs aimed at this population are highlighted. Alcohol use is emphasized because it is consistently cited as a critical problem among college students and because it has been studied more extensively than other substances. In most studies, college students are defined as individuals who are 1 to 4 years after high school and who are attending a 2-year or 4-year institution full time.[4]

EPIDEMIOLOGY OF SPECIFIC DRUGS IN COLLEGE STUDENTS

Although alcohol is the most commonly used substance among college students, a variety of other drugs are also used during this developmental period.[1] The following section describes the epidemiology of alcohol use, tobacco, marijuana, prescription medications, and other drugs. Statistics are largely gleaned from the 2014 report of the Monitoring the Future National Survey on Drug Use.[4] This nationally representative study surveyed eighth, tenth, and twelfth grade high school students, as well as college students and young adults in the United States.[4] Current statistics for past year, past month, and daily use (when available) can be found in **Table 1**.

Alcohol

Alcohol use is the greatest contributor to morbidity and mortality among college students.[1,9] It is associated with more than 1400 deaths, 600,000 assaults, 70,000 to 100,000 sexual assaults, and 500,000 injuries annually on college campuses.[8,10–12] These estimates are believed to be conservative.[11] Motor vehicle crashes represent a leading cause of death among people 15 to 24 years old and approximately half of these crashes are thought to be related to alcohol use.[11] Although there was an 8% proportional decline in the number of students who reported drinking and driving between 2002 and 2005,[13] 38.9% of college students reported riding in the past month with a driver who had consumed alcohol.[11]

Heavy drinking is normative during college.[14] In fact, most college students cite "getting drunk" as their primary reason for drinking,[15] with 60.5% of surveyed students reporting becoming drunk at least once in the past year.[4] Many students endorse heavy episodic (ie, binge) drinking,[16] which is defined as 5 or more drinks in a single drinking session for male students, and 4 or more drinks in a session for female students.[4,11] Binge drinking often results in dangerously high blood alcohol content due to ingesting large quantities of alcohol in short periods of time.[17] Researchers have estimated that 10% to 20% of first-year college students drink alcohol at levels twice that of the heavy drinking threshold.[18] Furthermore, engaging in binge drinking is associated with illicit drug use.[1,8] The more days per month a student engages in binge drinking, the higher the odds for using other substance use as well.[1] Binge drinking is associated with numerous individual characteristics, including male gender and white race.[1] Upwards of 31% of the 8 million current college students in the United States meet diagnostic criteria for alcohol abuse.[19]

Table 1
Prevalence of specific substance use among college students in 2014

	Past Year (%)	Past 30 Days (%)	Daily Use (%)
Alcohol	76.1	63.1	4.3
Binge Drinking	35.0	—	—
Any Illicit Drug	38.6	22.7	—
Not Including Marijuana	20.8	10.0	—
Marijuana	34.4	20.8	5.9
Synthetic Marijuana	0.9	0.0	—
Inhalants	1.3	0.3	—
Hallucinogens	4.0	1.0	—
LSD	2.2	0.5	—
Other than LSD	3.2	0.7	—
MDMA (Ecstasy)	5.0	1.4	—
Salvia	1.1	—	—
Cocaine	4.4	1.8	—
Crack	0.8	0.1	—
Other Cocaine	4.1	1.8	—
Heroin	0.0	0.0	—
Narcotics Other Than Heroin	4.8	1.2	—
OxyContin	1.3	—	—
Vicodin	2.8	—	—
Amphetamines	10.1	4.8	—
Ritalin	1.6	—	—
Adderall	9.6	—	—
Bath Salts	0.2	—	—
Methamphetamine	0.1	0.1	—
Crystal Methamphetamine	0.0	0.0	—
Sedatives (Barbiturates)	3.1	0.7	—
Tranquilizers	3.5	1.7	—
GHB	0.2	—	—
Ketamine	0.1	—	—
Cigarettes	22.6	12.9	5.2
E-Cigarettes	—	—	9.7
Steroids	0.5	0.0	—

Abbreviations: GHB, γ-hydroxybutyric acid; LSD, lysergic acid diethylamide; MDMA, 3,4-methylenedioxymethamphetamine.

Data from Johnston LD, O'Malley PM, Bachman JG, et al. Monitoring the future national survey results on drug use, 1975–2014: volume 2, college students and adults ages 19–55. Ann Arbor (MI): Institute for Social Research; The University of Michigan; 2015.

Most students tend to mature out of binge drinking behaviors,[20,21] evidenced by lower levels of binge drinking among graduate students[2] and a lower frequency of alcohol-related negative consequences after the first year of college.[22] Still, binge drinking during college is predictive of problematic drinking 7 years after college.[22] Use continues to escalate into adulthood for a sizable proportion of individuals.[23,24]

Tobacco

There has been an appreciable decline in cigarette smoking since 1997, with both annual and 30-day estimates declining in 2014 from the most recent peak of 31% 30-day prevalence in 1999.[4] Importantly, there is a strong relationship between the initiation of smoking and past year alcohol use.[25] White female students who are in their first year of college and have college-educated parents seem to be the most likely among college students to smoke cigarettes.[25] Use of cigarettes tends to persist over time, with 1 study finding that 62% of college men who endorsed smoking cigarettes during their freshman year still smoked in their senior year.[26] Likewise, this same study found that nearly 33% of college men who smoked also used smokeless tobacco products (eg, snus) and, though not statistically significant, the concurrent use of smokeless tobacco and cigarettes was associated with higher rates of continued cigarette use during participants' senior year.[26] Similarly, another recent study found that 49.4% of their college sample had tried some form of tobacco, with 38% endorsing the use of hookah.[27] Although alternative forms of tobacco, such as hookah and e-cigarettes, are increasingly popular, it does not seem that using these products increases the likelihood of use of cigarettes or smokeless tobacco.[27]

Marijuana

Although the overall prevalence of marijuana use among college students has somewhat unexpectedly declined since 1999, rates of daily marijuana use have increased over the past 7 years.[4] Marijuana use increases throughout college, with nearly 40% of students endorsing marijuana use before college, 50% using marijuana during their first year, and 60% using by their sophomore year.[8]

Illicit Drugs Other than Marijuana

The use of marijuana tends to drive statistics for illicit drug use among college students, causing overall rates of illicit drug use to seem quite high in this population.[4] Thus, it is necessary to examine other forms of illicit drug use separate from marijuana. See **Table 1** for a breakdown of annual and past 30-day use statistics for illicit drugs, including and excluding marijuana.

Prescription Drugs

Nonmedical use of prescription medications has become a significant problem in the United States,[4,5] with particularly high rates among college students.[28,29] A 2008 study reported that 19.6% of students had used prescription drugs (stimulants, analgesics, or both) nonmedically in their lifetime, and 15.6% had used these drugs in the past year.[5] Although nonmedical use of prescription analgesics is even more common in high school students, stimulants account for the most commonly misused prescription drug in college students.[8] One study found that more than 1 in 5 students have misused prescription stimulants by their sophomore year of college.[8] Nonmedical use of prescription stimulants is strongly correlated with use of other substances, such as cigarettes, alcohol, and illicit drugs,[29] and with engaging in other risk behaviors.[30] Following stimulants, narcotics are the next most commonly misused prescription medication, followed by tranquilizers and sedatives.[4]

A significant percentage of those who use prescription stimulants go on to develop both problem use and dependence.[31,32] Students often endorse nonmedical use of prescription drugs for the purposes of weight loss and pain control,[33] in addition to getting high and for experimentation.[29] One study found that high levels of academic strain, especially when associated with increased negative affect, was correlated with misuse of prescription drugs.[6] The nonmedical use of prescription medication is associated with engagement in binge drinking, use of ecstasy and marijuana,[34–39] being white and male gender,[30] having a higher family income,[29] attending a more competitive school, and being involved in fraternities or sororities.[30] Furthermore, nonmedical use of prescription stimulants and analgesics is also associated with academic disengagement, such as less time studying, skipping classes, and lower grade point averages.[5,30] Importantly, most college students report obtaining prescription medications from their peers and friends.[40]

COMPARING COLLEGE STUDENTS WITH PEERS NOT IN COLLEGE

A primary goal of the research exploring substance use among college students has been to determine whether these individuals deviate from their age-matched peers. Are late adolescence and emerging adulthood (typically defined as ages18 to 24 years) associated generally with increased substance use, or is there is a specific susceptibility associated with college attendance? Because both college students and their non–college-attending peers engage in heavy alcohol use, some have argued that substance use is a matter of life stage in this group.[41] However, there are aspects of use that distinguish college attendees from nonstudents.[10]

College students in the United States and in other parts of the world generally show lower levels of substance use compared with their non–college-attending peers, although findings have been mixed in some ways.[42] However, college students show higher rates of heavy alcohol consumption, such as binge drinking.[2,10,11,43] Although college students are not at greater risk for alcohol dependence than nonstudents, they suffer other consequences associated with binge drinking more frequently.[10] For example, study using a large representative national sample found that 18% of college students in the United States were suffering from clinically significant alcohol-related problems compared with 15% of their noncollege peers.[10] Notably, a recent study did not find any differences in the quantity or frequency of alcohol consumption between students and nonstudents.[7] Likewise, although nonstudents have historically had higher rates of daily drinking than students,[43] this trend was not sustained in 2014, with students and nonstudents drinking daily at similar rates (approximately 4%).[4] With regard to other substances, college students have consistently been found to use cigarettes, marijuana, and other illicit drugs at rates lower than that of their noncollege peers.[2,4,7]

DEVELOPMENTAL AND INDIVIDUAL CORRELATES OF SUBSTANCE USE

To better understand who is at highest risk for substance-related problems, individual characteristics and developmental factors associated with this behavior must be examined. Such efforts will aid in prevention and intervention efforts.

Transition from High School to College

Research indicates that the transition out of high school, rather than the transition into college, is associated with risk for substance use initiation.[7] Although increased risk for substance use is associated with moving out of high school generally, there are significant differences between those who enter a college setting versus those who do not. For some, exiting high school into an outside-college setting is associated with chronic substance use and associated consequences. In contrast, substance use associated with transitioning from high school into college is typically more time-limited.[7] In high school, college-bound students are less likely to use substances than their classmates who are not collegebound.[9,44] Nevertheless, after graduation, alcohol and marijuana use in college-bound students actually exceeds that of their nonstudent peers.[21] That said, high levels of alcohol consumption in high school are predictive of alcohol use during the first year of college.[45]

The move from high school to college represents a period of significant transition.[46,47] Adolescents often leave family and friends, develop new social networks,[48] live with increased independence, have more academic opportunities and demands, and have significantly less parental support and monitoring.[7] Major developmental tasks are occurring during this period and emerging adults are particularly susceptible to peer influence.[42] New environments and demands are associated with higher stress, depression, and lower self-esteem. Thus, students are at increased vulnerability for engagement in risky behaviors.[15] As such, this transition seems to be associated with increased substance use.[7]

Initiation of Drug Use in College

Initial exposure to and initiation of substance use often takes places in college, particularly in the first year.[8] Many students who either consumed alcohol minimally or abstained entirely during high school go on to increase their alcohol consumption after graduation.[49] Upwards of 40% to 50% of students who did not drink in high school will begin drinking during their first year of college.[49] Likewise, nearly 25% of student who abstained from binge drinking in high school will begin drinking at binge levels during their first year.[49] Beyond alcohol, a prospective study of 1253 college students found that nonmedical use of prescription stimulants was most likely to be initiated during college but that use often wanes with time. In contrast, marijuana is the drug most often initiated and maintained throughout the college years.[8] Students who endorse use of cocaine and nonmedical use of prescription stimulants also tend to show low rates of cessation.[8] Importantly, a large proportion of students cease drug use by their sophomore year of college,[8] indicating particular risk during the first year of college.

First-year College Students

Emerging adults are in a unique position of balancing their newfound independence and establishing social contacts while maintaining their safety.[7] Such priorities are often in competition. First-year students are most likely to socialize in contexts that include alcohol use because they make up the largest percentage of attendees at dormitory and fraternity parties.[50] Indeed, alcohol consumption increases substantially during the first year and many begin drinking heavily soon after arriving on campus.[9,16] First-year students are more likely than older students to participate in drinking games that are associated with high-volume alcohol consumption.[51] First-year college students are also most likely to engage in disruptive behaviors while drinking and visit the emergency room for alcohol-related injuries or illnesses.[9] Although first-year students typically make up approximately one-fourth of the student body, they represent one-third of all deaths on campus, many of which are related to alcohol consumption.[52]

Gender

By and large, men are more likely than women to engage in substance use and they also use with higher frequency.[4] Male college students tend to consume more alcohol during their first year of college, binge drink more often, and are at heightened risk for escalating alcohol use into adulthood compared with female college students.[2,9,16,53] College men are thought to suffer from alcohol-related problems at higher rates than women, with 1 study using a large representative national college sample finding that 24% of men and 13% of women endorsed such problems.[10] However, some studies have found that the gender divide is less pronounced in college students compared with their nonstudent peers. Some have reported that college men and women endorse equivalent levels of alcohol problems and similar levels of intoxication.[54–56] Regarding other substances, men generally use illicit drugs and misuse prescription stimulants at higher rates than women.[4,30] However, women are more likely to smoke cigarettes compared with men.[25]

Peer Influence

Peer influence is a significant factor affecting substance use in college students.[57] One study found that men who were randomly assigned to a roommate who also engaged in binge drinking in high school were most likely to engage in further binge drinking during college.[21] In addition to direct peer influence, perception of peers' substance use is equally influential. Indeed, the perception that substance use is normative increases risk for initiating and maintaining substance use in college students.[7] Unfortunately, students consistently overestimate both their peers' subjective approval of substance use and how much their peers actually use.[1,21,57,58] That said, substance use in college is typical, even if to a lesser extent than students' perception.[14] Not surprisingly peer norms are most influential for first-year college students.[59]

Many students use alcohol to facilitate social interactions, and using it for this purpose is associated with high levels of use.[7,9,60] Social motives for alcohol use (eg, fitting in, increasing one's sense of belonging) are strongly associated with drinking during the first year of college. Heavy drinking is associated with peer acceptance during freshman year.[9,61] Drinking games are popular during this developmental stage and, as stated previously, are associated consistently with higher levels of alcohol consumption.[51,62] Such games also correlated with first-year alcohol use and are understandably highly influenced by social context.[9]

Personality Characteristics

Numerous individual-level characteristics affect substance use behavior. Lower scores on the Big Five traits of conscientiousness and agreeableness have been found among college students who endorse heavy use of substances, as opposed to their moderately using and abstaining counterparts.[63] Likewise, the Behavioral Activation Scales subscales of Fun Seeking (desire for and impulsive approach to rewards) and, to a lesser extent, Drive (pursuit of goals) are associated with the number of illicit substances used, quantity of alcohol use, and the frequency of binge drinking.[64] Sensation seeking is also consistently related to heavy drinking in college (particularly the first year) and heightened alcohol use over time.[16,18] Ruiz and colleagues[65] provided a succinct personality profile of college students most likely to use alcohol, noting these individuals tend to be low in conscientiousness and high in impulsivity, sensation-seeking, and negative affect. Somewhat distinct personality trait constellations may be associated with drug preference. For example, high levels of novelty-seeking and lower levels of persistence are predictive of marijuana use in college students.[66]

From a trait perspective, emotional lability, impulsivity, and conditions characterized by high levels of these traits are associated with substance use problems.[67] Emotional instability and difficulties with affect regulation are associated with cigarette smoking,[25] as well as alcohol use, abuse, and dependence, in college students.[25,42] Among those who engage in suicidal and nonsuicidal self-injurious behaviors, higher rates of these behaviors are associated with higher levels of drug use (particularly marijuana), compared with those who engage in self-injury and binge drink but do not use other drugs, and those who self-injure but do not use drugs or binge drink.[68]

With regard to other characteristics associated with substance use, Borsari and colleagues[9] found that coping strategies correlate with alcohol use during the first year of college. Students who cited coping as a reason for drinking are more likely to engage in binge drinking and heavy alcohol use in general.[69,70] Interestingly, Magid and colleagues[71] found that coping motives may mediate the association between impulsivity and alcohol use, with impulsivity itself not influencing drinking behaviors in the absence of a need for quick relief from unpleasant circumstances or emotions. Additionally, negative self-image has been found to relate to heavy alcohol use in first-year college students[61] and negative life events predict alcohol use in first-year students.[72]

Interactions Between Other Psychiatric Conditions and Substance Use

Psychiatric conditions, such as mood and anxiety disorders, are highly comorbid with substance use disorders and existing mental health conditions often exacerbate substance use problems.[2,73] Substance use is often associated with more severe disorders that tend to be chronic in nature, place the individual at higher risk for suicide, and are associated with greater functional impairment.[2] Some scholars theorize that high rates of co-occurrence may reflect attempts to self-medicate.[74] For example, negative mood and major depression have been associated with frequent marijuana use, higher rates of cigarette smoking, and lower frequency of binge drinking.[2,25] Generalized anxiety disorder (GAD) and panic disorder are associated with high rates of cigarette smoking, and GAD is additionally associated with higher likelihood of binge drinking.[2] Incoming college students who acknowledged a history of panic attacks are more likely to report lifetime use of sedatives, stimulants, and opioids compared with their peers without panic disorder.[74] Finally, a childhood diagnosis of attention-deficit/hyperactivity disorder is associated with higher rates of substance use in general.[75]

Importantly, although Cranford and colleagues[2] found that 67% of college students in their sample engaged frequently in binge drinking, endorsed mental health problems, and perceived a need for psychological help, only 38% had obtained services in the year prior. This suggests that close to half of college students struggling with such problems are not receiving intervention.

Engagement in Other Risky Behaviors

Substance use during college is strongly associated with engagement in a variety of other risky behaviors,[76,77] particularly risky sexual choices. Male and female students who endorse heavy drinking are 2 to 3 times more likely than their peers who are not heavy drinkers to have multiple sexual partners.[78,79] Number of sexual partners is also related to higher rates of use of marijuana,[36] 3,4-methylenedioxymethamphetamine (MDMA),[38] and methamphetamine.[80] Level of alcohol use is predictive of sexual involvement. For example, the likelihood that a female college student is sexually active is predicted by whether or not he or she has ever been drunk.[77] The use of alcohol in sexual situations (eg, on a date) increases the likelihood that the student will have sex and decreases the likelihood of a conversation about risks and protection.[77] Risk for engaging in violence is also heightened by the use of both alcohol and methamphetamines.[80] In addition, heavy alcohol use has been found to moderate the relation between presence of a mood disorder and proneness to suicide.[81] Though not specific to college students, cigarette smoking is also associated with increased risk for completed suicide.[82]

SPECIAL POPULATIONS
Athletes

There is considerable evidence that college athletes use substances at higher rates than their nonathlete peers.[83] Though it can be argued that the potential for negative consequences is greater for student athletes than nonathletes (eg, random drug testing, negative effect on performance[84]), high levels of stress associated with college athletic involvement may increase the use of substances for coping purposes.[83] Studies suggest that cigarette smoking and illicit drug use is less likely to occur in college athletes,[83] yet binge drinking is significantly more common in this population.[85] Green and colleagues[84] found that athletes in Division I athletic teams endorsed the lowest levels of substance use; whereas athletes in Division III systems endorsed the highest levels of use of marijuana, alcohol, and amphetamines. This is perhaps unsurprising, given that higher division athletes likely have more to lose by substance use engagement.

Fraternity or Sorority Involvement

Greek membership during college is also associated with heightened engagement in binge drinking and more tolerant views regarding alcohol use.[1,9] Increased drinking is associated with joining a sorority or fraternity, although alcohol use decreases when students are no longer a part of these systems. Students involved in fraternities and sororities are more likely than those not involved in these groups to use alcohol as a means for social activity and establishing friendships.[9] Additionally, members of sororities and fraternities consistently report using nonmedical prescription stimulants and analgesics, as well as higher rates of other drugs.[30,36,39,86] The combination of choosing to be part of a Greek organization (ie, selection) and the social atmosphere of Greek systems seem to influence the phenomenon of high levels of substance use in fraternities and sororities.[45]

Sexual Minorities

Sexual minority status is generally associated with higher rates of substance use disorders and other mental disorders, such as depression, panic attacks, and generalized anxiety disorder.[42,87,88] This association is thought to be the result of a variety of factors, including minority stress,[89] experiences of heterosexism, and internalized homophobia.[90] Interestingly, a study found that female college students with a history of partners of both sexes were twice as likely as those with a history of opposite-sex or same-sex partners only to engage in cigarette smoking, binge drinking, and marijuana use.[91] In contrast, male college students with partners of both sexes were shown to be less likely to engage in heavy drinking compared with those with opposite-sex partners only. Coping with social stress or an increased tendency to experiment with risky behaviors were presented as possible interpretations of these findings.[91]

Racial and Ethnic Minorities

Research indicates that white students generally engage in higher levels of substance use compared with their racial and ethnic minority counterparts. White students are most likely to engage in binge drinking, followed by Hispanic students, with black students being the least likely to binge drink.[1] White students are also more likely than students of other races to smoke cigarettes.[25] Although Hispanic adolescents tend to initiate substance use earlier than those of other ethnicities, white adolescents and young adults use substances at the greatest level throughout the college years.[92]

There are, however, significant risk factors associated with racial and ethnic minority status. The experience of minority stress, which results from identifying as part of a stigmatized group that is subject to discrimination and prejudice, is a common experience among racial and ethnic minority students who attend predominantly White universities.[93] The experience of minority stress is associated with increased depressive symptoms[93] and perceived racism in general is associated with poorer mental health.[94] Indeed, 1 recent study found that higher numbers of microaggressions experienced was related to higher rates of binge drinking among ethnic minority college students.[95]

PROTECTIVE FACTORS FOR SUBSTANCE USE IN COLLEGE STUDENTS

Unfortunately, relatively little research has explored factors that protect against substance abuse among college students. Two consistently identified factors are religiosity or spirituality and effective parental involvement. Borsari and colleagues[9] found a negative correlation between degree of religiosity and alcohol consumption. Likewise, spirituality was found to affect the decision of whether or not to use alcohol (any consumption and binge drinking) and marijuana.[96] Importantly, depth of religious commitment (ie, living in accordance to one's religious beliefs) seems more predictive of reduced alcohol consumption than mere religious involvement (eg, church attendance).[97]

Although college students typically gain increased independence, parental influence remains important for substance use decisions.[9] Indeed, peers seem less influential over college students whose parents had previously set stringent rules around alcohol use[9] and for those who endorse feeling strongly influenced by their parents.[18,98] Likewise, attitudes regarding alcohol consumption and subsequent alcohol-related behaviors of college students correlate with parental attitudes and behaviors.[99,100] Importantly, fewer alcohol-related negative consequences are reported among students who have high quality parent-child relationships. This is particularly salient for father-son relationships.[101]

PREVENTION AND INTERVENTION

Given the high percentages of substance use among college students, effective prevention and intervention programs are clearly needed. Although numerous programs exist (for instance, all 747 university administrators surveyed in a study endorsed alcohol abuse prevention efforts on their campuses),[102] only 49% of students surveyed in a nationwide sample reported receiving prevention information about alcohol and other drug use from their university.[1] Although the literature in this area is relatively scant, prevention programs seem to struggle to effectively thwart substance use among college students. For example, e-TOKE is a computerized prevention program aimed at correcting norms and preventing marijuana use via assessment and feedback regarding students' risk factors and understanding of marijuana use norms.[103] Examination of this program found that, although norms were indeed corrected among participants, rates of marijuana initiation did not differ between the intervention group and controls who received only the assessment of risks but no feedback.[103] Similarly, although expectancy challenges have been used successfully in decreasing alcohol use (see later discussion), the same effect was not seen in a study examining nonmedical use of prescription stimulants.[104] As in the e-TOKE program, participants reported more negative expectancies associated with stimulant use, yet rates of use were comparable to those of a control group 6 months later.[104]

Meta-analyses of intervention programs targeted at alcohol use find that risk reduction programs generally result in less alcohol consumption and fewer alcohol-related negative consequences among college students.[102] Specifically, individual-level interventions focused on cognitive-behavioral skills and brief motivational interviews have been shown to be particularly efficacious.[105] Cognitive-behavioral skills-based interventions for alcohol use are wide-ranging, with some focusing exclusively on alcohol-related information and skills (eg, drink refusal), and others incorporating numerous additional components, such as general life skills (eg, time and stress management[105]). Alcohol-specific interventions, such as those implemented by Darkes and Goldman,[106,107] found that engaging heavy-drinking male college students in expectancy challenges significantly decreased alcohol use at 2-week[106,107] and 6-week[107] follow-ups. Likewise, studies that asked college student participants to self-monitor their drinking over various periods of time (eg, spring break[108]) found statistically significant decreases in alcohol consumption compared with controls in alcohol education groups[109] as well as fewer negative alcohol-related consequences compared with controls.[108]

Multicomponent interventions have shown particularly strong results.[110] Specifically, those interventions that contain 4 or more components, including personalized feedback, as well as strategies for moderating alcohol consumption, have been shown to be most effective in reducing consumption and problems associated with alcohol in first-year college students compared with other modes of intervention.[110] For example, reductions in alcohol use were seen when fraternity pledges engaged in self-monitoring and were educated regarding alcohol moderation and blood alcohol content, as well as trained in assertiveness skills such as drink refusal.[109] Similar results were seen among college students who took part in an intervention that included assertiveness training, life-balance skills, relaxation techniques, and psychoeducation regarding pacing and setting limits on alcohol consumption.[111]

Significant evidence points to the effectiveness of brief motivational interventions with regard to alcohol use in college students. Dimeff and colleagues[112] created a manualized treatment, Brief Alcohol Screening and Intervention for College Students (BASICS). This intervention includes approximately 2 weeks of tracking daily alcohol consumption before a 50-minute face-to-face interview in which participants are given feedback using a motivational interview style in which content is based on their personal alcohol consumption. Specifically, BASICS sessions include evaluation of alcohol use patterns, comparison of those patterns to actual and perceived campus alcohol use norms, and a review of the effects of alcohol, as well as the individual's experienced consequences from alcohol use, and a review of placebo and tolerance effects of alcohol. In addition, BASICS participants are given handouts with strategies for reduction of alcohol use and a card allowing them to estimate their blood alcohol content based on their gender and weight. Importantly, a recent study[113] found that both volunteer students and students mandated to treatment as a result of breaking campus substance use policies benefitted from BASICS participation. Specifically, results showed significant reductions in weekly alcohol consumption and peak alcohol consumption, and overall reduction in alcohol use and alcohol-related problems that were sustained for 12 months.[113] Earlier studies using similar protocols also found statistically significant reductions in alcohol consumption and alcohol-related negative consequences for up to 2 years.[114] Likewise, these programs have shown declines in heavy drinking episodes[115] and reduction in peak blood alcohol content among fraternity and sorority members.[116]

A similar intervention strategy aimed at reducing marijuana use among college students found similar results to those targeting alcohol use.[117] After completing a survey regarding marijuana use, students participated in a 1-hour in-person feedback session that included a graphic illustration of their individual marijuana use, which included information such as frequency, quantity, and timing of use, as well as a review of self-reported reasons for use, consequences in multiple life domains, estimates of the amount of money spent on marijuana and associated paraphernalia (as well as alternative uses of the same amount of money), costs and benefits of reducing or ceasing use, family history risk, and an exploration of the effect of marijuana use on the participant's social network as well as on his or her goals for the following year.[118] Compared with controls who received only the assessment but not the in-person feedback, target participants reported decreased weekly marijuana use at 3-month follow-up. Although these participants used marijuana for the same number of days as their control counterparts, they smoked fewer joints overall. However, observed differences were no longer evident at 6-month follow-up.

Overall, a recent meta-analysis[110] suggests that receiving personalized feedback, though higher in financial and time costs, is a particularly effective intervention component, as are providing strategies for moderating use and challenging expectancies. Importantly, a review found that interventions seem to be less effective for students in highest-risk groups, such as college athletics or fraternities and sororities.[102] Because alcohol and other substances may function uniquely in these groups (eg, more overtly social purposes),[117] they may require customized prevention and intervention efforts tailored more specifically to these students.[102]

SUMMARY

College is a time of increased risk for problem behaviors, including substance use. Indeed, college students in the United States engage in heavy alcohol consumption, marijuana use, and nonmedical use of prescription drugs at alarmingly high rates, along with lower but significant rates of other types of drugs. College substance use is associated with a host of negative consequences from legal problems and academic difficulties to increased rates of injury and death. Furthermore, drug and alcohol use are associated with engagement in other risky behaviors and worsening mental health problems. White male college students seem to be at particularly high risk for substance use, in addition to individuals who endorse high impulsivity and sensation-seeking traits. Sexual minority students, college athletes, those involved in the Greek systems, and students in their first year of college are also at increased risk for substance use. Although the rates of substance use are high in late adolescence and emerging adulthood generally, use is not equivalent between college students and their non–college-attending peers. Indeed, although college students tend to use fewer substances than those who are not students, overall, they are more likely to binge drink, which is associated with adverse consequences. Most college campuses provide prevention and intervention programs at the group and individual level, and meta-analyses suggest that many of these interventions, particularly those that are cognitive-behavioral skills-based and brief motivational in nature, are quite effective both in the short term and long term. However, it seems that these programs may not reach students at hoped-for rates. It is imperative that prevention and intervention efforts are continually honed for this high-risk population.

REFERENCES

1. Jones SE, Oeltmann J, Wilson TW, et al. Binge drinking among undergraduate college students in the United States: implications for other substance use. J Am Coll Health 2001;50(1):33–8.

2. Cranford JA, Eisenberg D, Serras AM. Substance use behaviors, mental health problems, and use of mental health services in a probability sample of college students. Addict Behav 2009;34(2):134–45.

3. Substance Abuse and Mental Health Services Administration. Results from the 2013 National Survey on Drug Use and Health: Summary of National Findings, NSDUH Series H-48, HHS Publication No. (SMA) 14–4863. 2014. Available at: http://www.samhsa.gov/data/sites/default/files/NSDUHresultsPDFWHTML2013/Web/NSDUHresults2013.pdf. Accessed October 23, 2015.

4. Johnston LD, O'Malley PM, Bachman JG, et al. Monitoring the Future national survey results on drug use, 1975-2014: volume 2, College students and adults ages 19–55. Ann Arbor (MI): Institute for Social Research, The University of Michigan; 2015.

5. Arria AM, O'Grady KE, Caldeira KM, et al. Nonmedical use of prescription stimulants and analgesics: associations with social and academic behaviors among college students. J Drug Issues 2008;38(4):1045–60.

6. Ford JA, Schroeder RD. Academic strain and non-medical use of prescription stimulants among college students. Deviant Behav 2008;30(1):26–53.

7. White HR, Labouvie EW, Papadaratsakis V. Changes in substance use during the transition to adulthood: a comparison of college students and their noncollege age peers. J Drug Issues 2005;35(2):281–306.

8. Arria AM, Caldeira KM, O'Grady KE, et al. Drug exposure opportunities and use patterns among college students: results of a longitudinal prospective cohort study. Subst Abuse 2008;29(4):19–38.

9. Borsari B, Murphy JG, Barnett NP. Predictors of alcohol use during the first year of college: implications for prevention. Addict Behav 2007;32(10):2062–86.

10. Slutske WS. Alcohol use disorders among US college students and their non-college-attending peers. Arch Gen Psychiatry 2005;62(3):321–7.

11. Hingson RW, Heeren T, Zakocs RC, et al. Magnitude of alcohol-related mortality and morbidity among U.S. college students ages 18-24. J Stud Alcohol 2002;63(2):136–44.

12. Hingson RW, Heeren T, Winter M, et al. Magnitude of alcohol-related morbidity and mortality among U.S. college age students 18–24: changes from 1998–2001. Annu Rev Public Health 2005;26:259–79.

13. Hingson RW, Zha W, Weitzman ER. Magnitude of and trends in alcohol-related mortality and morbidity among U.S. college students ages 18–24, 1998–2005. J Stud Alcohol Drugs Suppl 2009;(Suppl 16):12–20.

14. Chen K, Kandel DB. The national history of drug use from adolescence to the mid-thirties in a general population sample. Am J Public Health 1995;85(1):41–7.

15. Jessor R, Costa FM, Krueger PM, et al. A developmental study of heavy episodic drinking among college students: the role of psychosocial and behavioral protective risk factors. J Stud Alcohol 2006;67(1):86–94.

16. Del Boca FK, Darkes J, Greenbaum PE, et al. Up close and personal: temporal variability in the drinking of individual college students during their first year. J Consult Clin Psychol 2004;72(2):155–64.

17. Fournier AK, Ehrhart IJ, Glindemann KE, et al. Intervening to decrease alcohol use at university parties: differential reinforcement of intoxication level. Behav Modif 2004;28(2):167–81.

18. White AM, Kraus CL, Swartzwelder HS. Many college freshman drink at levels far beyond the binge threshold. Alcohol Clin Exp Res 2006;30(6):1006–10.

19. Knight JR, Wechsler H, Kuo M, et al. Alcohol abuse and dependence among U.S. college students. J Stud Alcohol 2002;63(3):263–70.
20. Covault J, Tennen H, Armeli S, et al. Interactive effects of the serotonin transporter 5-HTTLPR polymorphism and stressful life events on college student drinking and drug use. Biol Psychiatry 2007;61(5):609–16.
21. Duncan GJ, Boisjoly J, Kremer M, et al. Peer effects in drug use and sex among college students. J Abnorm Child Psychol 2005;33(3):375–85.
22. O'Neill SE, Parra GR, Sher KJ. Clinical relevance of heavy drinking during the college years: cross-sectional and prospective perspectives. Psychol Addict Behav 2001;15(4):350–9.
23. Jackson KM, Sher KJ, Gotham HJ, et al. Transitioning into and out of large-effect drinking in young adulthood. J Abnorm Psychol 2001;110(3):378–91.
24. Jennison KM. The short-term effects and unintended long-term consequences of binge drinking in college: a 10 year follow-up study. Am J Drug Alcohol Abuse 2004;30(3):659–84.
25. Reed MB, Wang R, Shillington AM, et al. The relationship between alcohol use and cigarette smoking in a sample of undergraduate college students. Addict Behav 2007;32(3):449–64.
26. Wolfson M, Suerken CK, Egan KL, et al. The role of smokeless tobacco use in smoking persistence among male college students. Am J Drug Alcohol Abuse 2015;41(6):541–6.
27. Meier EM, Tackett AP, Miller MD, et al. Which nicotine products are gateways to regular use? Am J Prev Med 2015;48(1):S86–93.
28. Babcock Q, Byrne T. Student perceptions of methylphenidate abuse at a public liberal arts college. J Am Coll Health 2000;49(3):143–5.
29. Teter CJ, McCabe SE, Boyd CJ, et al. Illicit methylphenidate use in an undergraduate student sample: prevalence and risk factors. Pharmacotherapy 2003;23(5):609–17.
30. McCabe SE, Knight JR, Teter CJ, et al. Non-medical use of prescription stimulants among US college students: prevalence and correlates from a national survey. Addiction 2005;100(1):96–106.
31. Zacny J, Bigelow G, Compton P, et al. College on Problems of Drug Dependence taskforce on prescription opioid non-medical use and abuse: position statement. Drug Alcohol Depend 2003;69(3):215–32.
32. Simoni-Wastila L, Strickler G. Risk factors associated with problem use of prescription drugs. Am J Public Health 2004;94(2):1084–8.
33. Quintero G, Peterson J, Young B. An exploratory study of socio-cultural factors contributing to prescription drug misuse among college students. J Drug Issues 2006;36(4):903–31.
34. Cashin JA, Presley CA, Meilman PW. Alcohol use in the Greek system: follow the leader? J Stud Alcohol 1998;59(1):63–70.
35. Wechsler H, Lee JE, Kuo M, et al. College binge drinking in the 1990s: a continuing problem. Results of the Harvard school of public health 1999 college alcohol study. J Am Coll Health 2000;48(5):199–210.
36. Bell R, Wechsler H, Johnston LD. Correlates of college student marijuana use: results of a US national survey. Addiction 1997;92(5):571–81.
37. Gledhill-Hoyt J, Lee H, Strote J, et al. Increased use of marijuana and other illicit drugs at US colleges in the 1990s: results of three national surveys. Addiction 2000;95(11):1655–67.
38. Strote J, Lee JE, Wechsler H. Increasing MDMA use among college students: results of a national survey. J Adolesc Health 2001;31(4):64–72.

39. Yacoubian GS Jr. Correlates of ecstasy use among students surveyed through the 1997 College Alcohol study. J Drug Educ 2003;33(1):61–9.

40. McCabe SE, Teter CJ, Boyd CJ. Medical use, illicit use and diversion of prescription stimulant medication. J Psychoactive Drugs 2006;38(1):43–56.

41. Jackson KM, Sher KJ, Park A. Drinking among college students: consumption and consequences. In: Galanter M, editor. Recent developments in alcoholism: alcohol problems in adolescents and young adults, vol. 17. New York: Springer; 2005. p. 85–117.

42. Karam E, Kypri K, Salamoun M. Alcohol use among college students: an international perspective. Curr Opin Psychiatry 2007;20(3):213–21.

43. O'Malley PM, Johnston LD. Epidemiology of alcohol and other drug use among American college students. J Stud Alcohol 2002;(Suppl 14):23–39.

44. Bachman J, Wadsworth K, O'Malley P, et al. Smoking, drinking and drug use in young adulthood: the impacts of new freedoms and responsibilities. Mahwah (NJ): Erlbaum; 1997.

45. Grekin ER, Sher KJ. Alcohol dependence symptoms among college freshman: prevalence, stability and person-environment interactions. Exp Clin Psychopharmacol 2006;14(3):329–38.

46. Compas BE, Wagner BM, Slavin LA, et al. A prospective study of life events, social support, and psychological symptomatology during the transition from high school to college. Am J Community Psychol 1986;14(3):241–57.

47. Conley CS, Kirsch AC, Dickson DA, et al. Negotiating the transition to college: developmental trajectories and gender differences in psychological functioning, cognitive-affective strategies, and social well-being. Emerg Adulthood 2014; 2(3):195–210.

48. Parker PD, Ludtke O, Trautwein U, et al. Personality and relationship quality during the transition from high school to early adulthood. J Pers 2012;80(4): 1061–89.

49. Weitzman ER, Nelson TF, Wechsler H. Taking up binge drinking in college: the influences of person, social group, and environment. J Adolesc Health 2003; 32(1):26–35.

50. Harford TC, Wechsler H, Seibring M. Attendance and alcohol use at parties and bars in college: a national survey of current drinkers. J Stud Alcohol 2002;63(6): 726–33.

51. Adams CE, Nagoshi CT. Changes over one semester in drinking game playing and alcohol use and problems in a college student sample. Subst Abuse 1999; 20(2):97–106.

52. David R, DeBarros A. In college, first year is by far the riskiest. USA Today 2006. Available at: http://usatoday30.usatoday.com/news/nation/2006-01-24-campus-deaths-cover_x.htm. Accessed October 25, 2015.

53. Bingham CR, Shope JT, Tang X. Drinking behavior from high school to young adulthood: differences by college education. Alcohol Clin Exp Res 2005; 29(12):2170–80.

54. Ham LS, Hope DA. College students and problematic drinking: a review of the literature. Clin Psychol Rev 2003;23(5):719–59.

55. Perkins HW. Surveying the damage: a review of research on consequences of alcohol misuse in college populations. J Stud Alcohol 2002;(Suppl 14):91–100.

56. White HR, Jackson K. Social and psychological influences on emerging adult drinking behavior. Alcohol Res Health 2005;28(4):182–90.

57. Borsari B, Carey KB. Peer influences on college drinking: a review of the research. J Subst Abuse 2001;13(4):391–424.

58. Borsari B, Carey KB. Descriptive and injunctive norms in college drinking: a meta-analytic integration. J Stud Alcohol 2003;64(3):331–41.
59. Turrisi R, Padilla KK, Wiersma KA. College student drinking: an examination of theoretical models of drinking tendencies in freshmen and upperclassmen. J Stud Alcohol 2000;61(4):598–602.
60. Rimal RN, Real K. How behaviors are influenced by perceived norms. Communic Res 2005;32(3):389–414.
61. Maggs JL. Alcohol use and binge drinking as goal-directed action during the transition to post-secondary education. In: Schulenberg J, Maggs JL, Hurrelman K, editors. Health risks and developmental transitions during adolescence. New York: Cambridge University Press; 1997. p. 346–71.
62. Gettleman J. As young adults drink to win, marketers join in. The New York Times 2005. Avaialable at: http://www.nytimes.com/2005/10/16/us/as-young-adults-drink-to-win-marketers-join-in.html?_r=0. Accessed October 25, 2015.
63. Walton KE, Roberts BW. On the relationship between substance use and personality traits: abstainers are not maladjusted. J Res Pers 2004;38(6):515–35.
64. Franken IHA, Muris P. BIS/BAS personality characteristics and college students' substance use. Pers Individ Dif 2006;40(7):1497–503.
65. Ruiz MA, Pincus AL, Dickinson KA. NEO PI-R predictors of alcohol use and alcohol-related problems. J Pers Assess 2003;81(3):226–36.
66. Hale RL, Whiteman S, Muehl K, et al. Tridimensional personality traits of college student marijuana users. Psychol Rep 2003;92(2):661–6.
67. Dennhardt AA, Murphy JG. Prevention and treatment of college student drug use: a review of the literature. Addict Behav 2013;38(10):2607–18.
68. Serras A, Saules KK, Cranford JA, et al. Self-injury, substance use, and associated risk factors in a multi-campus probability sample of college students. Psychol Addict Behav 2010;24(1):119–28.
69. Ichiyama MA, Kruse MI. The social contexts of binge drinking among private university freshman. J Alcohol Drug Educ 1998;44(1):18–33.
70. O'Connor RM, Colder CR. Predicting alcohol patterns in first-year college students through motivational systems and reasons for drinking. Psychol Addict Behav 2005;19(1):10–20.
71. Magid V, MacLean MG, Colder CR. Differentiating between sensation seeking and impulsivity through their mediated relations with alcohol use and problems. Addict Behav 2007;32(10):2046–61.
72. Rutledge PC, Sher KJ. Heavy drinking from the freshman year into early young adulthood: the roles of stress, tension-reducing drinking motives, gender and personality. J Stud Alcohol 2001;62(4):457–66.
73. Kendler KS, Prescott CA, Myers J, et al. The structure of genetic and environmental risk factors for common psychiatric and substance use disorders in men and women. Arch Gen Psychiatry 2003;60(9):929–37.
74. Valentiner DP, Mounts NS, Deacon BJ. Panic attacks, depression and anxiety symptoms, and substance use behaviors during late adolescence. J Anxiety Disord 2004;18(5):573–85.
75. Lee SS, Humphreys KL, Flory K, et al. Prospective association of childhood attention-deficit/hyperactivity disorder (ADHD) and substance use and abuse/dependence: a meta-analytic review. Clin Psychol Rev 2011;31(3):328–41.
76. Jessor R, Donovan JE, Costa FM. Beyond adolescence: problem behavior and young adult development. Cambridge (England): Cambridge University Press; 1991.

77. Cooper LM. Alcohol use and risky sexual behavior among college students and youth: evaluating the evidence. J Stud Alcohol 2002;(Suppl 14):101–17.

78. Wechsler H, Dowdall GW, Davenport A, et al. A gender-specific measure of binge drinking among college students. Am J Public Health 1995;85(7):982–5.

79. Graves KL. Risky behavior and alcohol use among young adults: results from a national survey. Am J Health Promot 1995;10(1):27–36.

80. Baskin-Sommers A, Sommers I. The co-occurrence of substance use and high-risk behaviors. J Adolesc Health 2006;38(5):609–11.

81. Dvorak RD, Lamis DA, Malone PS. Alcohol use, depressive symptoms, and impulsivity as risk factors for suicide proneness among college students. J Affect Disord 2013;149(1–3):326–34.

82. Li D, Yang X, Ge Z, et al. Cigarette smoking and risk of completed suicide: a meta-analysis of prospective cohort studies. J Psychiatr Res 2012;46(10):1257–66.

83. Lisha NE, Sussman S. Relationship of high school and college sports participation with alcohol, tobacco, and illicit drug use: a review. Addict Behav 2010;35(5):399–407.

84. Green GA, Uryasz FD, Petr TA, et al. NCAA study of substance use and abuse habits of college student-athletes. Clin J Sport Med 2001;11(1):51–6.

85. Martens MP, Dams-O'Connor K, Beck NC. A systematic review of college student-athlete drinking: prevalence rates, sport-related factors, and interventions. J Subst Abuse Treat 2006;31(3):305–16.

86. Wechsler H, Lee JE, Kuo M, et al. Trends in college binge drinking during a period of increased prevention efforts. Findings from 4 Harvard School of Public Health College Alcohol Study surveys: 1993-2001. J Am Coll Health 2002;50(5):203–17.

87. Cochran SD, Sullivan JG, Mays VM. Prevalence of mental disorders, psychological distress, and mental health services use among lesbian, gay, and bisexual adults in the United States. J Consult Clin Psychol 2003;71(1):53–61.

88. McCabe SE, Hughes TL, Bostwick WB, et al. Sexual orientation, substance use behaviors and substance dependence in the United States. Addiction 2009;104(8):1333–45.

89. Hatzenbuegler ML, Nolen-Hoeksema S, Erickson SJ. Minority stress predictors of HIV risk behavior, substance use, and depressive symptoms: results from a prospective study of bereaved gay men. Health Psychol 2008;27(4):455–62.

90. Weber G. Using to numb the pain: substance use and abuse among lesbian, gay, and bisexual individuals. J Ment Health Couns 2008;30(1):31–48.

91. Eisenberg M, Wechsler H. Substance use behaviors among college students with same-sex and opposite-sex experience: results from a national study. Addict Behav 2003;28(5):899–913.

92. Chen P, Jacobson KC. Developmental trajectories of substance use from early adolescence to young adulthood: gender and racial/ethnic differences. J Adolesc Health 2012;50(2):154–63.

93. Wei M, Liao KY, Chao RC, et al. Minority stress, perceived bicultural competence, and depressive symptoms among ethnic minority college students. J Couns Psychol 2010;57(4):411–22.

94. Pieterse AL, Todd NR, Neville HA, et al. Perceived racism and mental health among Black American adults: a meta-analytic review. J Couns Psychol 2012;59(1):1–9.

95. Blume AW, Lovato LV, Thyken BN, et al. The relationship of microaggressions with alcohol use and anxiety among ethnic minority college students in a historically White institution. Cultur Divers Ethnic Minor Psychol 2012;18(1):45–54.

96. Stewart C. The influence of spirituality on substance use of college students. J Drug Educ 2001;31(4):343–51.

97. Galen LW, Rogers WM. Religiosity, alcohol expectancies, drinking motives and their interaction in the prediction of drinking among college students. J Stud Alcohol 2004;65(4):469–76.

98. Wood MD, Read JP, Mitchell RE, et al. Do parents still matter? Parent and peer influences on alcohol involvement among recent high school graduates. Psychol Addict Behav 2004;18(1):19–30.

99. Sessa FM. The influence of perceived parenting on substance use during the transition to college: a comparison of male residential and commuter students. J Coll Student Dev 2005;46(1):62–74.

100. Standing L, Nicholson B. Models for student drinking and smoking: parents or peers? Soc Behav Personal 1989;17(2):223–9.

101. Turner AP, Larimer ME, Sarason IG. Family risk factors for alcohol-related consequences and poor adjustment in fraternity and sorority members: explaining the role of parent-child conflict. J Stud Alcohol 2000;61(6):818–26.

102. Carey KB, Scott-Sheldon LAJ, Carey MP, et al. Individual-level interventions to reduce college student drinking: a meta-analytic review. Addict Behav 2007; 32(11):2469–94.

103. Elliott JC, Carey KB. Correcting exaggerated marijuana use norms among college abstainers: a preliminary test of preventive intervention. J Stud Alcohol Drugs 2012;73(6):976–80.

104. Looby A, DeYoung KP, Earleywine M. Challenging expectancies to prevent nonmedical prescription stimulant use: a randomized, controlled trial. Drug Alcohol Depend 2013;132(1–2):362–8.

105. Larimer ME, Cronce JM. Identification, prevention, and treatment: a review of individual-focused strategies to reduce problematic alcohol consumption by college students. J Stud Alcohol Suppl 2002;(Suppl 14):148–63.

106. Darkes J, Goldman MS. Expectancy challenge and drinking reduction: experimental evidence for a mediational process. J Consult Clin Psychol 1993;61(2): 344–53.

107. Darkes J, Goldman MS. Expectancy challenge and drinking reduction: process and structure in the alcohol expectancy network. Exp Clin Psychopharmacol 1998;6(1):64–78.

108. Cronin C. Harm reduction for alcohol-use-related problems among college students. Subst Use Misuse 1996;31(14):2029–37.

109. Garvin RB, Alcorn JD, Faulkner KK. Behavioral strategies for alcohol abuse prevention with high-risk college males. J Alcohol Drug Educ 1990;36(1):23–34.

110. Scott-Sheldon LAJ, Carey KB, Elliott JC, et al. Efficacy of alcohol interventions for first-year college students: a meta-analytic review of randomized controlled trials. J Consult Clin Psychol 2014;82(2):177–88.

111. Kivlahan DR, Marlatt GA, Fromme K, et al. Secondary prevention with college drinkers: evaluation of an alcohol skills training program. J Consult Clin Psychol 1990;58(6):805–10.

112. Dimeff LA, Baer JS, Kivlahan DR, et al. Brief alcohol screening and intervention for college students (BASICS): a harm reduction approach. New York: Guilford Press; 1999.

113. Terlecki MA, Buckner JD, Larimer ME, et al. Randomized controlled trial of brief alcohol screening and intervention for college students for heavy-drinking mandated and volunteer undergraduates: 12-month outcomes. Psychol Addict Behav 2015;29(1):2–16.
114. Marlatt GA, Baer JS, Kivlahan DR, et al. Screening and brief intervention for high-risk college student drinkers: results from a two-year follow-up assessment. J Consult Clin Psychol 1998;66(4):604–15.
115. Borsari B, Carey KB. Effects of a brief motivational intervention with college student drinkers. J Consult Clin Psychol 2000;68(4):728–33.
116. Larimer ME, Turner AP, Anderson BK, et al. Evaluating a brief alcohol intervention with fraternities. J Stud Alcohol 2001;62(3):370–80.
117. Resnicow K, Soler R, Braithwaite RL, et al. Cultural sensitivity in college substance use prevention. J Community Psychol 2000;28(3):271–90.
118. Lee CM, Kilmer JR, Neighbors C, et al. Indicated prevention for college student marijuana use: a randomized controlled trial. J Consult Clin Psychol 2013;81(4): 702–9.

Technology-based Interventions for Preventing and Treating Substance Use Among Youth

Lisa A. Marsch, PhD*, Jacob T. Borodovsky, BA

KEYWORDS

- Youth • Substance use disorders • Prevention • Treatment • Technology

KEY POINTS

- Technology-based interventions are effective for preventing and treating substance use disorders.
- Technology is particularly suited to youth.
- Technology-based interventions are relevant at any stage in the development of a substance use disorder.
- Technology-based interventions provide solutions to extant problems of traditional interventions.

INTRODUCTION

Substance use and substance use disorders among youth pose unique developmental and clinical challenges for families, providers, and youth themselves. Close to 40% of high school seniors have used an illicit drug in the last year, and 20% of high school seniors have used an illicit drug other than cannabis in the last year.[1] Youth who use substances are at risk for sexually transmitted diseases,[2] impaired cognitive functioning,[3] major depressive episodes,[4] poor educational attainment,[5]

The preparation of this article was partially supported by NIDA/NIH P30DA029926 (L.A. Marsch: PI) and NIDA/NIH T32DA037202-02 (J.T. Borodovsky). In addition to her academic affiliation, Dr L.A. Marsch is affiliated with HealthSim, LLC, a health-promotion software development organization that developed a few of the web-based tools referenced in this article. Dr L.A. Marsch has worked extensively with her institutions to manage any potential conflict of interest. All research data collection, data management, and statistical analyses were conducted by individuals with no affiliation to HealthSim, LLC.
Center for Technology and Behavioral Health, Dartmouth College, 46 Centerra Parkway EverGreen Center, Suite 315, Lebanon, NH 03766, USA
* Corresponding author.
E-mail address: Lisa.A.Marsch@dartmouth.edu

Child Adolesc Psychiatric Clin N Am 25 (2016) 755–768
http://dx.doi.org/10.1016/j.chc.2016.06.005
1056-4993/16/$ – see front matter © 2016 Elsevier Inc. All rights reserved.

involvement in the criminal justice system,[6] and having a substance use disorder later in life.[7,8]

Substance use disorder development takes time and is influenced by various risk factors and behaviors. Intervening during this development process plays a vital role in redirecting a young person's life trajectory. Intervention strategies along this trajectory include universal prevention, selective prevention, and treatment.[9,10] The goal of universal prevention is to prevent substance use initiation (ie, prevent youth from trying a drug for the first time). Selective prevention involves identifying high-risk youth and intervening to stop problematic substance using behaviors that may escalate into a diagnosable disorder. The goal of treatment is to intervene with individuals who meet diagnostic criteria for a substance use disorder.

Numerous implementation barriers hinder our ability to deliver evidence-based universal prevention, selective prevention, and treatment interventions for youth.[11-14] Clinician-delivered treatment is expensive with variable adherence to intervention fidelity. Unfortunately, less than one-third of substance abuse treatment facilities offer adolescent-specific programs,[15] and only 10% to 15% of youth who could benefit from treatment actually receive it.[14] Interventions that leverage computer, mobile, and Web technologies are appealing to youth,[16] require minimal cost,[13,17] deliver therapeutic content in a consistent and standardized manner,[17] minimize burden on staff,[18] and can be tailored to different individuals and treatment settings.[17,19] Technology is well suited as a means of providing universal prevention,[20] selective prevention,[21] and treatment[22] interventions that can fully or partially replace face-to-face interactions with prevention or therapeutic staff (thereby reducing costs and freeing staff to attend to more patients) or augment standard services under a clinician extender model that increases access and availability of evidenced-based practices outside clinical settings.[23]

The widespread use of technology among youth underscores the opportunity for delivering these interventions to this cohort. Approximately 80% of youth in the United States have a cell phone (many of these are smartphones)[24] and more than 90% have access to a computer and the Internet.[24] Abroad, Internet and smartphone access and use are increasing among younger age groups.[25] Given technology's prevalence and acceptance among youth and its ability to enhance cost effectiveness and fidelity to psychotherapeutic models, technology-based interventions fill critical gaps for preventing and treating substance use among youth.

This article provides an overview of the current research on the use of technology-based substance use prevention (universal and selected) and treatment interventions for youth. Directions for future research are also identified and discussed. Web site links to more information about specific interventions are provided in **Table 1**.

TECHNOLOGY-BASED UNIVERSAL PREVENTION

Technology-based universal prevention interventions generally target youth between ages 10 and 18 who self-report never having used alcohol or other substances. These interventions often consist of interactive, digital, activities designed to increase drug-related knowledge and alter attitudes and normative beliefs around substance use[26] to prevent or delay the onset of substance use. These interventions can be adapted from empirically supported interventions and delivered via computer.[27] Early studies have used CD-ROM technology to deliver interventions, but many studies have shifted to Internet and mobile technologies. The following section summarizes the patterns of findings from scientific evaluations of

Table 1	
Technology-based universal, selective, and treatment interventions	
Universal Prevention	
CLIMATE	http://www.climateschools.com/
Head On	http://www.preventionsciencemedia.com
Thinking Not Drinking	http://www.childtrends.org/?programs=thinking-not-drinking
RealTeen	http://socialwork.columbia.edu/research/research-scientists/traci-schwinn
Refuse to Use	http://www.orcasinc.com/
Selective Prevention	
Alcohol 101+	http://responsibility.org/college-students-and-drinking/alcohol-101/
Alcohol Edu	https://everfi.com/higher-education/alcoholedu/
Check Your Drinking	http://www.checkyourdrinking.net
CDCU	http://www.collegedrinkerscheckup.com/
E-CHUG	http://www.echeckuptogo.com/usa/programs/coll_alcohol.php
E-TOKE	http://www.echeckuptogo.com/usa/programs/coll_mj.php
THRIVE	http://lamp.health.curtin.edu.au/thrive/baselinetest.php
Treatment	
ARISE	http://www.liebertonline.com/g4h
MicroCog	http://www.pearsonclinical.com/
MOMENT (presentation)	http://www.nattc.org/userfiles/file/Shrier_L(1).pdf
TES	http://www.sudtech.org

technology-based universal prevention interventions in 3 settings: primary care, schools, and homes.

Primary Care Settings

To our knowledge, Walton and colleagues[28] (2014) have conducted the only published randomized, controlled study showing the use of a technology-based universal prevention (ie, no study subjects with lifetime substance use) intervention in a primary care medical setting. This randomized, controlled trial evaluated the effectiveness of a computer-delivered brief intervention designed to prevent cannabis use onset among a sample of 714 adolescents (ages 12–18) who reported no lifetime cannabis use. Youth were randomly assigned to 1 of 3 conditions in a large urban pediatric practice setting: computer-delivered brief intervention, therapist-delivered brief intervention, or control (educational brochure about cannabis use). The computer-delivered intervention consisted of animated scenarios presenting different risks for substance use and modeled positive choices. The 2 primary outcome measures in this study were initiation and frequency of cannabis use. A secondary outcome was frequency of other drug use. The computer-delivered brief intervention resulted in a lower cumulative proportion of cannabis use initiation 12 months after intervention compared with the educational brochure control (17% vs 24%), lower frequency of cannabis use at 3 and 6 months, and lower use of other drugs at 6 months. The therapist-delivered intervention showed no significant difference from the educational control in terms of cumulative proportion of cannabis use initiation 12 months after the intervention (21% vs 24%). The study was not powered to compare the therapist brief intervention with the computer brief intervention.[28]

School Settings

CLIMATE

Multiple randomized, controlled trials have confirmed that The CLIMATE (Clinical Management and Treatment Education) intervention consistently produces positive prevention outcomes.[13,29] CLIMATE provides 6 lessons based primarily on social influence theories via CD-ROM and the Web. Lessons include information about the prevalence and consequences of substance use and ways to avoid substance use and associated risks. After the computer activity, students and teachers (who require no training) collaborate in role playing, group discussion, decision making and problem-solving activities, and skill rehearsal.[30] The CLIMATE intervention is more effective than standard health class curricula (eg, unstructured social influence and harm minimization materials delivered by a teacher) at enhancing primary outcomes such as alcohol-related knowledge and reducing positive expectations around alcohol,[30] cannabis,[31] and Ecstasy use.[31]

HeadOn

The HeadOn intervention is a substance abuse prevention program designed for youth in grades 6 through 8. HeadOn is delivered via CD or the Internet and consists of interactive, simulated scenarios that require students to engage in substance-related decision making. Youth have the opportunity to explore 10 topics related to substance use (eg, consequences of drug use, drug-refusal skills training, social skills training) and earn skills cards for mastering each topic. Youth use these skill cards to engage in an electronic card game designed to reinforce the substance abuse knowledge they have acquired.

The HeadOn intervention was evaluated in 2 schools for 15 sessions over 1 school year. Two additional schools (serving as the control group) received the empirically validated Life Skills Training substance abuse prevention program.[32] Students in both the HeadOn and the Life Skills Training intervention had positive outcomes in terms of self-reported use of cigarettes and alcohol, intentions to use these substances, acquisition of knowledge about drug use, and attitudes about drug use. However, students in the HeadOn intervention had more accurate responses to questions evaluating knowledge of substance abuse than those in the Life Skills Training Program. Youth also reported that the HeadOn intervention was interesting, fun, and useful.[33] These findings were replicated using a modified version of HeadOn developed for a younger age group. In a similarly structured randomized trial of more than 500 youth in grades 3 to 5, the HeadOn intervention increased self-esteem, problem-solving skills, and substance use prevention knowledge among youth.[34]

Home Setting

Schinke and colleagues[35] have led a systematic line of research to develop technology-based interventions that can be delivered at home. By delivering technology-based interventions in home settings (usually in the form of a Web site accessed via a home computer) youth can engage with the intervention and their parent(s) at the same time. Thus, intervention modules grounded in family interaction theories can be effectively used. These interventions offer the opportunity for parents to reinforce new behaviors and beliefs to foster healthy relationships by, for example, teaching mothers how to communicate with daughters to build their self-esteem and set rules and consequences for substance use.[35] This method helps youth develop better conflict management and substance refusal skills, better self-efficacy, and less alcohol, cannabis, prescription drug, and inhalant use.[35–37]

A recent exemplary intervention—informed by years of prior work[38]—is called *Real-Teen*. RealTeen is a Web-based intervention that is easily accessible from home. Youth create a username and password to access the intervention and can receive email reminders to complete modules. This intervention is designed to mitigate drug use risk factors to prevent or delay the onset of substance use by enhancing mediators of substance use prevention. It does this by using interactive skills-building sessions that place youth in realistic drug use scenarios designed to improve cognitive and social skills. These scenarios help young girls avoid drug use by teaching them to cope with stress and set goals.[38,39] In a study conducted to evaluate this intervention, 236 seventh-, eighth-, and ninth-grade girls were randomly assigned to RealTeen or a control (assessment-only) group. At the 6-month follow-up, intervention participants had lower rates of past 30-day alcohol, marijuana, and polydrug use and total drug use.[38]

TECHNOLOGY-BASED SELECTIVE PREVENTION

Selective prevention models such as the screening, brief intervention, and referral to treatment (SBIRT) model, identify at-risk adolescents across a range of treatment settings and patient populations,[17] help them re-evaluate their substance use, and provide first steps for seeking treatment.[40] (See Borus J, Parhami I, Levy S: Screening, Brief Intervention and Referral to Treatment, in this issue).

Technology-based selective prevention interventions fit the SBIRT model well. These interventions often contain therapeutic content adapted from validated screening tools like the CRAFFT (Car, Relax, Alone, Forget, Friends, Trouble)[41] and deliver this content via a computer or tablet. Many of these interventions tailor their content based on an individual's responses.

In contrast to universal prevention interventions (predominantly school-based and focused on younger children with no lifetime substance use), few technology-based selective prevention interventions have been tested in school-age youth.[42] Most selective prevention interventions are SBIRT interventions that target youth who have already begun using substances and are primarily between the ages of 18 and 25. These interventions are primarily used in medical (primary care and emergency room) or university settings.

Medical Settings

Primary care

The Harris Primary Care Trial was a multisite, international trial (with sites in New England and the Czech Republic) aimed at evaluating a computer-facilitated screening and brief advice system (cSBA) in a primary care setting.[43] Youth (ages 12–18) attending routine primary care were eligible for the study. The trial evaluated both substance use initiation and cessation (making this a universal and selective prevention trial). The cSBA system is based on the CRAFFT tool and requires participants to complete a questionnaire about their substance use. The cSBA system uses this information to calculate a risk score and automatically provide the physician with tailored talking points on substance-related health risks and advice on how to promote conversation with the participant about substance use. Participants in the control group received treatment as usual specific to the clinic providing care. At 12 months, the cSBA system produced better alcohol initiation and cessation outcomes at the New England sites and better cannabis initiation and cessation outcomes at the Czech Republic sites.[43]

Emergency room

Approximately one-fourth of youth in emergency departments screen positive for risky drinking behaviors.[44] Additionally most college drinkers sent to university emergency departments are willing to receive a brief alcohol use screening—half of whom will screen positive for alcohol use problems and are open to receiving counseling.[45] Laptop interventions delivered in emergency room settings help high-risk youth think more about their alcohol use, require little assistance to operate, and are rated favorably among youth.[46] Compared with giving risky alcohol-using youth a brochure to review, computer-based interventions that use therapeutic constructs such as personalized normative feedback (PNF), improve perceptions concerning the importance of cutting down on alcohol use and the likelihood they will actually do so.[44]

University Setting

Colleges and universities struggle with identifying and managing risky alcohol use among students.[47] Universities typically provide alcohol counseling to a student after an alcohol-related incident[47] (ie, mandated students). Universities also deliver preventative interventions to large groups of non-mandated students (eg, freshman orientation or student health center) by screening the whole student population, identifying heavy-drinking students, and then providing an intervention to the heavy-drinking students. Technology-based interventions can effectively serve both of these needs. These interventions address the needs of students across the spectrum of alcohol use severity[48] and provide immediate access to different types of content related to alcohol use.[49] These interventions use a mix of education, skill development, motivational techniques, and personalized normative feedback.[49]

Personalized normative feedback and technology

PNF is a crucial component of any technology-based intervention aimed at reducing college students' alcohol use and related negative consequences.[50,51] College students often use alcohol heavily and have skewed perceptions of alcohol use norms and risk.[52] PNF delivered via computer, changes student perceptions of norms and their alcohol use by providing corrective information about normative drinking among peers.[53]

A variety of PNF-based interventions effectively address alcohol use among students. For example, compared with education-based interventions, checkyourdrinking.net reduces mandated students' amount and frequency of alcohol use and estimates of alcohol use among peers.[54] The Web site does this by providing summary information about a student's drinking habits and helps the student visually compare (via graphs) their habits with normative drinking patterns among their peers. Technology-based screening and brief interventions can also be used in non-mandated student populations. Used in this context, these inventions are easy to implement, appeal to youth, and reduce risky drinking compared with educational controls.[55] Compared with assessment-only controls, the College Drinkers Check-Up (CDCU) reduces drinking among high-risk college students up to 1 year after the intervention.[56] CDCU is Web-based and contains brief motivational techniques and PNF-based modules such as the Get Feedback module (normative behavior feedback).[56] The Electronic CHECKUP TO GO (e-CHUG) intervention also incorporates personalized feedback and has been evaluated in multiple randomized, controlled trials for high-risk drinkers. e-CHUG lowers weekly alcohol consumption and psychosocial consequences related to their alcohol use.[51] e-CHUG also reduces university sanctions among incoming freshmen with risky drinking behaviors.[57]

Other drugs in university settings

Technology-based interventions in college settings have also been used for substances other than alcohol. Technology-based interventions increase the rate of tobacco abstinence by close to 50%.[58] Few studies, however, have evaluated technology-based interventions focused on marijuana among college students.[58] Technology-based interventions can be geared towards changing perceptions of marijuana use norms. For example, the Web-based Marijuana E-Checkup (E-Toke) intervention helps students weigh pros and cons of marijuana use and uses PNF to correct beliefs about marijuana use norms.[59]

TECHNOLOGY-BASED TREATMENT

The scientific community has made significant progress developing and testing different psychotherapies for youth with substance use disorders. However, although treatment mitigates psychological,[60] medical,[61] and legal problems[60] associated with substance use, our current models for delivering that treatment are fraught with problems.[11,14] Few treatment facilities offer adolescent-specific programs,[15] and only 10% to 15% of youth who may benefit from treatment actually receive it.[14] Community-based treatment programs with limited finances, staff, and resources, struggle to provide evidenced-based treatment in the context of shifting payment and reimbursement models.[11,62] Although treatment reduces substance use,[63] the effects typically diminish after 3 to 6 months.[63] Youth who complete treatment struggle to maintain sobriety on their own; thus, posttreatment therapeutic support is critical.[14] (See Robinson Z, Riggs PD: Co-occurring Psychiatric and Substance Use Disorders, in this issue).

The Institute of Medicine report used to generate the intervention categories in this article (universal, selected, treatment) emphasized a distinction between "indicated prevention" and "treatment." Specifically, interventions that focus on individuals with a specific diagnosed disorder are deemed *treatment* rather than *indicated prevention*.[64]

Technology-based interventions are cost-effective[65] and adhere to evidence-based psychotherapeutic principles such as motivational interviewing, cognitive-behavioral paradigms,[23] or community reinforcement approaches.[66,67] These interventions provide effective posttreatment support[68] and are effective in treating adults with substance use disorders[65] as stand-alone,[66] partial replacement[69] and clinician extender interventions.[70] These interventions are commonly implemented via a computer or mobile phone. However, few studies have explored the use of technology-based interventions for treating youth with substance use disorders. Attitude and focus group data suggest that youth in treatment view these technologies (particularly mobile phone texting) as potentially useful components of treatment and posttreatment relapse prevention treatment.[71–73]

Therapeutic Education System

The Therapeutic Education System (TES) is a Web-based intervention. It is an interactive program designed to help individuals with substance use disorders develop skills emphasized in cognitive-behavioral therapy and relapse prevention training. TES contains human immunodeficiency virus (HIV)-related modules that have been found, in 2 randomized clinical trials, to be an effective in HIV prevention among youth with substance use disorders.[74,75]

Step Up

The Web-based Step Up intervention comprises 21 modules completed over 12 sessions. The intervention is designed to help users develop assertiveness and communication skills and is based on the Adolescent Community Reinforcement Approach.[76] Users complete modules at their own pace and receive tailored content based on their responses. Step Up was recently evaluated in a randomized, controlled trial. Youth (ages 12–18) entering a substance use treatment program were randomly assigned to standard treatment or standard treatment with parts replaced by Step Up. Results showed that replacing components of standard treatment with Step Up allows youth to achieve similar reductions in substance use and mental health outcomes compared with treatment as usual. Additionally, Step Up was rated as highly acceptable to youth.[77]

Identifying Therapeutic Opportunities: Ecological Momentary Assessment

Ecological Momentary Assessment (EMA) "…involves repeated sampling of subjects' current behaviors and experiences in real time, in subjects' natural environments."[78] Mobile phone–based EMA provides the ability to collect real-time data and obtain an accurate profile of the temporal relationship between behaviors and outcomes. This method allows us to identify where, when, and why youth are most vulnerable and develop interventions that target these windows of vulnerability.[79] In terms of clinical applications, the EMA paradigm is well suited to serve in a clinician extender capacity that can augment treatment in 2 potential ways. First, EMA can serve to inform functional analysis (eg, identifying different emotional or peer influence triggers) that therapists may use in the context of cognitive behavioral therapy. Second, EMA can address the poor posttreatment relapse rates common among youth with substance use disorders.[14,63,80,81] To date, a handful of studies have evaluated treatment of youth with substance use disorders using EMA data, all with promising results.

Educating and Supporting Inquisitive Youth in Recovery

Educating and Supporting Inquisitive Youth in Recovery (ESQYIR) is an EMA program that uses mobile phone technology to help youth maintain sobriety after leaving treatment. ESQYIR's text message content and delivery schedule are programmed based on focus group data from youth in substance use treatment programs.[72] ESQYIR provides 2 daily text messages (eg, self-monitoring and recovery tips) and social support resource information on weekends.[68] ESQYIR titrates content of text messages based on real-time feedback provided by youth. For example, youth receive monitoring questions to assess current challenges (eg, mood issues). Youth then provide a numeric response indicating the severity of the problem. Based on this information, youth are classified under a risk of relapse category and specific text message content (previously vetted and matched to this level of severity) is sent.[68]

In a pilot study, individuals were randomly assigned to receive ESQYIR or aftercare as usual (ie, 2 monthly phone calls for recovery monitoring). Youth who received ESQYIR were half as likely to relapse as those who received treatment as usual during the 12-week study period and at the 3-month follow-up. Youth who use ESQYIR also have fewer severe problems related to substance use and show active participation in their recovery (ie, attendance in recovery groups).[68] Notably, youth who participate in this intervention are significantly less likely to test positive for substances at 6- and 9-month follow-up assessments.[82]

Momentary Self-Monitoring and Feedback Motivational Enhancement

The Momentary Self-Monitoring and Feedback Motivational Enhancement (MOMENT) intervention is another EMA intervention that uses mobile technology to intervene with cannabis-using youth. Youth first meet with counselors for 2 brief motivational interviewing sessions to discuss their top 3 triggers for using cannabis. Over the next 2 weeks, youth report their triggers, cravings, and actual cannabis use with their mobile phone. Participants receive text messages to help them cope with the previously identified triggers. Researchers have found that MOMENT can be successfully implemented in treatment settings and is acceptable to youth. Preliminary effectiveness data suggest that using MOMENT lowers frequency of marijuana use compared with baseline levels of use.[83]

SUMMARY AND FUTURE DIRECTIONS

Technology-based interventions offer us the ability to rapidly expand access and availability of evidence-based preventative and treatment interventions for youth. These interventions have the potential to address gaps in existing clinical services such as recovery support services or continuing care. These interventions offer a variety of advantages over traditional interventions and may be used as adjuncts to traditional interventions or as stand-alone interventions.

Across universal prevention, selective prevention, and treatment interventions, technology-based solutions are not only effective but also remedy many implementation problems associated with traditional interventions, including an insufficient workforce to deliver evidence-based interventions, time constraints for delivering evidence-based interventions in many systems of care, and cost of person-delivered interventions. Technology allows one to tailor interventions to different subgroups, adapt content in real time, and facilitate rapid dissemination to large groups with minimal effort. Technology also allows for anytime/anywhere access to evidence-based therapeutic support in a wide array of settings. And, as the temporal trends in various substance preferences among youth shift in new directions, many use technology-based interventions to respond quickly and effectively to provide a scalable response.

One promising and currently underutilized potential new direction in addressing substance use among youth is social media. About 95% of 12- to 17-year-olds use the Internet, and 81% use social networks.[84] Popular sites among youth include Instagram, Twitter, Snapchat, Facebook, Tumblr, Google+, and Pinterest.[85] Given the ubiquity of social media use among youth, the opportunities to harness social media for delivering preventative and therapeutic interventions to a large end-user base are substantial and undertapped. Social media offers the potential to provide new avenues for delivering individual or group-based preventative and treatment interventions that have yet to be explored scientifically.

Overall, the research literature to date, although limited, underscores the promise of using technology in the prevention and treatment of substance use disorders among youth. Technology-based interventions may serve as important tools to reach youth at a population level. As the scientific community learns more about mechanisms of therapeutic change and how to translate them into digital formats, technology's influence and clinical applications in addressing substance use among adolescents will become more prolific.

REFERENCES

1. Johnston LD, O'Malley PM, Miech RA, et al. Monitoring the future national survey results on drug use: 1975-2014: overview, key findings on adolescent drug use. Ann Arbor (MI): Institute for Social Research, The University of Michigan; 2015.
2. Dembo R, Belenko S, Childs K, et al. Gender differences in drug use, sexually transmitted diseases, and risky sexual behavior among arrested youths. J Child Adolesc Subst Abuse 2010;19(5):424–46.

3. Hanson KL, Medina KL, Padula CB, et al. Impact of adolescent alcohol and drug use on neuropsychological functioning in young adulthood: 10-year outcomes. J Child Adolesc Subst Abuse 2011;20(2):135–54.
4. Ali MM, Dean D Jr, Lipari R, et al. The mental health consequences of nonmedical prescription drug use among adolescents. J Ment Health Policy Econ 2015;18(1):3–15.
5. Chatterji P. Illicit drug use and educational attainment. Health Econ 2006;15(5):489–511.
6. Lennings CJ, Kenny DT, Nelson P. Substance use and treatment seeking in young offenders on community orders. J Subst Abuse Treat 2006;31(4):425–32.
7. Jefferis BJMH, Power C, Manor O. Adolescent drinking level and adult binge drinking in a national birth cohort. Addiction 2005;100(4):543–9.
8. McCarty CA, Ebel BE, Garrison MM, et al. Continuity of binge and harmful drinking from late adolescence to early adulthood. Pediatrics 2004;114(3):714–9.
9. Gordon RS Jr. An operational classification of disease prevention. Public Health Rep 1983;98(2):107–9.
10. Mrazek PJ, Haggerty RJ. Reducing risks for mental disorders: Frontiers for preventive intervention research. Washington, DC: National Academies Press; 1994.
11. McLellan AT, Meyers K. Contemporary addiction treatment: a review of systems problems for adults and adolescents. Biol Psychiatry 2004;56(10):764–70.
12. Botvin GJ, Griffin KW. School-based programmes to prevent alcohol, tobacco and other drug use. Int Rev Psychiatry 2007;19(6):607–15.
13. Hopson L, Wodarski J, Tang N. The effectiveness of electronic approaches to substance abuse prevention for adolescents. J Evid Inf Soc Work 2015;12(3):310–22.
14. Belendiuk KA, Riggs P. Treatment of adolescent substance use disorders. Curr Treat Options Psychiatry 2014;1(2):175–88.
15. Mericle AA, Arria AM, Meyers K, et al. National trends in adolescent substance use disorders and treatment availability: 2003-2010. J Child Adolesc Subst Abuse 2015;24(5):255–63.
16. Bosworth K. Application of computer technology to drug abuse prevention. Handbook of Drug Abuse Prevention. Boston: Springer; 2006. p. 629–48.
17. Lord S, Marsch L. Emerging trends and innovations in the identification and management of drug use among adolescents and young adults. Adolesc Med State Art Rev 2011;22(3):649.
18. Bishop D, Bryant KS, Giles SM, et al. Simplifying the delivery of a prevention program with web-based enhancements. J Prim Prev 2006;27(4):433–44.
19. Marsch LA, Gustafson DH. The role of technology in health care innovation: a commentary. J Dual Diagn 2013;9(1):101–3.
20. Champion KE, Newton NC, Barrett EL, et al. A systematic review of school-based alcohol and other drug prevention programs facilitated by computers or the internet. Drug Alcohol Rev 2013;32(2):115–23.
21. Donoghue K, Patton R, Phillips T, et al. The effectiveness of electronic screening and brief intervention for reducing levels of alcohol consumption: a systematic review and meta-analysis. J Med Internet Res 2014;16(6):e142.
22. Marsch LA, Dallery J. Advances in the psychosocial treatment of addiction: the role of technology in the delivery of evidence-based psychosocial treatment. Psychiatr Clin North Am 2012;35(2):481–93.
23. Marsch LA, Carroll KM, Kiluk BD. Technology-based interventions for the treatment and recovery management of substance use disorders: a JSAT special issue. J Subst Abuse Treat 2014;46(1):1–4.

24. Madden M, Lenhart A, Duggan M, et al. Teens and technology 2013, Pew research center's Internet & American life project. Washington, DC: PEW; 2013.
25. Poushter J. Emerging, developing countries gain ground in the tech revolution. 2016. Available at: http://www.pewresearch.org/fact-tank/2016/02/22/key-takeaways-global-tech/#. Accessed February 26, 2016.
26. Rodriguez DM, Teesson M, Newton NC. A systematic review of computerised serious educational games about alcohol and other drugs for adolescents. Drug Alcohol Rev 2014;33(2):129–35.
27. Williams C, Griffin KW, Macaulay AP, et al. Efficacy of a drug prevention CD-ROM intervention for adolescents. Subst Use Misuse 2005;40(6):869–78.
28. Walton MA, Resko S, Barry KL, et al. A randomized controlled trial testing the efficacy of a brief cannabis universal prevention program among adolescents in primary care. Addiction 2014;109(5):786–97.
29. Newton NC, Vogl LE, Teesson M, et al. CLIMATE Schools: alcohol module: cross-validation of a school-based prevention programme for alcohol misuse. Aust N Z J Psychiatry 2009;43(3):201–7.
30. Vogl L, Teesson M, Andrews G, et al. A computerized harm minimization prevention program for alcohol misuse and related harms: randomized controlled trial. Addiction 2009;104(4):564–75.
31. Newton NC, Andrews G, Teesson M, et al. Delivering prevention for alcohol and cannabis using the Internet: a cluster randomised controlled trial. Prev Med 2009; 48(6):579–84.
32. Botvin GJ, Baker E, Dusenbury L, et al. Long-term follow-up results of a randomized drug abuse prevention trial in a white middle-class population. JAMA 1995; 273(14):1106–12.
33. Marsch LA, Bickel WK, Grabinski MJ. Application of interactive, computer technology to adolescent substance abuse prevention and treatment. Adolesc Med State Art Rev 2007;18(2):342–56, xii.
34. Marsch LA. The Application of Technology to the Prevention and Treatment of Substance Use Disorders: Research Findings, Opportunities, and Future Directions. American Psychological Association 120th Annual Meeting. Orlando, FL, August 2, 2012.
35. Schinke SP, Fang L, Cole KC, et al. Preventing substance use among Black and Hispanic adolescent girls: results from a computer-delivered, mother-daughter intervention approach. Subst Use Misuse 2011;46(1):35–45.
36. Schinke SP, Cole KC, Fang L. Gender-specific intervention to reduce underage drinking among early adolescent girls: a test of a computer-mediated, mother-daughter program. J Stud Alcohol Drugs 2009;70(1):70.
37. Schinke SP, Fang L, Cole KC. Computer-delivered, parent-involvement intervention to prevent substance use among adolescent girls. Prev Med 2009;49(5): 429–35.
38. Schwinn TM, Schinke SP, Di Noia J. Preventing drug abuse among adolescent girls: outcome data from an internet-based intervention. Prev Sci 2010;11(1): 24–32.
39. Schwinn TM, Hopkins JE, Schinke SP. Developing a web-based intervention to prevent drug use among adolescent girls. Res Soc Work Pract 2016;26(1):8–13.
40. Mitchell SG, Gryczynski J, O'Grady KE, et al. SBIRT for adolescent drug and alcohol use: current status and future directions. J Subst Abuse Treat 2013; 44(5):463–72.
41. Knight JR, Shrier LA, Bravender TD, et al. A new brief screen for adolescent substance abuse. Arch Pediatr Adolesc Med 1999;153(6):591–6.

42. Doumas DM. Web-based personalized feedback: is this an appropriate approach for reducing drinking among high school students? J Subst Abuse Treat 2015;50:76–80.
43. Harris SK, Csemy L, Sherritt L, et al. Computer-facilitated substance use screening and brief advice for teens in primary care: an international trial. Pediatrics 2012;129(6):1072–82.
44. Walton MA, Chermack ST, Blow FC, et al. Components of brief alcohol interventions for youth in the emergency department. Subst Abus 2015;36(3):339–49.
45. Helmkamp JC, Hungerford DW, Williams JM, et al. Screening and brief intervention for alcohol problems among college students treated in a university hospital emergency department. J Am Coll Health 2003;52(1):7–16.
46. Gregor MA, Shope JT, Blow FC, et al. Feasibility of using an interactive laptop program in the emergency department to prevent alcohol misuse among adolescents. Ann Emerg Med 2003;42(2):276–84.
47. Lenk KM, Erickson DJ, Winters KC, et al. Screening services for alcohol misuse and abuse at four-year colleges in the U.S. J Subst Abuse Treat 2012;43(3): 352–8.
48. Walters ST, Neighbors C. College prevention: a view of present (and future) web-based approaches. Alcohol Res Health 2011;34(2):222–4.
49. Walters ST, Miller E, Chiauzzi E. Wired for wellness: e-interventions for addressing college drinking. J Subst Abuse Treat 2005;29(2):139–45.
50. Cronce JM, Bittinger JN, Liu J, et al. Electronic feedback in college student drinking prevention and intervention. Alcohol Res 2015;36(1):47–62.
51. Walters ST, Vader AM, Harris TR. A controlled trial of web-based feedback for heavy drinking college students. Prev Sci 2007;8(1):83–8.
52. Kypri K, Hallett J, Howat P, et al. Randomized controlled trial of proactive web-based alcohol screening and brief intervention for university students. Arch Intern Med 2009;169(16):1508–14.
53. Neighbors C, Larimer ME, Lewis MA. Targeting misperceptions of descriptive drinking norms: efficacy of a computer-delivered personalized normative feedback intervention. J Consult Clin Psychol 2004;72(3):434–47.
54. Doumas DM, McKinley LL, Book P. Evaluation of two Web-based alcohol interventions for mandated college students. J Subst Abuse Treat 2009;36(1):65–74.
55. Kypri K, Saunders JB, Williams SM, et al. Web-based screening and brief intervention for hazardous drinking: a double-blind randomized controlled trial. Addiction 2004;99(11):1410–7.
56. Hester RK, Delaney HD, Campbell W. The college drinker's check-up: outcomes of two randomized clinical trials of a computer-delivered intervention. Psychol Addict Behav 2012;26(1):1–12.
57. Doumas DM, Nelson K, DeYoung A, et al. Alcohol-related consequences among first-year university students: effectiveness of a web-based personalized feedback program. J Coll Counsel 2014;17(2):150–62.
58. Gulliver A, Farrer L, Chan JK, et al. Technology-based interventions for tobacco and other drug use in university and college students: a systematic review and meta-analysis. Addict Sci Clin Pract 2015;10:5.
59. Elliott JC, Carey KB. Correcting exaggerated marijuana use norms among college abstainers: a preliminary test of a preventive intervention. J Stud Alcohol Drugs 2012;73(6):976–80.
60. Hser YI, Grella CE, Hubbard RL, et al. An evaluation of drug treatments for adolescents in 4 US cities. Arch Gen Psychiatry 2001;58(7):689–95.

61. Joshi V, Hser Y-I, Grella CE, et al. Sex-related HIV risk reduction behavior among adolescents in DATOS-A. J Adolesc Res 2001;16(6):642–60.
62. Sterling S, Weisner C, Hinman A, et al. Access to treatment for adolescents with substance use and co-occurring disorders: challenges and opportunities. J Am Acad Child Adolesc Psychiatry 2010;49(7):637–46 [quiz: 725–6].
63. Winters KC, Tanner-Smith EE, Bresani E, et al. Current advances in the treatment of adolescent drug use. Adolesc Health Med Ther 2014;5:199–210.
64. O'Connell ME, Boat T, Warner KE. Preventing mental, emotional, and behavioral disorders among young people: progress and possibilities. Washington, DC: National Academies Press; 2009.
65. Bickel WK, Christensen DR, Marsch LA. A review of computer-based interventions used in the assessment, treatment, and research of drug addiction. Subst Use Misuse 2011;46(1):4–9.
66. Bickel WK, Marsch LA, Buchhalter AR, et al. Computerized behavior therapy for opioid-dependent outpatients: a randomized controlled trial. Exp Clin Psychopharmacol 2008;16(2):132–43.
67. Budney A, Higgins S. A community reinforcement plus vouchers approach: treating cocaine addiction (NIDA Publication No. 98–4309 ed). Rockville (MD): National Institute on Drug Abuse; 1994.
68. Gonzales R, Ang A, Murphy DA, et al. Substance use recovery outcomes among a cohort of youth participating in a mobile-based texting aftercare pilot program. J Subst Abuse Treat 2014;47(1):20–6.
69. Marsch LA, Guarino H, Acosta M, et al. Web-based behavioral treatment for substance use disorders as a partial replacement of standard methadone maintenance treatment. J Subst Abuse Treat 2014;46(1):43–51.
70. Campbell AN, Nunes EV, Matthews AG, et al. Internet-delivered treatment for substance abuse: a multisite randomized controlled trial. Am J Psychiatry 2014;171(6):683–90.
71. Trudeau KJ, Ainscough J, Charity S. Technology in treatment: are adolescents and counselors interested in online relapse prevention? Child Youth Care Forum 2012;41(1):57–71.
72. Gonzales R, Douglas Anglin M, Glik DC. Exploring the feasibility of text messaging to support substance abuse recovery among youth in treatment. Health Educ Res 2014;29(1):13–22.
73. Shrier LA, Rhoads AM, Fredette ME, et al. "Counselor in Your Pocket": youth and provider perspectives on a mobile motivational intervention for marijuana use. Subst Use Misuse 2013;49(1–2):134–44.
74. Marsch LA, Grabinski MJ, Bickel WK, et al. Computer-assisted HIV prevention for youth with substance use disorders. Subst Use Misuse 2011;46(1):46–56.
75. Marsch LA, Guarino H, Grabinski MJ, et al. Comparative effectiveness of web-based vs. educator-delivered HIV prevention for adolescent substance users: a randomized, controlled trial. J Subst Abuse Treat 2015;59:30–7.
76. Godley SH, Smith JE, Passetti LL, et al. The Adolescent Community Reinforcement Approach (A-CRA) as a model paradigm for the management of adolescents with substance use disorders and co-occurring psychiatric disorders. Subst Abus 2014;35(4):352–63.
77. Acosta MC, Marsch LA, Xie H, et al. The Step up Program: development and evaluation of a web-based psychosocial treatment for adolescents with substance use disorders. Under Review. 2016.
78. Shiffman S, Stone AA, Hufford MR. Ecological momentary assessment. Annu Rev Clin Psychol 2008;4:1–32.

79. Shrier LA, Walls CE, Kendall AD, et al. The context of desire to use marijuana: momentary assessment of young people who frequently use marijuana. Psychol Addict Behav 2012;26(4):821–9.

80. Acri MC, Gogel LP, Pollock M, et al. What adolescents need to prevent relapse after treatment for substance abuse: a comparison of youth, parent, and staff perspectives. J Child Adolesc Subst Abuse 2012;21(2):117–29.

81. King S, McChargue D. Adolescent substance use treatment: the moderating effects of psychopathology on treatment outcomes. J Addict Dis 2014;33(4): 366–75.

82. Gonzales R, Hernandez M, Murphy DA, et al. Youth recovery outcomes at 6 and 9 months following participation in a mobile texting recovery support aftercare pilot study. Am J Addict 2016;25(1):62–8.

83. Shrier LA, Rhoads A, Burke P, et al. Real-time, contextual intervention using mobile technology to reduce marijuana use among youth: a pilot study. Addict Behav 2014;39(1):173–80.

84. Lenhart A. Teens, Social Media & Technology Overview. 2015. Available at: http://www.pewinternet.org/2015/04/09/teens-social-media-technology-2015/. Accessed January 6, 2016.

85. Piper Jaffray & Co. Taking Stock with Teens. 2015. Available at: http://www.piperjaffray.com/3col.aspx?id=3631. Accessed February 26, 2016.

Integrated Care for Pediatric Substance Abuse

Rebecca P. Barclay, MD[a],*, Robert J. Hilt, MD[b]

KEYWORDS

- Delivery of health care • Integrated • Substance-related disorders
- Patient-centered care • Mental health services • Pediatrics

KEY POINTS

- Integrated care is in focus as a way to improve the prevention, identification, and treatment of mental health difficulties, including substance abuse, in pediatric care.
- The pediatrician's access, expertise in typical development, focus on prevention, and alignment with patients and families can allow successful screening, early intervention, and referral to treatment.
- Although scientific evidence for benefit from integrated care of substance abuse in adults is well-established, in children and teens, a comprehensive body of evidence is still emerging.
- Successful integrated substance abuse care for youth is challenged by current reimbursement systems, information exchange, and provider role adjustment issues, but these are being addressed as comfort with this care form and resources to support its development grow.

INTRODUCTION: INTEGRATED CARE FOR PEDIATRIC SUBSTANCE ABUSE—TIMELY AND DEFINED

Integrated care, or the systematic coordination of general and behavioral health care, is an exciting and expanding area on the national stage, which is influencing the way substance abuse care is or will be delivered to children and teens. When primary care providers (PCPs), child and adolescent psychiatrists (CAPs), and other mental health specialists partner with children and families (within primary care settings, behavioral health settings, health homes, via televideo or the Web), pediatric mental health problems can be prevented, identified earlier, and more effectively managed. Collaboration improves safety and effectiveness of treatment.[1,2] It maximizes both the pediatric and psychiatric caregivers' capabilities and time, ideally overcomes reimbursement constraints, increases care access, and strengthens connections with families.[1]

This is an opportune time for the growth of integrated medical, substance abuse, and behavioral health care, both because of increasing knowledge of the value of

[a] Child Psychiatry, Seattle Children's Hospital, M/S CPH, PO Box 5371, Seattle, WA 98145, USA;
[b] Department of Psychiatry, University of Washington, Seattle Children's Hospital, Seattle, WA 98145, USA
* Corresponding author.
E-mail address: rebecca.barclay@seattlechildrens.org

Child Adolesc Psychiatric Clin N Am 25 (2016) 769–777
http://dx.doi.org/10.1016/j.chc.2016.05.007   childpsych.theclinics.com
1056-4993/16/$ – see front matter © 2016 Elsevier Inc. All rights reserved.

this approach and because of greater system allowances for integrated care via changes in reimbursement structures. Reimbursement incentives started to change in 2008 with the Mental Health Parity and Addiction Equity Act, which elevated insurance coverage for substance abuse and behavioral health disorders, and continued with the 2010 Patient Protection and Affordable Care Act, which incentivizes integration through care coordination, health homes, and multidisciplinary practitioner teams.[3,4] These laws set the stage for broad health system changes that are still playing out today.

Many national policy and research institutions (**Box 1**) have offered suggestions for catalyzing better care coordination, redesigning funding pathways, arranging for national conferences, and using more targeted screening instruments, training handbooks, and performance measures to encourage successful care integration of substance abuse treatment.[5–9] The widespread transition to electronic medical records and the use of common procedural terminology (CPT) codes for identifying and treating substance use problems in primary care offers further opportunity to nurture the shift in the field.[5,10]

Professional organizations also encourage well-implemented integrated care for pediatric mental health issues, creating important guidelines on the topic. The American Academy of Pediatrics (AAP) has been a long-standing advocate for the medical home as the place where accessible, continuous, comprehensive, culturally competent, and family-focused care may best occur.[1] The American Academy of Child and Adolescent Psychiatry (AACAP) has described the core care components of integration:

- Screening/early detection
- Triage/referral to appropriate behavioral health treatment
- Ready access to CAP consultation
- Care coordination to enhance service delivery and collaboration
- Access to specialty treatment for those with moderate-to-severe psychiatric issues
- Monitoring outcomes on the individual and system levels[11]

THE ROLE OF PEDIATRIC PRIMARY CARE

The pediatrician's traditional role in caring for the health of children and adolescents aligns well with preventing and treating substance abuse concerns. With their

---

Box 1
Policy, research and professional organizations that endorse integrated care

- Agency for Healthcare Research and Quality
- Substance Abuse and Mental Health Services Administration (SAMHSA)
- Office of National Drug Control Policy
- Surgeon General
- Institute of Medicine
- AAP
- AACAP
- American Medical Association
- Many others…

expertise in typical development and well-established relationships with children and families, pediatricians are able to identify troubles early (**Box 2**).[12] As the AAP states, "Primary care practitioners are ideally suited for preventing problem behaviors and consistently screening for them, including the development of mental health disorders and psychosocial problems, among which are substance abuse and addiction."[13]

Pediatricians view prevention, keeping kids safe, and reducing accidents and injuries as important parts of their therapeutic role. When pediatricians address substance abuse, this fits this mission well around reducing the risk of adverse outcomes including death by overdose, suicide, and motor vehicle crash, infection with HIV or hepatitis, teen pregnancy, violence exposure (victim and aggressor), and criminality.[12,14] Pediatric primary care providers also play an important role in promoting healthy habits early in life. Habits such as exercise, quality and quantity of food intake, and substance misuse once established in childhood will commonly affect a lifetime.[1,12] The age at first substance use inversely correlates with a lifetime risk of developing a substance use disorder.[13,14]

Too often, initial referrals for substance abuse treatment come through the juvenile justice system, but pediatricians are poised to intervene long before that level of severity is approached.[15] The passive method of waiting for patients to seek treatment limits the potential of early intervention efforts.[14] Although teens dealing with substance abuse often do not seek out mental health treatment, half of all teens who have used an illicit substance at least once by high school graduation present regularly to their pediatrician's office for sports physicals, birth control, and annual examinations. These are unique opportunities for the pediatrician to identify broader difficulties and offer help.[14]

Among teens with substance use disorder, 66% to 76% also have other comorbid psychiatric difficulties.[5,15] Shared risk factors may be at work or increased vulnerability to substance abuse in those already experiencing mental health problems. A pediatrician's early involvement and referral for treatment may reduce the severity of co-occurring mental health issues and the expense and intensity of needed treatment later on.[15]

Another advantage of the pediatrician's potential role in addressing substance abuse is his or her relationship with the family. Although many families may resist engaging in a physically separated specialty mental health system due to stigma or hassle, pediatricians are accessible and approachable.[16] They can educate and motivate patients and families to be more open to engaging in mental health care. Increased engagement from families improves outcomes for substance abusing teens.[15]

PUTTING INTEGRATION INTO PRACTICE: SCREENING, BRIEF INTERVENTION, AND REFERRAL TO TREATMENT

The AAP states, "As a group, adolescents are at the highest risk of experiencing substance use-related acute and chronic health consequences, so they are also the age

---

Box 2
Some assets of the pediatrician to care integration

- Experts in typical development
- Focused on prevention and fostering healthy growth
- Can magnify power of intervention through early access
- Respected and trusted by families

group likely to derive the most benefit from universal SBIRT (screening, brief intervention, and referral for treatment)."[13] The National Institutes of Health (NIH), Substance Abuse and Mental Health Services Administration (SAMHSA), and most major medical organizations endorse the integrated care process, SBIRT, in pediatrics for its potential to screen many children/teens promptly, identify difficulties that might have been overlooked as well as problematic substance use in early stages, intervene efficiently, motivate patients and families to accept treatment, and close the access gap.[5,14,17]

Screening

Routine or every office visit screenings for substance abuse among adolescents is the ideal starting point for triggering integrated care services. Despite being well placed to screen for substance abuse and intervene as well as being encouraged by national and professional organizations to use SBIRT in primary care pediatrics, pediatricians' current screening and intervention rates are low, and what does occur is often not based on evidence-based guidelines.[5] For example, the CRAFFT, a verbally administered, simple-to-score, and easy-to-remember screening tool for substance abuse in teens, is 1 aspect of SBIRT with a good evidence base to date that is underutilized.[5,18] When a substance abuse screening tool like the CRAFFT is administered routinely and results indicate further help for a child's substance abuse is needed, the CRAFFT authors themselves highlight that "new intervention strategies for those who screen positive are urgently needed."[18] Referral to specialty substance abuse care may be appropriate for positive screens, but office-delivered brief interventions in that moment are more reliably received.

Brief Intervention

Motivational interviewing is a prominent brief intervention strategy that can be widely employed under a variety of circumstances. This consists of a conversation between patient and provider that focuses on eliciting the patient's own motivation and getting him or her to talk about reasons to change, rather than trying to impose external motivation and play the usual doctor role of "telling" a patient what to do. In order to utilize this approach effectively, providers often need to learn to use new skills such as eliciting change talk from their patients. For instance, instead of making a didactic statement "You need to stop using marijuana," one may say something else like, "If because of the problems we have been talking about you were to decide to stop using marijuana, how would you go about it?" The goals are usually to motivate change, accept treatment, and enable talking about the problem more openly with family. There is evidence for motivational interviewing's efficacy in a broad context—for those at-risk who need brief advice to those with severe symptoms for whom accepting treatment is essential.[13,14] Still, it too is underutilized.[5]

Referral to Treatment

Although both screening and brief intervention are not employed in practice in the community as often as recommended, there are even more difficulties with resource availability to fulfill the referral portion of SBIRT. Despite CAP workforce challenges, the AAP states, "Adolescent patients with alcohol or other drug use disorders should be managed collaboratively (or comanaged) with child and adolescent mental health or addiction specialists whenever possible and scheduled for medical home office visits throughout the recovery process."[13]

The evidence is growing to endorse the efficacy, effectiveness, and feasibility of SBIRT at producing positive outcomes, including reduced substance use and severity, driving after drinking, smoking and emergency department utilization.[5]

Despite the challenges of helping pediatricians become accustomed to routinely employing the SBIRT process and increasing needed resource availability, more providers are becoming knowledgeable about aspects of SBIRT.[19]

CHALLENGES AND OPPORTUNITIES
Information Exchange

For providers to work collaboratively together, mechanisms must be in place for easy sharing of clinical care information (**Box 3**). Although President Barrack Obama made computerizing patients' medical records a priority of his administration, this has not yet resulted in the ability of providers to easily exchange patient data electronically.[20] Efforts are still underway to make information sharing more possible and convenient, which would smooth the course of collaboration and integration.[20,21]

Health Insurance Portability and Accountability Act (HIPAA) law allows for the exchange of mental health care information contained in a medical record between treating providers without a signed patient release for such communication. However, HIPAA law also says that any other federal or state laws that are more restrictive about information exchange would supersede these regulations.[22] With specific relevance to substance abuse treatment, providers should be aware that the 42 Code of Federal Regulations (CFR) Part 2 is one of these areas of greater information restrictions, and applies to information sharing by federally funded alcohol or drug abuse programs.[23] Under that portion of the legal code, clinical information exchange relevant to a patient's substance use treatment that is maintained by a federally funded substance abuse program cannot occur without a written patient consent, which could limit the timely exchange of clinical information between primary care and specialty care settings.

State and local regulations also impact exchange of information, and providers practicing integrated care are challenged with maintaining familiarity with these policies.[13] For example, in Washington State, where the authors practice, teens beginning at 13 years of age may restrict the sharing of mental health treatment information with their parents. The integrated care ideal of the provider working to help a teen while involving the family system to improve outcomes may in some cases be limited by age of consent in the state.

Box 3
Challenges

- Information exchange potential challenge examples
  - Electronic data sharing barriers
  - 42 Code of Federal Regulations limits substance abuse diagnosis sharing
  - Adolescent age of consent

- Financial challenges
  - Nonfinancially quantifiable outcomes difficult to measure in dollars
  - Fee-for-service may not reward consultative and coordination activities

- Role challenges
  - Primary care discomfort with mental health diagnoses and treatment
  - Inadequate time, training, knowledge of resources, and specialty access

- Evidence base challenges
  - Lack of data about comprehensive integrated care in children
  - Evidence that exists suggests benefit, but limited study number and strength of outcomes

Financial Challenges

Under-recognition and treatment of substance abuse issues may result in fewer patients receiving services. Although there is a common sense inherent cost to the individual and society from inadequate identification and management of substance abuse problems, producing quantifiable cost savings outcome from interventions that yield many nonfinancial benefits can be a challenge (see **Box 3**).

Positive outcomes of treatment may include increased school attendance; reduced juvenile delinquency; improved parental employment attendance; growth in patient, family and provider satisfaction; improved ability for child and teen to function in his or her developmentally appropriate role; and decreased future burden of the child on the family and society. Models that study the economics of integrated care struggle to measure these long-term impacts to children, families, and society.

Fee-for-service models often do not support consultative and care-coordination activities, which also can be a barrier to collaboration. For example, provider visits with a young person's parents without the patient present are often excluded from insurance reimbursement, or result in lower reimbursement rates. Consultation time between different care providers about a shared patient is rarely compensated, such as a PCPs consulting with a CAP by phone. Integrated care, which stresses the importance of collaboration and care management, would be encouraged if these consultative and coordination tasks were universally incentivized and reimbursed similar to other health care benefits.[11]

Role Challenges

Although pediatricians are ideally suited to put integrated care for pediatric substance abuse issues into practice and the American Medical Association's *Guidelines for Adolescent Preventive Services* recommend that providers ask all adolescent patients annually about substance use, adherence to universal screening has been low.[18] Role tensions may be a factor in pediatricians' underuse of SBIRT to date (see **Box 3**).

PCPs report feeling they lack comfort and familiarity with making mental health diagnoses and recommending treatment.[1,18] They cite insufficient time, training, knowledge of resources, specialty access, and teamwork across specialties as challenges.[11,16] That said, PCPs experience improved comfort, knowledge, and ability to diagnose and treat mental health problems when employing collaborative care.[1]

Evidence Base Challenges

There is good evidence for benefit from care integration in adults, but a disparity exists relative to the amount of research that has been done regarding integrated care in pediatrics.[14,16,24–26] Of the studies that have occurred, differences between their designs make meta-analysis challenging, and no 1 study incorporates all the elements of integrated care described by SAMHSA and professional associations (see **Box 3**).[14]

Despite the lack of robust data for pediatric integrated care of substance abuse, the data from individual studies that do exist are fairly positive. Most studies address screening and brief intervention; no studies examine referral to treatment.[14] There is solid evidence for the reliability and validity of screening using the CRAFFT.[14,26] Brief intervention for alcohol use in teens and transitional age youths has demonstrated effectiveness.[14] A study of case management for youth with co-occurring mental health issues demonstrated reduced hospitalizations, hospital days, and symptoms, as well as increased time in the community and improved functioning.[15]

A 2015 meta-analysis demonstrated an advantage for integrated care relative to usual care on all behavioral health outcomes for children and adolescents. Based on this meta-analysis, an individual child has a 66% probability of experiencing a better outcome after receiving an integrated behavioral health intervention than for usual care. If the child experienced collaborative care (with PCP, care manager, and mental health specialist working together), the randomly selected youth would have a 73% probability of experiencing a better outcome than treatment as usual.[12]

But within that meta-analysis, there were few substance abuse-specific trials. Only 6 of the included studies were regarding substance abuse prevention, and 4 studies addressed treatment.[12] The beneficial effect of prevention was weak and not significant (d = 0.07, -0.13–0.28, P = .49), and treatment was mild (d = 0.17, -0.18–0.52, P = .35). That said, 1 large individual substance abuse prevention trial showed good benefit.[27] Clearly, there is a need for additional studies to clarify whether evidence will strongly support integrated care, but what evidence does exist to date points toward some benefit from portions of the SBIRT continuum in pediatric substance abuse.

SUMMARY

Integrated care for substance abuse in children and teens is an important and growing area, receiving significant attention as a critical area for growth by national governmental and professional organizations. It promises to deliver efficient, just-in-time, collaborative and specific treatment for children at risk for substance abuse and its consequences.

From a practical as well as a systems perspective, the integration of pediatric substance abuse care into primary practice is a commonsense approach to improving the potential health and well-being of children by protecting them from the all-too-common consequences of substance misuse in pediatric years, consequences that can extend across a lifetime. Integrated care also promises to improve provider contentment with the ability to more effectively and comfortably intervene to protect the health of children.

Despite the promise, there are barriers that have prevented its widespread implementation to date, but they are being met with momentum from many domains (policy, research, professional, and economic) in order to see this promising care form utilized broadly. The emerging evidence suggests integrated care offers real benefits to children and teens and to provider's satisfaction in preventing and minimizing harm to children from substance abuse.

REFERENCES

1. Committee on Collaboration with Medical Professionals. A guide to building collaborative mental health care partnerships in pediatric primary care. Washington, DC: American Academy of Child & Adolescent Psychiatry; 2010. Available at: https://www.aacap.org/App_Themes/AACAP/docs/clinical_practice_center/guide_to_building_collaborative_mental_health_care_partnerships.pdf. Accessed October 15, 2015.
2. What is integrated care? SAMHSA-HRSA Center for Integrated Health Solutions. Available at: http://www.integration.samhsa.gov/about-us/what-Is-integrated-care. Accessed October 13, 2015.
3. Paul Wellstone and Pete Domenici Mental Health Parity and Addiction Equity Act of 2008. Available at: https://www.cms.gov/Regulations-and-Guidance/Health-Insurance-Reform/HealthInsReformforConsume/downloads/MHPAEA.pdf. Accessed October 7, 2015.

4. The Affordable Care Act. U.S. Department of Health & Human Services. Available at: http://www.hhs.gov/healthcare/rights/law/index.html. Accessed October 7, 2015.

5. Sterling S, Valkanoff T, Hinman A, et al. Integrating substance use treatment into adolescent health care. Curr Psychiatry Rep 2012;14:453–61.

6. Integrating behavioral health and primary care. Agency for Healthcare Research and Quality. Available at: http://integrationacademy.ahrq.gov/. Accessed October 7, 2015.

7. Croghan TW, Brown JD. Integrating mental health treatment into the patient centered medical home. Rockville, MD: AHRQ Publication; 2010. Available at: https://pcmh.ahrq.gov/sites/default/files/attachments/Integrating%20Mental%20Health%20and%20Substance%20Use%20Treatment%20in%20the%20PCMH.pdf. Accessed October 7, 2015.

8. Integrate treatment for substance use disorders into mainstream health care and expand support for recovery. Office of National Drug Control Policy. Available at: https://www.whitehouse.gov/ondcp/chapter-integrate-treatment-for-substance-use-disorders. Accessed October 7, 2015.

9. Health Care Systems, Insurers, and Clinicians. National prevention strategy partners in prevention. Washington, DC: National Prevention Council; 2010. Available at: http://www.surgeongeneral.gov/initiatives/prevention/resources/npc_factsheet_healthcare_508.pdf. Accessed October 13, 2015.

10. Paying for primary care and behavioral health services provided in integrated care settings. SAMHSA-HRSA Center for Integrated Health Solutions. Available at: http://www.integration.samhsa.gov/financing/billing-tools. Accessed October 7, 2015.

11. Martini R, Hilt R, Marx L, et al. Best principles for integration of child psychiatry into the pediatric health home. Washington, DC: American Academy of Child & Adolescent Psychiatry; 2012. Available at: https://www.aacap.org/App_Themes/AACAP/docs/clinical_practice_center/systems_of_care/best_principles_for_integration_of_child_psychiatry_into_the_pediatric_health_home_2012.pdf?WebsiteKey=a2785385-0ccf-4047-b76a-64b4094ae07f&=404%3bhttps%3a%2f%2fwww.aacap.org%3a443%2faacap%2fApp_Themes%2fAACAP%2fdocs%2fclinical_practice_center%2fsystems_of_care%2fbest_principles_for_integration_of_child_psychiatry_into_the_pediatric_health_home_2012.pdf. Accessed October 15, 2015.

12. Asarnow JR, Rozenman M, Wiblin J, et al. Integrated medical-behavioral care compared with usual primary care for child and adolescent behavioral health. JAMA Pediatr 2015;169(10):929–37.

13. American Academy of Pediatrics Policy Statement. Substance use screening, brief intervention, and referral to treatment for pediatricians. Pediatrics 2011;128(5):e1330–40.

14. Mitchell SG, Gryczynski J, O'Grady KE, et al. SBIRT for adolescent drug and alcohol use: current status and future directions. J Subst Abuse Treat 2013;44:463–72.

15. Hawkins EH. A tale of two systems: co-occurring mental health and substance abuse disorders treatment for adolescents. Annu Rev Psychol 2009;60:197–227.

16. Raney LE. Integrated care: interface of primary care and behavioral health. Arlington (VA): American Psychiatric Publishing; 2014. p. 67–98.

17. Levy S, Knight JR. Screening, brief intervention, and referral to treatment for adolescents. J Addict Med 2008;2(4):215–21.

18. Knight JR, Sherritt L, Shrier LA, et al. Validity of the CRAFFT substance abuse screening test among adolescent clinic patients. Arch Pediatr Adolesc Med 2002;156:607–14.
19. Schwartz RP. Motivational interviewing. Performing preventive services: a bright future handbook. Available at: http://www2.aap.org/oralhealth/docs/appendixf_mi.pdf. Accessed October 14, 2015.
20. Pear R. Tech rivalries impede digital medical record sharing. New York Times 2015;26:A15.
21. Clancy CM, Anderson KM, White PJ. Investing in health information infrastructure: can it help achieve health reform. Health Aff 2009;28(2):478–82.
22. Hilt RJ. HIPAA: still misunderstood after all these years. Pediatr Ann 2014;43(7): 249.
23. Electronic code of federal regulations. Part 2-confidentiality of alcohol and drug abuse patient records. Available at: http://www.ecfr.gov/cgi-bin/text-idx?rgn=div5;node=42%3A1.0.1.1.2. Accessed October 13, 2015.
24. Unutzer J, Harbin H, Schoenbaum M, et al. The collaborative care model: an approach for integrating physical and mental health care in Medicaid Health Homes. Center for Health Care Strategies Brief May 2013. Available at: http://www.medicaid.gov/State-Resource-Center/Medicaid-State-Technical-Assistance/Health-Homes-Technical-Assistance/Downloads/HH-IRC-Collaborative-5-13.pdf. Accessed September 23, 2015.
25. Archer J, Bower P, Gilbody S, et al. Collaborative care for depression and anxiety problems. Cochrane Database Syst Rev 2012;(10):CD006525.
26. Pilowsky DJ, Wu L. Screening instruments for substance use and brief intervention targeting adolescents in primary care: a literature review. Addict Behav 2013; 38:2146–53.
27. Pbert L, Flint AJ, Fletcher KE, et al. Effect of a pediatric practice-based smoking prevention and cessation intervention for adolescents: a randomized, controlled trial. Pediatrics 2008;121(4):e738–47.

Index

Note: Page numbers of article titles are in **boldface** type.

Child Adolesc Psychiatric Clin N Am 25 (2016) 779–787
http://dx.doi.org/10.1016/S1056-4993(16)30092-X
1056-4993/16/$ – see front matter

childpsych.theclinics.com

UNITED STATES POSTAL SERVICE®

Statement of Ownership, Management, and Circulation
(All Periodicals Publications Except Requester Publications)

1. Publication Title	2. Publication Number	3. Filing Date
CHILD AND ADOLESCENT PSYCHIATRIC CLINICS OF NORTH AMERICA	011 – 368	9/18/2016

4. Issue Frequency	5. Number of Issues Published Annually	6. Annual Subscription Price
JAN, APR, JUL, OCT	4	$297.00

7. Complete Mailing Address of Known Office of Publication (Not printer) (Street, city, county, state, and ZIP+4®)

ELSEVIER INC.
360 PARK AVENUE SOUTH
NEW YORK, NY 10010-1710

Contact Person
STEPHEN R. BUSHING
Telephone (Include area code)
215-239-3688

8. Complete Mailing Address of Headquarters or General Business Office of Publisher (Not printer)

ELSEVIER INC.
360 PARK AVENUE SOUTH
NEW YORK, NY 10010-1710

9. Full Names and Complete Mailing Addresses of Publisher, Editor, and Managing Editor (Do not leave blank)

Publisher (Name and complete mailing address)

ADRIANNE BRIGIDO, ELSEVIER INC.
1600 JOHN F KENNEDY BLVD. SUITE 1800
PHILADELPHIA, PA 19103-2899

Editor (Name and complete mailing address)

LAUREN ELISE BOYLE, ELSEVIER INC.
1600 JOHN F KENNEDY BLVD. SUITE 1800
PHILADELPHIA, PA 19103-2899

Managing Editor (Name and complete mailing address)

PATRICK MANLEY, ELSEVIER INC.
1600 JOHN F KENNEDY BLVD. SUITE 1800
PHILADELPHIA, PA 19103-2899

10. Owner (Do not leave blank. If the publication is owned by a corporation, give the name and address of the corporation immediately followed by the names and addresses of all stockholders owning or holding 1 percent or more of the total amount of stock. If not owned by a corporation, give the names and addresses of the individual owners. If owned by a partnership or other unincorporated firm, give its name and address as well as those of each individual owner. If the publication is published by a nonprofit organization, give its name and address.)

Full Name	Complete Mailing Address
WHOLLY OWNED SUBSIDIARY OF REED/ELSEVIER, US HOLDINGS	1600 JOHN F KENNEDY BLVD. SUITE 1800 PHILADELPHIA, PA 19103-2899

11. Known Bondholders, Mortgagees, and Other Security Holders Owning or Holding 1 Percent or More of Total Amount of Bonds, Mortgages, or Other Securities. If none, check box ☐ None

Full Name	Complete Mailing Address
N/A	

12. Tax Status (For completion by nonprofit organizations authorized to mail at nonprofit rates) (Check one)
The purpose, function, and nonprofit status of this organization and the exempt status for federal income tax purposes:
☐ Has Not Changed During Preceding 12 Months
☐ Has Changed During Preceding 12 Months (Publisher must submit explanation of change with this statement)

13. Publication Title	14. Issue Date for Circulation Data Below
CHILD AND ADOLESCENT PSYCHIATRIC CLINICS OF NORTH AMERICA	JULY 2016

15. Extent and Nature of Circulation			Average No. Copies Each Issue During Preceding 12 Months	No. Copies of Single Issue Published Nearest to Filing Date
a. Total Number of Copies (Net press run)			298	377
b. Paid Circulation (By Mail and Outside the Mail)	(1)	Mailed Outside-County Paid Subscriptions Stated on PS Form 3541 (Include paid distribution above nominal rate, advertiser's proof copies, and exchange copies)	138	160
	(2)	Mailed In-County Paid Subscriptions Stated on PS Form 3541 (Include paid distribution above nominal rate, advertiser's proof copies, and exchange copies)	0	0
	(3)	Paid Distribution Outside the Mails Including Sales Through Dealers and Carriers, Street Vendors, Counter Sales, and Other Paid Distribution Outside USPS®	45	62
	(4)	Paid Distribution by Other Classes of Mail Through the USPS (e.g., First-Class Mail®)	0	0
c. Total Paid Distribution (Sum of 15b (1), (2), (3), and (4))			183	222
d. Free or Nominal Rate Distribution (By Mail and Outside the Mail)	(1)	Free or Nominal Rate Outside-County Copies Included on PS Form 3541	53	70
	(2)	Free or Nominal Rate In-County Copies Included on PS Form 3541	0	0
	(3)	Free or Nominal Rate Copies Mailed at Other Classes Through the USPS (e.g., First-Class Mail)	0	0
	(4)	Free or Nominal Rate Distribution Outside the Mail (Carriers or other means)	0	0
e. Total Free or Nominal Rate Distribution (Sum of 15d (1), (2), (3) and (4))			53	70
f. Total Distribution (Sum of 15c and 15e)			236	292
g. Copies not Distributed (See Instructions to Publishers #4 (page #3))			62	85
h. Total (Sum of 15f and g)			298	377
i. Percent Paid (15c divided by 15f times 100)			78%	76%

* If you are claiming electronic copies, go to line 16 on page 3. If you are not claiming electronic copies, skip to line 17 on page 3.

16. Electronic Copy Circulation	Average No. Copies Each Issue During Preceding 12 Months	No. Copies of Single Issue Published Nearest to Filing Date
a. Paid Electronic Copies ▲	0	0
b. Total Paid Print Copies (Line 15c) + Paid Electronic Copies (Line 16a) ▲	183	222
c. Total Print Distribution (Line 15f) + Paid Electronic Copies (Line 16a) ▲	236	292
d. Percent Paid (Both Print & Electronic Copies) (16b divided by 16c × 100) ▲	78%	76%

☒ I certify that 50% of all my distributed copies (electronic and print) are paid above a nominal price.

17. Publication of Statement of Ownership
☒ If the publication is a general publication, publication of this statement is required. Will be printed
in the OCTOBER 2016 issue of this publication.
☐ Publication not required.

18. Signature and Title of Editor, Publisher, Business Manager, or Owner

STEPHEN R. BUSHING - INVENTORY DISTRIBUTION CONTROL MANAGER

Date 9/18/2016

I certify that all information furnished on this form is true and complete. I understand that anyone who furnishes false or misleading information on this form or who omits material or information requested on the form may be subject to criminal sanctions (including fines and imprisonment) and/or civil sanctions (including civil penalties).

PS Form 3526, July 2014 (Page 3 of 4) PSN: 7530-01-000-9931   PRIVACY NOTICE: See our privacy policy on www.usps.com.

PS Form 3526, July 2014 (Page 1 of 4 (see instructions page 4))   PSN: 7530-01-000-9931   PRIVACY NOTICE: See our privacy policy on www.usps.com.

Moving?

Make sure your subscription moves with you!

To notify us of your new address, find your **Clinics Account Number** (located on your mailing label above your name), and contact customer service at:

Email: journalscustomerservice-usa@elsevier.com

800-654-2452 (subscribers in the U.S. & Canada)
314-447-8871 (subscribers outside of the U.S. & Canada)

Fax number: 314-447-8029

Elsevier Health Sciences Division
Subscription Customer Service
3251 Riverport Lane
Maryland Heights, MO 63043

*To ensure uninterrupted delivery of your subscription, please notify us at least 4 weeks in advance of move.

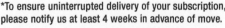
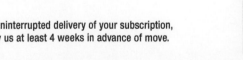

Printed and bound by CPI Group (UK) Ltd, Croydon, CR0 4YY

03/10/2024

01040395-0003